The Cytotoxics Handbook

Second Edition

Edited for
The Cytotoxics Services Working Group by

Michael Allwood

BPharm, PhD, MRPS, Director, Medicines Research Unit,
Derbyshire Institute of Health and Community Studies,
University of Derby

and

Patricia Wright

BPharm, MPhil, MRPS, Principal Pharmacist,
West Middlesex University Hospital, Isleworth, Middlesex

RADCLIFFE MEDICAL PRESS
OXFORD

© 1993 Radcliffe Medical Press Ltd
15 Kings Meadow, Ferry Hinksey Road, Oxford OX2 0DP

First edition 1990
Second edition 1993

British Library Cataloguing in Publication Data

A catalogue record for this book is available from the British Library

ISBN 1 870905 04 0

Typeset by Advance Typesetting Ltd, Oxfordshire
Printed and bound in Great Britain

Contents

PART ONE

Cytotoxic Services

PART TWO

Drug Monographs: Compendium of Intravenous Drugs in Cancer Chemotherapy

The past 20 to 25 years have witnessed impressive changes in the drug treatment of cancer.

A better understanding of the nature of neoplastic disease has led to the development of cancer chemotherapeutic drugs, encompassing a wide spectrum of chemical compounds, which kill or impair susceptible tumour cells by blocking a drug-sensitive biochemical or metabolic pathway. The ability to use a number of agents in combination has improved clinical outcome in a variety of conditions and increasingly complex regimens continue to be developed.

However, cytotoxic therapy has its limitations: poor selectivity between neoplastic and normal cells, especially in the bone marrow and reproductive organs, can produce severe side-effects; many of the agents are carcinogens and mutagens and have been implicated in causing secondary neoplasms in patients being treated for cancer and most agents cause local damage to skin and mucous membranes due to their irritant, vesicant or allergenic action.

The obvious toxicity of these drugs has led to concern over their possible hazard to healthcare workers who prepare and administer the drugs and care for patients during treatment. In response to a number of reports indicating skin absorption and droplet inhalation of cytotoxics prepared in uncontrolled environments, guidelines for the safe handling of antineoplastic drugs have been drawn up by a number of countries. All make the same basic recommendations: controlled handling procedures; a high level of staff training and, where practicable, centralized reconstitution of IV cytotoxics in pharmacy departments with suitable controlled working areas.

The development of centralized pharmacy cytotoxic services in many countries has occurred in a non-uniform manner depending on local requirements, legislation, the availability of funding and the existing service commitments. The diversity of services, both within some countries and between countries, is still significant. Where services have been established, much time has been spent researching the literature for information on drug stability, designing documentation, establishing training programmes and ensuring that facilities comply with Health and Safety requirements. That services have been established is commendable considering the general lack of information on the safe handling and stability of IV cytotoxics and the divergent and conflicting views of much published work.

In response to the obvious need for more practical information on the procedures involved in setting up and running such units, a group comprising pharmacists and technicians in the UK met for informal, 'round table' discussions during the winter of 1987–88. All members had a substantial interest and expertise in cancer chemotherapy and the development of pharmacy-based hospital cytotoxic services and represented hospital pharmacy, pharmaceutical industry and academic interests. Early in the discussions, it was agreed that the Cytotoxic Services Working Group would produce, as quickly as possible: a manual on how to set up and operate pharmacy-based cytotoxic services, with specific detail on equipment, facilities, Health and Safety, documentation and training; and a compendium of cytotoxic drugs detailing their pharmaceutical properties, reconstitution details and stability in secondary packaging systems based on an informed review of the literature. This in-house edition was printed in late 1988.

An extensively updated and expanded, first complete edition was published in 1990. In this, the manual and compendium were combined into a single handbook designed primarily for use by pharmacists wishing to establish or update centralized cytotoxic services, but also aimed at other healthcare workers in this speciality.

This second edition has been further updated and is now geared towards a more international readership. Contributions from the USA and Europe have now been included. Much superfluous and overlapping information has been removed to aid information retrieval and all information pertaining to stability is now contained within the individual monographs.

Part one is divided into 11 chapters, each giving detailed information on a specific topic related to cytotoxic services. The information given is representative of the current 'state of the art' cytotoxic reconstitution services and reflects international recommendations and the contributors' own experience. A new chapter on clinical monitoring and control of side-effects of cancer chemotherapy has been added.

Part two is a compendium of monographs on injectable cytotoxic drugs. These monographs have been prepared for specific use by those hospital pharmacists and experienced pharmacy technicians who have responsibility for the provision of reconstituted and ready-to-administer cytotoxic drugs. Information on stability refers to preparation in controlled environments, where the sterility of the final product can be assured. The object of each monograph is to provide the basic information relevant to the preparation; stability on storage in the primary container; stability in secondary packaging systems; administration and disposal of the drugs. Use of the monographs should obviate the need for extensive literature searching and interpretation of data. The author of each monograph is named and can be consulted on specific queries.

Interferon, interleukins and granulocyte-stimulating factors are now included in the handbook for completeness. Although they do not have a direct cytotoxic action and can be handled safely, they are increasingly being incorporated as part of complex cytotoxic regimens and there is little information on their stability in clinical practice.

The section on investigational agents has been updated. However, readers are referred to the National Cancer Institute book of Investigational Drugs (available from The Pharmaceutical Resources Branch, NCI, Executive Plaza North, Suite 818, Bethesda, Maryland 20892, USA) and specialist oncology centres for further information.

Authors and Contributors

Michael C. Allwood
Director
Medicines Research Unit
University of Derby
Mickleover
Derby

Rosamund M. Baird
Consultant in Pharmaceutical Microbiology
Pharmacy Department
Yeatman Hospital
Sherborne
Dorset

Nigel Blackburn
Product Manager, GCSP
Roche Products Ltd
Welwyn Garden City
Hertfordshire

Kay A. Buttars
Chief Technician
Pharmacy Department
Addenbrookes Hospital
Cambridge

Yaacob Cass
Pharmacy Department
Hadassah University Hospital
Jerusalem
Israel

Christine L. Chard
Oncology Business Manager
ASTA Medica Ltd
168, Cowley Road
Cambridge

Alan Crossley
Pharmacy Department
St James Hospital
Leeds

Carol Davis
Senior Medical Information Officer
Lederle Laboratories Ltd
Fareham Road
Gosport
Hampshire

Karen S. Davis
Business Development Manager
Unicare Medical Services Ltd
Cambridge Road
Harlow
Essex

Susanne Foy
Technical Support Manager
David Bull Laboratories
Spartan Close
Tachbrook Park
Warwick

Monica Francomb
Principal Pharmacist
Pharmacy Department
Royal Liverpool Hospital
Liverpool

Sally Gardner
Pharmacy Department
Nottingham General Hospital
Nottingham

Ian J. Goss
Director of Operational Services
Pharmacy Department
Leeds General Infirmary
Leeds

Nigel M. Goulding
Principal Pharmacist
Pharmacy Department
Charing Cross Hospital
London

Pauline E. Heath
Commercial Development Manager
Bristol-Myers Squibb Pharmaceuticals Ltd
Hounslow
Middlesex

Dora Kan
Pharmacy Department
The Royal Marsden Hospital
London

Jeff Koundakjin
Pharmacy Department
Clatterbridge Hospital
Bebington
Wirral

Jane W. Kwan
Co-ordinator, Pharmacy Alternate Delivery Programs
MD Anderson Cancer Center
Houston
Texas

A. Paul Launchbury
Technical Director
Farmitalia Carlo Erba Ltd
St Albans
Hertfordshire

M. Gerard Lee
Regional Quality Controller
Pharmacy Department
Mersey Regional Health Authority
Liverpool

Susan Mahoney
Marketing Services Manager
Amgen Ltd
Featherstone
Staffordshire

Tony C. Moore
Principal Pharmacist, Technical Services
Pharmacy Department
Royal Hallamshire Hospital
Sheffield

Richard J. Needle
Pharmacy Technical Support Manager
Pharmacy Support Unit
Colchester General Hospital
Colchester

Margaret Nicolson
Pharmacy Department
Christie Hospital
Manchester

Jonathan M. Oakes
Principal Pharmacist
Pharmacy Department
Countess of Chester Hospital
Chester

Nutan Patel
Chief Technician
Pharmacy Department
The Royal Marsden Hospital
London

Tim R. Root
Chief Pharmacist
Pharmacy Department
The Royal Marsden Hospital
London

Graham J. Sewell
Principal Pharmacist and Senior Lecturer in
    Biomedical Sciences
Department of Pharmacy
Royal Devon and Exeter Hospital
Exeter

Robert J.S. Shaw
Regional Quality Controller
East Anglian Regional Pharmaceutical Services
Norfolk and Norwich Hospital
Norwich

Andrew P. Stanley
District Oncology Pharmacist
St Chads Unit
Dudley Road Hospital
Birmingham

Helen R. Streeter
Pharmacist, Bone Marrow Transplant Services
Pharmacy Department
University Hospital of Wales
Cardiff

Max Summerhayes
Principal Pharmacist
Pharmacy Department
Guy's Hospital
London

Ted Thom
Regional Quality Controller
Regional Quality Control Centre
Edgware General Hospital
Edgware
Middlesex

M. Jayne Wood
Assistant Director (Clinical Services)
Pharmacy Department
Hope Hospital
Salford

M. Patricia Wright
Principal Pharmacist
Pharmacy Department
West Middlesex University Hospital
Isleworth
Middlesex

PART ONE: Cytotoxic Services

CHAPTER 1

Setting up a Cytotoxic Reconstitution Service

The reconstitution of cytotoxic chemotherapy in a safe and effective manner is an essential component in the treatment of patients suffering from cancer. Chemotherapy must be prepared in a way that assures the quality of the product and also protects the operator and the working environment.

A cytotoxic reconstitution service can address these issues by ensuring reconstitution takes place in an appropriately controlled environment.

This chapter provides a structured framework to assist the decision-making process. It examines the key aspects to be considered when evaluating the need for the cytotoxic reconstitution service, and also how the type and level of service may be determined. Suggestions on achieving these objectives, and the role of a cytotoxics working party, are also included.

IS THERE A NEED FOR SUCH A SERVICE?

1 Range of Service and Projected Workload

It will be necessary to establish the following.

The number and type of individual cytotoxic doses administered per annum and whether new types of therapy (eg continuous domiciliary) are likely to change workload patterns.

Who prescribes cytotoxic chemotherapy; where and when is it administered and by whom (eg are certificated nurses available to administer parenteral chemotherapy)?

Is the workload continuous or does it fluctuate; at what time of day/week are particular regimens commenced?

Is bolus injection (manual or via syringe pump) or intravenous infusion the preferred method of administration?

2 Health and Safety Considerations

Where is cytotoxic reconstitution currently being carried out and by whom? Are these arrangements satisfactory and appropriate from a patient safety and operator protection point of view?

3 Cost

What is the current capital and revenue expenditure on cytotoxic chemotherapy (drugs, equipment, facilities and staff)?

Are significant amounts of medical and nursing time, that would be better utilized providing direct patient care, being devoted to the preparation of cytotoxic chemotherapy?

Will centralization of cytotoxic reconstitution produce economies of scale and reduce revenue expenditure?

4 Consultation

All interested parties (medical, nursing, administrative and pharmaceutical) should be approached for information and opinions. The choice of a formal or informal approach will depend on local circumstances and relationships.

5 Commitments and Resources

The present level of commitments and resources should be examined before proceeding further. A centralized reconstitution service is a major development and will require either additional resources, or the redeployment of existing resources. An awareness of strategic plans is vital at this stage to ensure that an appropriate balance of commitments to resources is achieved.

6 Collecting and Testing Data

A pilot scheme is an effective mechanism for collecting data, canvassing opinions and testing logistics and procedures. Such a scheme should have clear objectives, a fixed timescale and an agreed endpoint when the results can be evaluated without prejudice. A decision to proceed or not can then be made, based on actual local experience.

Before starting a pilot study a multidisciplinary working party should be established with a nominated co-ordinator.

SETTING UP A CYTOTOXICS WORKING PARTY

1 Membership

Membership of the working party should include:

Clinicians	Oncologists
	Haematologists
	Radiologists
	Radiotherapists
Nurses	Nurse managers
	Tutors
	Specialists
	Community/homecare
Pharmacy staff	Pharmacists
	Technicians
Management	General manager or representative
Occupational health	Senior representative

2 Objectives

▼ to establish and co-ordinate a pilot study in accordance with previously agreed aims and objectives
▼ to assess the capital and revenue implications of the service and allocate resources as appropriate
▼ to monitor the performance of the service.

It is desirable that a smaller working party should continue to meet in the longer term to formulate policy and provide advice on relevant issues.

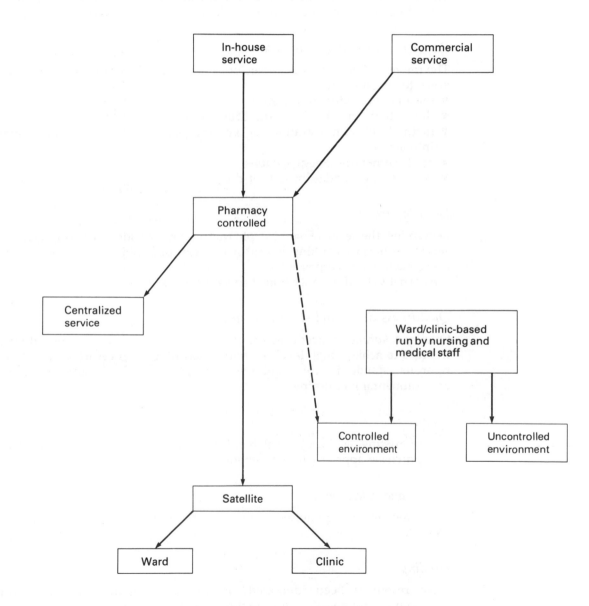

Figure 1.1: *Flow chart summarizing service selection criteria*

WHAT TYPE OF SERVICE IS REQUIRED?

An option appraisal is useful in determining the type of service required. Areas for consideration are outlined in Figure 1.1.

1 Service Selection Criteria

Workload

The volume of work, measured as individual patient doses per annum, and annual expenditure on cytotoxic chemotherapy are key considerations.

Range and presentation of doses

The range and pattern of cytotoxic prescribing needs to be determined. The key areas to consider are:
▼ the range of cytotoxics used
▼ the stability in solution of the drugs used
▼ methods of administration (eg bolus injections, infusions and continuous infusions)
▼ are treatment regimens established?
▼ is there any standardization of doses?

Level of service

Determine the level of service pharmacy can provide. Will this give a total service in normal working hours? If not, can prescribing habits be changed to make such a service possible?
   Alternatively, does a 24 hour service need to be established?

Quality assurance and sterility assurance

Quality assurance procedures should be agreed, documented and adhered to. In order to achieve high levels of sterility assurance, procedures should include rigorous standards for equipment maintenance, operator training and environmental monitoring.

Facilities

Utilize existing facilities if available. If these are not available, convert facilities and purchase appropriate equipment.

Health and safety needs

Local and national guidelines must be adhered to (*see* Chapter 6, Health and Safety).

Funding

Have resources been identified? If not, can potential savings on drug expenditure and medical and nursing time be utilized?
   What other developments are underway or being planned and what is the order of priority?

Personnel

Are there staff available and what is their level of expertise? Are funds available for recruitment and training?

Logistics

Points for consideration:

▼ the physical geography of the site/sites
▼ is more than one site being serviced?
▼ location of in-patients and out-patients within the same site in relation to pharmacy
▼ communication and transport systems
▼ consultants' prescribing habits.

Clinical commitment

The level of clinical involvement by pharmacy can be enhanced by providing a service. This level of involvement with patient care should not detract from the efficiency of the service and will depend on the attitudes of local personnel and their managers.

DECIDING ON THE LEVEL OF SERVICE

Some of the advantages and disadvantages of each type of service are shown in Table 1.1.

Table 1.1: *Advantages and Disadvantages of Possible Service Options*

Service	Advantages	Disadvantages
Pharmacy controlled centralized unit	Existing facilities.	Potential large capital cost if using cleanroom technology.
	High sterility/stability assurance.	Extended lines of communication between pharmacy/nurse/doctor.
	Cost/efficiency savings on a high workload.	Problems of distribution to clinical areas and off-site locations.
	Planned workload.	Slower reaction/lead times.
	Suitably trained, skilled staff.	Out of hours service may not be provided.
	High level of operator/product protection.	Potential long-term pharmacy staff exposure.
	Easier supervision.	High level of long-term pharmacy commitment.
	Standardization of presentation of doses.	Loss of expertise at ward level.
	Comprehensive documentation.	Deployment of staff away from pharmacy, with the potential for increased staff requirements and labour costs.
Pharmacy controlled satellite unit	Workload centralized in designated hospital areas.	

Table 1.1: *continued.*

Service	Advantages	Disadvantages
	Short lines of communication.	Increased stock holdings.
	Reduced distribution problems.	Potential for greater wastage.
	Increased inter-professional contact.	Fragmentation of pharmacy service.
	Ability to respond more quickly to requests.	Negotiating space within another department.
	Cost/efficiency savings on high workload.	May also be required to supply oral medication and adjuvant therapy.
	High sterility/stability assurance.	Potential long-term pharmacy staff exposure.
	Easier to provide an extended hours service.	
	Potential for access by non-pharmacy staff out of hours (working to strict pharmacy procedures).	
	High level of operator/product protection.	
Ward/clinic based in an uncontrolled environment (nurse/ doctor operated)	Status quo.	Health and safety aspects/ operator protection.
		No product protection.
		High level of wastage.
		High stock holdings.
		Limited pharmacy control.
		No record of preparation process; therefore no recall traceability.
		Possibility of untrained staff preparing doses.
Ward/clinic based in a controlled environment (nurse/ doctor operated)	Reduced pharmacy labour costs.	High nursing and medical staff turnover, leading to increased training requirements.
	Rapid response, 24-hour service.	Less time for direct patient care.
		Decreased assurance of sterility/stability.
	Short lines of communication.	Higher level of wastage.
	No distribution or delivery problems.	
		Limited pharmacy control.
		No record of preparation process; therefore no recall traceability.

Table 1.1: *continued.*

Service	Advantages	Disadvantages
		Increased stock holdings.
		Difficult to maintain high standard of quality assurance.
		Pharmacy activity undertaken by non-pharmacy staff.
		Management responsibilities and levels of control poorly defined.
		Formal accrediting/validation system would be required, which would lead to increased quality assurance costs.
Commercial service	No additional capital or staff costs (full off-site service).	Potential for increased revenue expenditure.
	Provision of a full range of drugs in a ready-to-use form.	
	Health and safety aspects of local reconstitution eliminated.	Communication and supply logistics (if service off-site).
	Standardization of presentation of doses.	Further distribution of drugs from a central delivery point to the ward/clinic.
	Planned workload.	
	Comprehensive documentation.	
	Minimal stock holdings.	
	Reduced wastage.	
	High sterility/stability assurance.	

CHAPTER 2

Facilities

INTRODUCTION

The selection of equipment and working environment is dependent on a number of factors:

▼ expected workload
▼ existing facilities and commitments
▼ resources available (capital/revenue, personnel, accommodation).

The following flow chart (Figure 2.1) identifies options to be considered in the decision-making process.

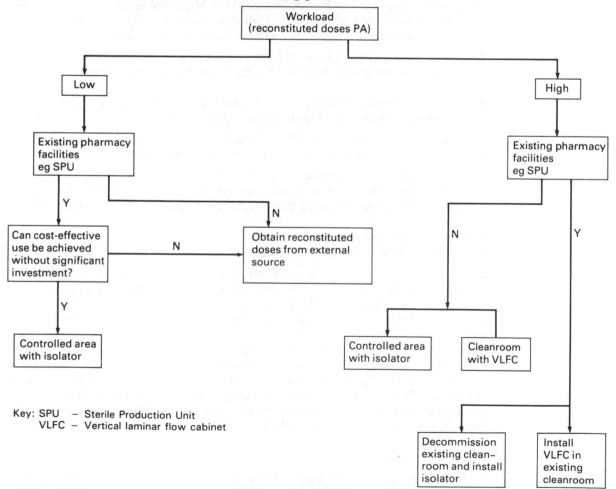

Figure 2.1: *Flow chart of options to be considered when selecting equipment and working environment*

VERTICAL LAMINAR FLOW CABINETS AND ISOLATORS

The risks associated with the handling and administration of cytotoxic drugs have resulted in the widespread use of safety cabinets for the preparation and dispensing of these products. Such cabinets must achieve a balance between operator and product protection in order to provide adequate levels of safety for both the patient and the staff preparing and administering the drug. Vertical laminar flow cabinets (VLFC) with similar operating characteristics to Class II microbiological safety cabinets have been used, but the limitations of these cabinets have led to an increased use of isolators (totally enclosed glove boxes). These have an advantage over cleanrooms in that they do not require an expensive air handling plant nor do they need costly and time-consuming gowning procedures.

1 Vertical Laminar Flow Cabinets

1.1 Standards

There are no nationally agreed standards in the UK for vertical laminar flow drug safety cabinets. The British Standard for Microbiological Safety Cabinets, BS 5726,[1] makes reference to vertical laminar flow protection cabinets, but this Standard is not readily applicable to hazardous drugs because:

▼ bacteria have a defined mass or bulk and are of known particle size, whereas cytotoxic contaminants will be of variable size and may be solid, liquid or gaseous
▼ for the materials handled in microbiological safety cabinets, operator protection is more critical than product protection.

The Australian Standard, AS 2567, 1982[2] has been written to apply only to cytotoxic cabinets. Some of the features of this Standard are:

▼ all potentially contaminated zones are under negative pressure
▼ all filter seals which may come into contact with potentially hazardous material are under negative pressure with respect to the uncontaminated zones
▼ stainless steel construction
▼ incorporation of carbon exhaust filter.

In Germany a 'cytostatic work station' is defined in a document describing principles of operation and test procedures, GS-GES-04, published by the Professional Association of Health Service and Welfare Care[3] (GS DIN 12590). Filters are tested to DIN standard 24184 and are of 99.99% efficiency. These work stations are, in essence, compact laminar downflow cabinets with a front visor having two apertures for the worker to access the work zone. Whilst manufacturers vary the machine dimensions and number of filters used, the principles and tests in GS-GES-04 are common to all. In the USA, the American Society of Hospital Pharmacists have produced guidelines on cytotoxic drug handling.[4] Laminar downflow safety cabinets which comply with US National Sanitation Foundation Standards[5] are described.

1.2 Operating principles

A vertical downflow of laminar-flow air, filtered through a HEPA filter (efficiency 99.997% in UK, 99.99% in Germany), passes over the work surface.

The air then passes through vents at the front and back of the cabinet, and is recirculated. Depending on the manufacturer there may be one or more filters in the recirculation and exhaust air flows. Approximately 30% of the recirculated air is exhausted from the cabinet and, to compensate for this, air is drawn in through the front opening. This creates a negative pressure within the cabinet. The balance between the cabinet downflow and the air drawn in at the front of the cabinet produces an air curtain, which is the basis of the operator and product protection properties of the cabinet. The air exhausted from the cabinet may be recirculated into the room or ducted to the outside.

1.3 Cabinet details

Cytomat (Medical Air Technology Ltd)

Cabinet dimensions (w × d × h (mm)) 1200 × 695 × 2135

Tray area (w × d (mm)) 1075 × 450

Filters The Cytomat is available in two formats. The fixed format has a downflow HEPA filter, 1100 mm × 500 mm × 150 mm and an exhaust HEPA filter, 1000 mm × 450 mm × 300 mm. The movable format has an additional in-line exhaust HEPA filter, 825 mm × 375 mm × 75 mm. Filters are sealed on both the upstream and downstream faces.

Design characteristics The manufacturer states that this machine is built to AS 2567,[2] but it does not fully comply as the working chamber tank is not entirely of stainless steel construction. The air flow through the cabinet is generated by a fan in the terminal exhaust duct; therefore the cabinet and exhaust system will be under negative pressure. The ducting is fitted with anti-blowback flaps. The filter case forms the walls of the air ducts; therefore air cannot bypass the filter. The exhaust duct can be fitted with either a carbon or an HEPA exhaust filter.

Figure 2.2 shows the airflow pattern for the total dumping (exhaust) and recirculating versions of this cabinet.

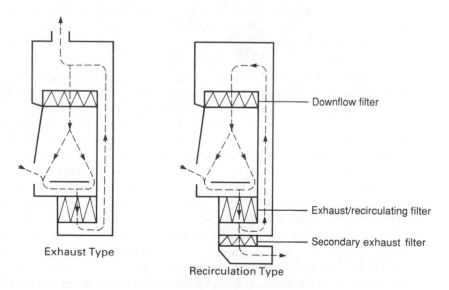

Exhaust Type

Recirculation Type

Downflow filter

Exhaust/recirculating filter

Secondary exhaust filter

Figure 2.2: *M.A.T. Cytomat airflow diagram*

Cytogard (Gelman Hawkseley Ltd)

Cabinet dimensions (h × w × d (mm))

model CG 900 – 2310 × 1180 × 768
model CG 120 – 2310 × 1340 × 770
model CH 180 – 2310 × 1950 × 770

Tray area (CG 900) (w × d (mm)) 875 × 590

Filters Filters are Gelman microseal 7531 series (dimensions not stated). One downflow HEPA filter and one exhaust HEPA filter is fitted, plus an activated carbon bed in the exhaust. The exhaust filter is sealed on the upstream face.

Design characteristics This cabinet complies with AS 2567.[2] The cabinets are bulkier and taller than the Cytomat. They have no normal provision for exhaust ducting, but this can be done. Manometers are optional and do not allow measurement downstream of the main filter.

Figure 2.3 shows the airflow pattern for this type of cabinet.

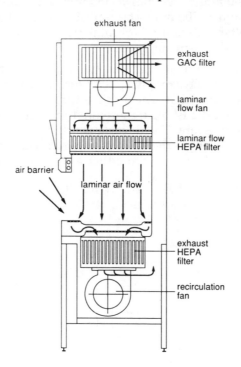

Figure 2.3: *Gelman, Cytogard airflow diagram*

1.4 General comments on VLFCs

A carbon exhaust filter is not a true filter but a gas absorption cell which can be subject to channelling. It can release carbon particles into the room and it is not possible to test the adsorption capacity non-destructively. There seems little need for a carbon exhaust filter, particularly if the air exhaust is ducted to the outside.

Where cabinets are sited in aseptic suites, product protection is simplified because the cabinet itself is in a Class E/F environment.[6] If situated in a dispensary or on a ward, local air turbulence will be a more critical determining factor of operator and product protection than the cabinet's design.

It should be borne in mind that the UK, USA, Australian and German cabinets are not strictly comparable and that it is necessary to ensure that the equipment complies with regulatory requirements in the country of use.

2 Isolators

2.1 Standards

There are no standards in the UK for isolators to be used for aseptic dispensing. BS 5726[1] includes a reference to Class III containment, microbiological safety cabinets.

2.2 Operating principles

Isolators are totally enclosed work stations supplied with filtered air which should meet BS 5295, Class E/F.[6] Operators use either glove ports, or a half-suit arrangement to access the working area. Materials are introduced either through an air lock or using an access port and docking device. During operation the cabinet is totally sealed from the outside. Isolators can be of a rigid or a flexible structure and their design can have a considerable impact upon their potential uses and upon operating, monitoring and disinfection procedures.

2.3 Flexible film isolators (Envair UK Ltd, La Calhene Ltd, Cambridge Isolation Technology (CIT), MDH Ltd)

The dimensions and configurations of flexible isolators are variable as there are a large number of working, bank, transfer and sterilization chambers marketed. Companies will meet the design needs of the customer.

Design characteristics Flexible film isolators have an enclosure made entirely of flexible PVC film supported on a chrome or stainless steel framework. Sizes can vary and two, three or four-glove port models, half-suit or double half-suit designs are available. Inlet and outlet air is HEPA filtered (99.997%) and the air supply can be so designed that the working environment is under positive or negative pressure. The air supply is not laminar flow and normally provides the contained unit with approximately 20 air changes per hour. Rapid transfer ports on the sides of the isolator enable enclosed containers to be locked on. In connecting the two together the lid from the container locks onto the port door. The contaminated surface of the isolator door and container lid are therefore sealed together and are not exposed to the isolator when the lid is removed to allow access to the container.

The half-suit systems offer greater flexibility and all-round movement but appear at first to be claustrophobic. The suits are double layered and are fed with an air supply which both inflates and lifts the suit so that it does not press against the operator while providing a flow of air across the face and body. By their very nature, flexible isolators are more easily damaged and require care during use.

For cytotoxic reconstitution, isolators must be under negative pressure. Extra support frames are required for this and the relative pressures may cause ingress of contaminated air if the PVC canopy is pin-holed. Monitoring procedures must be capable, therefore, of detecting pin-hole leaks.

La Calhene Ltd appear to have the more sophisticated range and they offer a wider choice of transfer containers but they are also the most expensive.

2.4 Rigid isolators

The walls of the cabinet are rigid with a totally enclosed working area. The inlet and outlet air supply is HEPA filtered (99.997%) and the air can be turbulent or laminar flow. The front panel is a clear plastic and is fitted with up to four glove ports. Materials are transferred into and out of the cabinets via air locks or enclosures.

Amercare Cytotoxic Drug Handling Suite (Amercare Ltd)

A large range of units is available.

Filters Inlet filters are cylindrical, 244 mm diameter × 305 mm long. Separate filters supply the entry enclosure and chamber. Exhaust filters are not fitted as standard but can be fitted to customer requirements.

Design characteristics These cabinets are of rigid steel construction comprising entry/exit enclosures together with a main processing enclosure. The inlet air supply is via HEPA filters (99.997%).

Enclosures are under negative pressure, air being drawn in via the HEPA filter located in the bench below the enclosure. The pressure is such that if the system is in any way compromised, eg by a door opening or a glove becoming damaged, air is extracted from the enclosure at a sufficient rate to give a safe inward velocity of air through the opening, allowing the negative pressure to be maintained. Air inlet and extraction is via vertical distribution tubes at the back of each enclosure. The exhaust air is ducted outside the building. The air velocity is such that it provides the cabinet with 250 air changes per hour.

There is an electromechanical interlock between the doors on the entry and working chambers.

Figure 2.4 shows the airflow pattern in a typical suite.

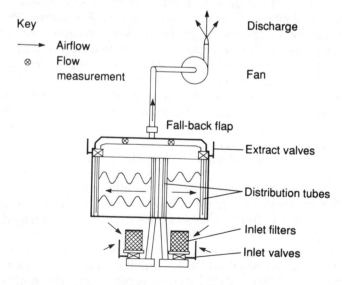

Figure 2.4: *Amercare Cytotoxic Drug Handling Suite airflow diagram*

Containair Dispensing Cabinet (Envair UK)

Cabinet dimensions (w × d × h (mm)) 2432 × 695 × 1300, not including stand which is fitted to customer requirements.

Filters Downflow HEPA, 1220 mm × 508 mm × 150 mm;
Main (primary exhaust) HEPA, 1130 mm × 456 mm × 203 mm;
Secondary exhaust HEPA, 590 mm × 420 mm × 66 mm;
(Minipleat), hatch HEPAs 460 mm × 320 mm × 66 mm;
Prefilter 600 mm × 180 mm × 25 mm.
The exhaust filters are sealed on the upstream and downstream faces.

Design characteristics The Containair is a rigid, steel cabinet. Two glove ports are fitted into the front viewing panel which is hydraulically assisted and may be lifted to allow the installation of large pieces of equipment. The cabinet is supplied with vertical laminar flow HEPA filtered air (99.997%) and is fitted with dual exhaust HEPA filters. The air supply provides approximately 20 air changes per hour.

Transfer ports are fitted on the side panels of the cabinet and are independently flushed with HEPA filtered air.

Figure 2.5 shows the airflow pattern for the work zone. Transfer hatch ventilation is not shown.

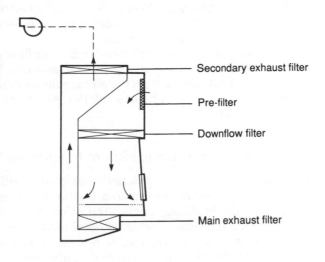

Figure 2.5: *Envair Containair airflow diagram*

Peteric Cytotoxic Drug Isolators (Peteric Ltd)

A range of two, four and eight-glove machines is available in a number of configurations.

Filters Inlet and exhaust filters, plus filters on the top and bottom of transfer hatches. Two configurations of exhaust filter can be supplied to allow sealing on the dirty side or on both sides before removal.

Design characteristics These isolators are rigid steel, and operate at negative pressure. Air flow at about 0.35 m/s produces a change of chamber air every three seconds. Transfer hatches are interlocked. Machines are normally ducted to exhaust, but can be made for recycling, when a second exhaust HEPA filter is fitted. Gauntlets or glove sleeve systems can be supplied.

Microflow/CIT Microtox Isolators (MDH Contamination Control)

A range of two and four-glove isolators is available.

Dimensions (h × w × d (mm)) 750 × 1200 × 650 or 750 × 1620 × 650. (Plus stand which can be supplied to adjustable height.)

Filters HEPA inlet and exhaust filters (99.997% efficiency) fitted with a prefilter sheet. Both filters are standard 305 mm² Minipleat. Transfer hatches (lock-chambers) are fitted with HEPA filters on inlet and exhaust.

Design characteristics This is a computer controlled system where chamber working pressure is monitored and controlled. The chambers are of epoxy coated mild steel. The work tray is stainless steel. Air flow is vertical laminar downflow. Air flow rate and chamber pressure is displayed digitally and high and low set pressure alarms are provided. Filters are changed from within the isolator using a safe change bagging technique. Power supplies can be fitted to the chamber. Sterilization and disinfection can be achieved with formaldehyde, Citanox® or by alcoholic surface treatment.

2.5 General comments on isolators

The rigid containment cabinets are relatively easy to clean and disinfect using hard surface disinfectants. Since they are designed to be used in an uncontrolled environment and will operate under negative pressure, high efficiency seals on all cabinet openings are essential.

In addition, those units with non-laminar air flow may have dead spots within the Class E/F area[6] and purging of contaminants from the cabinets will, to a large extent, be dependent on the air turbulence created within the cabinet. The greater number of air changes of the Amercare cabinets produce a more turbulent air flow.

3 Sterilization and Sanitization of Internal Surfaces

Gaseous sterilization is a practical means of sterilization of large flexible film isolators. This requires the filtered output air to be ducted outside and above the roof of the building, or that the exhaust air is passed through a suitable chemisorbant filter pack, which adds considerably to the cost.

It is possible to link together two or more flexible isolators via the transfer ports. Components, containers and equipment can be surface sterilized, by gaseous sterilization, in one isolator overnight then transferred the following day to the adjoining isolator prior to use.

Formaldehyde and peracetic acid are the usual sterilants. Peracetic acid is reported to be the more effective and easier to use but is also the more toxic. Formaldehyde will be absorbed by the PVC and therefore time must be allowed for the gas to desorb from the canopy. Cytanox®, a gaseous sterilant developed by Cambridge Isolation Technology (CIT) is available, but there is little information on its use.

It must be stressed that gaseous sterilization cannot be recommended for the surface sterilization of articles within an isolator unless the user can fully validate the system with respect to gas desorption from packaging, closures, syringes, etc. Equally it should be noted that there is a risk of gas entry into drug or diluent containers if stress cracks are present or if the closures of individual containers are not guaranteed impervious to gas ingress.

In the UK, COSHH regulations[7] would enforce the view that a safe and effective means of gas desorption, removal and disposal must be included in any sterilization equipment and protocol for use.

Sanitization of small flexible film isolators by hard surface disinfectants is not precluded but the effect of the alcoholic sprays on PVC film needs to be evaluated. Chlorhexidine-containing alcoholic sprays should be used with caution or not at all, as a film of chlorhexidine residue will build up on surfaces, potentially causing contamination of solutions.

For rigid isolators, surface sanitization with an alcoholic solution is the simplest and quickest option, but it should be noted that some manufacturers do not advocate the practice. However, direct questioning has revealed that the reservations expressed relate to long-term soaking in alcohol solutions leading to crazing of some types of clear plastic. The routine use of alcohol solutions by swab or spray application with subsequent rapid evaporation is not seen as problematic.

Both Amercare and Envair recommend the use of either gaseous sterilization or hard surface sanitization.

4 Glove Ports and Gauntlets (*see also* Chapter 3)

All isolators, whether they be rigid, flexible film or half-suit isolators, are accessed via a glove port. These are glove/sleeve arrangements which are designed to maintain the aseptic environment within the isolator. Several types of gauntlets and glove/sleeve systems, made from various materials are available and careful selection will be necessary.

4.1 Gauntlets

These are one piece, full-arm-length gloves. They are available in a range of materials. Pinholes are not uncommon since manufacturers are not always aware of the need for stringent testing for perforations during manufacturing.

They are usually changed on a weekly (or longer) basis due to the high cost, resulting in a potential risk of drug penetration and poor general hygiene, as a number of operators will use the same gloves. For these reasons, double-gloving is generally used. However, as gauntlets do not fit well, particularly under conditions of negative pressure, operator sensitivity will be reduced.

Gauntlets are usually thicker than surgeons' latex gloves, which may offset risk of drug penetration to a degree. They are not normally available pre-sterilized.

4.2 Glove/sleeve systems

These are multi-component systems consisting generally of a replaceable sleeve piece, a connecting cuff piece and the glove. The sleeve should be mechanically strong enough to remain in position without deterioration for a number of weeks. It should not be too rigid for comfortable working and should be resistant to chemical attack. The cuff piece should allow an easy, safe, aseptic glove change-over.

The glove/sleeve system allows gloves of an appropriate specification, particularly with respect to perforations and pinholes, to be used. It will, if correctly designed, allow the individual operator to fit and change gloves of correct size as frequently as required and enable the glove material to be altered without jeopardy to the isolator environment. Risk of drug penetration can be minimized in this way and general hygiene is improved as each operator can fit a fresh sterile pair of gloves each time the equipment is used.

5 Monitoring

The aseptic preparation facilities in hospitals enable the preparation of injections in controlled environments with greater assurance of sterility. The British Pharmacopoeia currently recommends that unpreserved injections, prepared aseptically from sterile ingredients, should have a 24-hour shelf life; furthermore, the product licences of lyophilized injections often restrict their shelf lives to 24 hours after reconstitution. The overriding reason for the 24-hour shelf life is the risk of microbial contamination of the product during preparation or reconstitution. However, in centralized cytotoxic dispensing facilities, where a licensed sterile product is used for the preparation of sterile medication, and is prepared under conditions of good manufacturing/dispensing practice in suitably monitored and audited premises, then the shelf life may be extended beyond 24 hours, provided the microbiological integrity of the process has been validated and the physicochemical stability of the product justifies it.

It is essential, therefore, that a monitoring programme is implemented which confirms that the aseptic dispensing facilities meet continuously their performance requirements, and which indicates and identifies system breakdown before product sterility is affected. Such a programme will include physical tests of the cabinets and isolators and the environment in which they are sited, together with active and passive microbial sampling of the controlled environment.

The extent and frequency of monitoring will depend upon the design of the facilities and upon the workload and frequency of use of the service. A suggested programme of monitoring for aseptic cytotoxic dispensing facilities is given in Table 2.1. Testing of VLFCs is similar to that for horizontal LFCs, but in addition to particle counts and filter challenge tests, operator protection factors should be measured regularly. Particle counts and filter challenge tests are equally applicable to isolators. In addition, there is a need to monitor for pinholes and defects in gloves, and in the canopies of flexible isolators, so regular leak tests are also required. Daily passive microbiological monitoring of the aseptic working environment will produce the most immediate indication of loss of microbial control. More rigorous testing is recommended on a weekly basis together with active monthly sampling of airborne viable organisms. Suggested limits for the monitoring results are given in Table 2.2. These limits are based on those in BS 5295[6] and on those in the Parenteral Society's technical monograph on environmental microbiological contamination in controlled environments.[8] Because of the imprecision of the methods, the expected low levels of contamination and the natural variability of the levels, the microbiological data require most careful analysis.

It is recommended that the levels given in Table 2.2 are regarded as target levels. Exceeding target levels on isolated occasions may not require more action than examination of control systems. However, the frequency of exceeding the limit should be examined and should be low. If the frequency is high or shows an upward trend, then action should be taken.

Table 2.1: *Environmental monitoring: frequency of testing*

	Controlled Areas	Laminar Flow	Isolators
Daily	Check pressure differential readings.	Check pressure differential across filter. Settle plates during procedure.	Check pressure differential readings. Settle plates during dispensing procedure.
Weekly	Check pressure alarms. Record pressure differentials. Settle plates at marked sites.	Visual examination of HEPA filter. Record pressure differentials. Settle plates at marked sites.	Check pressure alarms. Leak test (where possible). Record pressure differentials. Settle plates at marked sites in isolator and transfer hatch.
Monthly	No. of air changes. Airborne viable organisms. Surface swabs at marked sites.	Laminar air flow velocity. Airborne viable organisms. Surface swabs at marked sites.	Laminar air flow velocity. No. of air changes (turbulent flow). Airborne viable organisms. Surface swabs, at marked sites in isolator and transfer hatch.
Quarterly	Check calibration of manometers. Airborne particulate test.	Airborne particulate test.	Airborne particulate counts. Airborne viable organisms in transfer hatch.
Annual	Installation leak test. Filter efficiency.	Installation leak test. Filter efficiency. Operator protection test.	Installation leak test. Filter efficiency.

Notes: The number of settle plates and swabs will depend on the size and construction of the aseptic facility, and should be determined during commissioning studies.

Table 2.2: *Environmental monitoring: centralized cytotoxic dispensing services – limits for physical testing and target microbiological levels*

	Controlled Areas		Laminar Flow	Isolators	
	Filling Room	Change Area		Work Station	Transfer Hatch
Pressure	>10 Pa between classified area and adjacent area of lower classification				
	>15 Pa between classifed and unclassified area				
Airborne particle counts*					
>0.5 μ	3500	350 000	3500	3500	350 000
>5 μ	0	2000	0	0	2000
>10 μ	0	450	0	0	450
Air flow velocity/ exchange rate	>20 air changes/h		Horizontal: 0.45±0.1 m/s Vertical: 0.30±0.5 m/s	Turbulent flow >60 changes/h Vertical LF: 0.3±0.5 m/s	
Installation leak test			Max. conc. 0.001%	Max. conc. 0.001%	
Settle plates	5	20	1 per 2 plates	1 per 2 plates	5
Surface swabs	No growth	No growth	No growth	No growth	No growth
Airborne viable counts (cFu/m^3)	5	5	<1	<1	5

*Max. no. particles/m^{-3}

Notes: 1. The target limits for settle plates are based on a two-hour exposure time.
 2. It is not possible to quantify limits for surface sampling–limits should be defined locally.

6 Summary

Isolators offer significant advantages over cleanrooms for small-scale aseptic operations. They can be housed in a socially clean room and a minimum of gowning is required. Revenue and maintenance costs are substantially less than conventional cleanrooms. Rigid isolators are generally fairly compact and not designed for industrial-scale use. However, these cabinets are very suitable for small scale operations and particularly for one-off aseptic dispensing operations, since sanitization is quick and easy and materials can be introduced very simply.

Flexible isolators address the problem of space but create other problems, such as the detection of pinholes (particularly when under negative pressure), sanitization, and loading ready for use. Ideally they need to be loaded for a complete session of work and rapid, aseptic transfer of items that have been omitted is not easy.

The problems of turbulence, due to the immediate environment or the operator, limit the effectiveness of VLFCs as cytotoxic dispensing cabinets. Isolators offer a totally enclosed work area. Aseptic transfer into and out of isolators is more complicated than for VLFCs since there is no simple front aperture. In this respect the transfer hatches of the rigid isolators have an advantage over docking ports.

Isolators should be sited within a designated room or a designated area within the pharmacy department. When installing VLFCs and isolators with external ducting, there may be problems of filtration of the air supply to the cabinet and in balancing air pressures within the room in which the cabinet is sited. Adequate consideration should also be given to the discharge of the exhaust duct.

Gaseous sterilization should only be used on those cabinets fitted with external ducting or other appropriate means of removal of the toxic sterilant gas. Those isolators which lend themselves to sanitization with hard-surface disinfectants and do not require fumigation with formaldehyde or peracetic acid, are preferred by users and allow more flexibility. Also, air locks rather than access ports are preferred.

For very large scale operations and for batch manufacturing, a traditional cleanroom may be preferable because of the flexibility it allows, but the costs of operation will be higher and the increased risk potential should be recognized.

Choice of gloves and glove changing procedures are an important practical consideration and these should be thoroughly investigated before purchasing decisions are made.

It should be possible to change gloves without loss of Class E/F conditions within the isolator.

FACILITIES FOR NON-STERILE CYTOTOXIC DRUG MANIPULATION

Cytotoxic chemotherapy regimens often include oral cytotoxic preparations, and healthcare personnel should be aware of the potential hazards when handling them. Care in the supply and administration of solid dosage forms is essential to ensure that staff and, when appropriate, patients and their carers, are given suitable advice on the safe handling of cytotoxic drugs.

Developments in paediatric oncology have resulted in more babies and young children receiving cytotoxic chemotherapy. The treatment regimens for these patients can result in doses being prescribed that cannot be administered in commercially available solid oral dosage forms. In addition, liquid oral preparations are often required for babies and children, and also for adult patients who are unable to swallow solid dosage forms.

The extemporaneous preparation of medicines containing cytotoxic drugs must be avoided whenever possible. In addition, any manipulation of dosage forms on wards which may cause release of a drug into the atmosphere should be discouraged.

Any dosage manipulation or extemporaneous preparation must be restricted to the pharmacy department.

The extemporaneous preparation of liquid oral or any other non-parenteral cytotoxic drug should be performed in such a way that the operator is protected from dust from capsules, tablets and powders, and from aerosols of liquids.

Facilities for non-sterile manipulation of cytotoxic preparations need to provide satisfactory levels of operator protection, but product protection is less critical since product sterility is no longer necessary.

The use of appropriate personal protective clothing is essential, and the preparation should be carried out in fume cupboards or containment enclosures:

Fume Cupboards

Fume cupboards and exhaust hoods with a negative air inflow and a filtered or ducted exhaust air flow will provide suitable working environments. In the UK, fume cupboards should comply with the British Standard for fume cupboards BS 7258, 1990.[9] This standard, in its various parts, covers safety and performance, design and installation and use and maintenance of laboratory fume cupboards. An ancillary document, BS DD191,[10] describes methods for testing such equipment. However, such installations are not always appropriate to hospital pharmacy departments, since they are bulky, of fixed construction, and require ducted exhaust air flow. Some smaller bench top designs are now available which have a filtered air outlet but the size and bulk of these can still be a problem.

Enclosed Work Stations

Another option is the use of glove box containment cabinets. These are simplified, smaller designs of isolators with sealed glove ports. Inlet and outlet air supplies are HEPA filtered and they may also have activated carbon exhaust filters. Such cabinets are available from: Amercare Ltd, Miller-Howe, and Alvic Scientific. They can be free-standing or bench top units. They are, however, bulky typically (l × w × d (mm)) 800 × 600 × 600, expensive, and not easily moved, and their class F environment is an unnecessary luxury for handling non-sterile cytotoxic manipulations.

Portable Containment or Extraction Systems

Bench top, negative pressure extract systems which are portable or moveable and allow flexibility, are preferred. They should have a filtered exhaust air supply and the velocity of the inlet air flow should give satisfactory operator protection. Systems are available which provide a localized contained work station or localized extraction at low cost. Details of these are given on page 22.

Safetech Fume Bubble FX1 (Gelman Sciences) (Figure 2.6)

Dimensions (h × w × d (mm)) 580 × 500 × 600

Weight 15 kg

Volume 0.053 m³

Work surface area 1500 cm²

Filters Exhaust filter cartridges are available as either HEPA, activated carbon, or a combination of both. Filter cartridges have a 5 μ pre-filter. The HEPA filter efficiency is 99.997%.

Design characteristics This safety cabinet is a spherical, clear, acrylic construction with two hand ports. Air is drawn through the hand ports and is exhausted via the filter. The minimum negative air velocity at the hand ports is 0.7 m/s.

Nederman 2000 Extractor (Nederman Ltd) (Figure 2.7)

Dimensions (h × w × d (mm)) 272 × 385 × 175

Weight 10 kg

Filters The filter comprises a particle filter and an activated carbon filter, size (h × w × l (mm)) 285 × 288 × 388. The particle filtration efficiency is 99.97%.

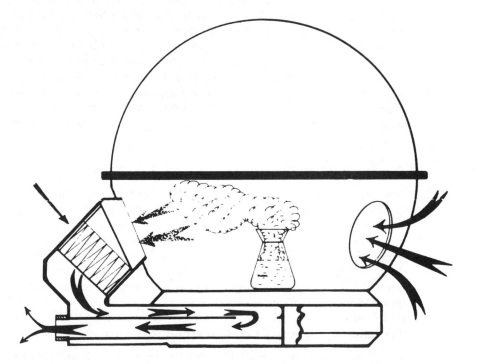

Figure 2.6: *Safetech Fume Bubble FX1 (Gelman Sciences)*

Design characteristics The extractor is a multi-component system. An aluminium, rectangular hood, which covers the work area, clips onto a polypropylene extraction arm; the extraction arm is clamped to the working surface and can be pivoted about its foot for manoeuvrability. It is connected, via a 2.5 m pvc flexible hose, to the fan which is attached to the exhaust filter. The fan fits directly onto the filter element and the total height of the fan and filter is 555 mm.

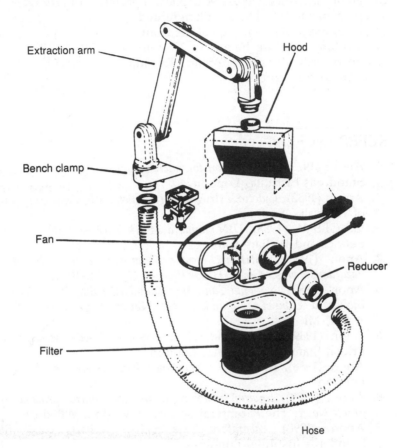

Extraction arm

Hood

Bench clamp

Fan

Reducer

Filter

Hose

Figure 2.7: *Nederman 2000 Extractor (Nederman Ltd)*

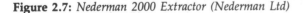

Alsident System (Industri Filter UK)

Work surface area Dome 350 mm diameter; canopy 150 × 200 mm

Filters Available both as a two-stage filter, which comprises a pre-filter and a HEPA filter, and a three-stage filter, which has a carbon filter as well as a pre-filter and HEPA filter.

Design characteristics A filter unit is connected by flexible tubing to an extraction tube. This comprises short lengths of 50 mm diameter, rigid, aluminium or polypropylene tubes connected together with polypropylene swivel joints. The extraction tube is clamped onto the work surface and terminates in a circular extraction dome or a rectangular extraction canopy.

Astecair 500 (Astec Environmental Systems)

Dimensions (h × w × d (mm)) 800 × 610 × 580

Weight 30 kg

Filters HEPA filter or activated carbon filter; (h × w × l (mm)) 50 × 250 × 500; weight 2.2 kg. Two identical filters per unit.

Design characteristics The Astecair 500 is a portable, filtration fume cabinet. It has an epoxy painted steel head unit mounted on a clear acrylic canopy. This canopy has an aperture 180 mm high at the front, with a flap opening that can increase the working aperture height to 275 mm. It is fitted with two filters and an electrostatically charged pre-filter. The input air velocity is 0.5 m/s or 0.3 m/s with the lower flap open.

REFERENCES

1. Anon. (1979). *Specification for microbiological safety cabinets, BS 5726.* British Standards Institute, London.
2. Anon. (1982). *Cytotoxic drug safety cabinets, AS 2567.* Standards Association of Australia, Sydney.
3. GS-GES-04. (1988). *DIN standard 24184.* Professional Association of Health Service and Welfare Care.
4. Anon. (1990). *ASHP technical assistance bulletin on handling cytotoxic and hazardous drugs. Am. J. Hosp. Pharm.* **47**, 1033–1049.
5. Anon. (1987). *National Sanitation Foundation Standard: Class II (laminar flow) Biohazard Cabinetry. Standard 49.* National Sanitation Foundation, Ann Arbor, MI.
6. Anon. (1989). *Environmental cleanliness in enclosed spaces, Parts 1,2,3, BS 5295.* British Standards Institute, London.
7. Anon. (1988). *The control of substances hazardous to health regulations.* HMSO, London.
8. Anon. (1989). *Environmental contamination control practice. Technical Monograph No. 2.* The Parenteral Society, Swindon, Wiltshire.
9. Anon. (1990). *Laboratory fume cupboards, Parts 1,2,3, BS 7258.* British Standards Institute, London.
10. Anon. (1990). *Method for delimination of the containment value of laboratory fume cupboards, BS DD191.* British Standards Institute, London.

CHAPTER 3

Protective Clothing

INTRODUCTION

Protective clothing should be worn at all times when handling cytotoxics. The degree of protection required will depend on the perceived exposure risk to the operator/handler and should be based on local or nationally agreed guidelines, if available.

Protective clothing is required to minimize exposure due to inhalation of drug powder or droplets, or direct skin or eye contact. It is not a substitute for adequate training in all aspects of cytotoxic handling; preparation in contained workstations using aseptic techniques; and adherence to strict hygiene and cleanliness procedures.

Table 3.1 summarizes the minimum requirements for the handling of cytotoxic drugs in various situations.

PROTECTIVE CLOTHING

1 Gowns, Cleanroom Suits and Armlets

In general these should be:

▼ lightweight
▼ low-linting
▼ of a low permeability, disposable or conventional fabric.

Gowns and suits should have:

▼ a solid front with covered fastenings
▼ long sleeves which are cuffed at the wrists.

Most commercially available fabrics for use in aseptic preparation areas are permeable to cytotoxic drugs and additional protection is required if gowns/suits made of these materials are worn.

Laidlaw et al.[1] investigated the permeability of four disposable protective clothing materials to seven antineoplastic drugs over a four-hour period. The materials tested were Saranex-laminated Tyvek, polyethylene-coated Tyvek, non-porous Tyvek and Kaycel.

All of the materials evaluated afforded protection from occupational exposure to antineoplastic drugs, whereas laboratory coats and disposable isolation gowns were completely absorbent. Saranex-laminated Tyvek and polyethylene-coated Tyvek afforded almost complete protection from the drugs. Non-porous Tyvek and Kaycel did allow some drug permeation, although the maximum permeation over a four-hour exposure time was 3.3% of the applied drug dose.

Table 3.1: *Minimum requirements to protect staff when handling cytotoxic drugs in various situations*

Activity	Protective measures
Preparation	
Controlled environment (contained workstation)	Sterile/non-sterile gown, suit or laboratory overall Gloves of a suitable quality Non-absorbent armlets
Uncontrolled environment	As above, plus: Plastic apron or non-absorbent overall Eye protection Dust or respirator mask
Checking	Laboratory overall or long-sleeved uniform Gloves of a suitable quality
Transport	No special protection required provided drugs are transported in a suitable transport container and the messenger is aware of the potential hazards
Dealing with spills	Non-absorbent overall or laboratory overall and plastic apron Heavy duty gloves Eye protection Dust or respirator mask
Administration/ handling patient waste	Long-sleeved uniform or non-absorbent armlets Plastic apron Gloves of a suitable quality Eye protection

As a general recommendation it is suggested that Saranex-laminated or polyethylene-coated Tyvek armlets be worn over standard cleanroom clothing for preparation of cytotoxics in a downward displacement, laminar air flow, cytotoxic cabinet where the arms of the operator are exposed throughout. These armlets should also be worn when preparing drugs in an isolator cabinet, as the rubber sleeves may not protect the operator from gross contamination.

Where disposable gowns are used, these should be made of Saranex-laminated Tyvek or polyethylene-coated Tyvek for maximum operator protection. However, these materials allow little air flow and tend to be uncomfortable to wear for an extended period of time. Non-porous Tyvek or Kaycel garments are more comfortable to wear but operators should be made aware of the lower degree of protection. Non-porous Tyvek armlets are suitable for all administration and waste disposal procedures.

2 Masks

Standard surgeons' masks are suitable for most procedures carried out in a 'contained environment'. If there is a possibility of inhalation and a drug is not handled in a 'contained environment' a suitable dust mask should be worn, eg a disposable 'bra cup' type to BS 6016.[2] A respirator mask may be required for dealing with large-scale spills or contamination.

3 Eye Protection

Eye protection to BS 2092C[2] is required for handling cytotoxic drugs if the material is not being handled in a suitable cabinet. Goggles should fully enclose the eyes to protect against dust and splashes.

4 Aprons

These provide a protective, water-resistant barrier to accidental spills or sprays. They can be ethylene oxide sterilized if required. Saranex-laminated or Tyvek aprons provide added protection for use in an uncontrolled environment (*see* Section 1, page 25).

5 Gloves

Disposable gloves should be worn at all times when preparing, checking and administering cytotoxic drugs.

The suitability of a wide range of commercially available gloves for cytotoxic handling has been investigated.[3-9] However, there is no consensus about which glove material offers the best protection.

A variety of techniques for determining permeation have been employed including a spectrophotometric method,[4] radiolabelling,[5] mutagenicity testing[6] and chromatographic analysis.[8] Permeation under static and flexed conditions has also been determined.[9] None of the studies considered the effect of solubility of the drug in the collection medium, yet Ehntholt *et al.*,[10] in an evaluation of protective glove materials in agricultural pesticide operations, found the collection medium to be a significant determinant of degree of break-through measured.

Several of these studies also determined the inter- and intra-batch variability in glove thickness and the surface characteristics.[4,11] Thomas and Fenton-May,[4] found that glove thickness varied considerably, with a tenfold difference between the extremes in the range. Variation in thickness within the same batch was also considerable for some manufacturers. Kotilainen *et al.*[11] used scanning electron microscopy to examine the surfaces of both PVC and latex gloves. They found that the surface was extremely irregular with multiple pits and defects, some up to 10 μ wide.

On the basis of these studies, it can be concluded that no glove material is completely impermeable to every cytotoxic agent. Although glove thickness is a major factor affecting drug permeation, molecular weight of the drug, lipophilicity, nature of the solvent in which the cytotoxic is dissolved, and glove material composition all affect permeation rates.

When selecting gloves for use with cytotoxics, the user must be assured that the glove material is of a suitable thickness and integrity to maximize protection whilst maintaining manual dexterity. Manufacturers should be asked to supply information on material composition, thickness (both mean and variation in) and durability. The use of poor quality, low cost gloves is neither cost-effective nor safe because multiple glove changes are required to ensure integrity.

The practice of double-gloving should be unnecessary provided gloves with appropriate qualities are used and the gloves are changed regularly during each work session, or immediately following known contact with a cytotoxic, or if punctured.

Industrial thickness gloves (>0.45 mm thick) made from latex with neoprene, nitrile synthetic rubber or similar materials should be used to clean up large-scale spills.

REFERENCES

1. Laidlaw, J.L. *et al.* (1985). Permeability of four disposable protective-clothing materials to seven antineoplastic drugs. *Am. J. Hosp. Pharm.* **42**, 2449–2454.
2. Glass, D.C. *et al.* (1989). *The control of substances hazardous to health. Guidance for the initial assessment in hospitals.* HMSO, London.
3. Oldcorne, M.A. *et al.* (1987). Handling cytotoxic drugs. *Pharm. J.* **238**, 488.
4. Thomas, P.H. and Fenton-May, V. (1987). Protection offered by various gloves to carmustine exposure. *Pharm. J.* **238**, 775–777.
5. Slevin, M.L. *et al.* (1984). The efficiency of protective gloves used in the handling of cytotoxic drugs. *Cancer Chemother. Pharmacol.* **12**, 151–153.
6. Laidlaw, J.L. *et al.* (1984). Permeability of latex and polyvinyl chloride gloves to 20 antineoplastic drugs. *Am. J. Hosp. Pharm.* **41**, 2618–2623.
7. Anon. (1987). Working Party Report – Guidelines for the handling of cytotoxic drugs: amendment. *Pharm. J.* **238**, 414.
8. Corlett, S.A. *et al.* (1991). Permeation of ifosfamide through gloves and cadaver skin. *Pharm. J.* **247**, R39.
9. Colligan, S.A. and Horstman, S.W. (1990). Permeation of cancer chemotherapeutic drugs through glove materials under static and flexed conditions. *Appl. Occup. Environ. Hyg.* **5**, 848–852.
10. Ehntholt, D.J. *et al.* (1990). A test method for the evaluation of protective glove materials used in agricultural pesticide operations. *Am. Ind. Hyg. Assoc. J.* **51**, 462–468.
11. Kotilainen, H.R. *et al.* (1989). Latex and vinyl examination gloves. Quality control procedures and implications for healthcare workers. *Arch. Intern. Med.* **149**, 2749–2753.

CHAPTER 4

Disposables

INTRODUCTION

Despite the range of items available for drug reconstitution, transport and disposal, the overriding aim when selecting disposables for use with cytotoxic drugs should be suitability, safety and simplicity. Devices listed in this chapter meet all three criteria, although choice of particular items will depend on the level of service provided. The cost of many of the devices may seem prohibitive but their use can be justified for health and safety reasons. No one particular manufacturer is recommended; the choice is left to each individual. Most hospital supplies departments stock a wide range of disposables.

SYRINGES AND ADMINISTRATION SYSTEMS

It is recommended that syringes used for cytotoxic drugs be luer-lock and made of polypropylene, as the material is chemically inert.[1,2] Styrene syringes are specifically not recommended for cytotoxic drugs. Standards for syringes are given in BS 5081, part 1 (1987)[3] and ISO 7886.[4]

Syringes are usually made in three parts–the barrel and piston of plastic materials and the plunger of rubber (Figure 4.1). Certain grades of rubber have been found to release water-soluble materials on prolonged contact with drug solutions.[5,6] Hence, chemical interactions between rubber extractives and the drugs are possible. If it is intended to store drugs in a particular brand of syringe for prolonged periods, it is advisable to check that there is no such interaction. Two-piece polypropylene luer-lock syringes are available, overcoming the possibility of an interaction between plunger and drug. In addition to ensuring that a drug is stable on storage, it is necessary to check that there is not an unacceptable degree of water loss from the syringe.[7]

Syringes must be fitted with blind hub closures, not needles, when prepared in the pharmacy. The blind hubs should be luer-lock, must be a good fit and not permit leakage. They must be of a suitable size to be easy for medical and nursing staff to remove safely.

Instillations of cytotoxic drugs are better presented in syringes or containers with catheter tips (Figure 4.1). Many bladder syringes have luer-lock connections in addition to the usual catheter tip. However, the addition of a luer-lock fitting to a bladder irrigation container may be potentially hazardous as it could facilitate IV administration of the bladder irrigation solution. Devices are made specifically for the instillation of fluids into the bladder. In certain countries, a fitting for converting a mini-bag into a bladder instillation device is available.

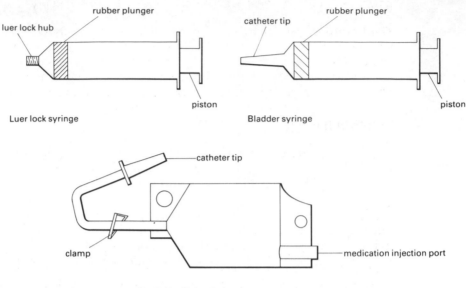

Figure 4.1: *Disposable administration systems*

NEEDLES AND FILTRATION SYSTEMS

1 Needles and Quills

When removing solutions from vials or ampoules, it is essential to use as wide a bore needle as possible to prevent undue pressure building up in the system. This is particularly important with viscous solutions such as etoposide. Specifications for needles are included in BS 5081, part 1 (1987)[3] and ISO 7886.[4] The length of the needle used will depend on the nature of the procedure being carried out.

Butterfly needles, which consist of a winged needle attached to a length of tubing with a luer-lock connector at the end, are useful for multiple additions or withdrawals from infusion bags or vials. They are available in standard needle sizes.

Quills are useful for drawing up solutions from ampoules, the rate of flow being greater than with a needle.

2 Filtration Systems

Sterilizing filters are not recommended for use with solutions of cytotoxic drugs because of the risk of pressurizing the system (*see* section on Reconstitution Devices and Air Vents). If a solution requires clarification, a filter with a pore size of not less than 5 µm can be used but with great caution. Filter straws are quills with a 5 or 10 µm filter attached. Filters are not recommended for use with etoposide as there is a potential chemical interaction with the material of which most filters are made.[8]

RECONSTITUTION DEVICES AND AIR VENTS

The hazard of aerosol production during the preparation of cytotoxic drugs is well recognized. To prevent the risk of exposure to individuals carrying out cytotoxic drug reconstitution, substantial positive or negative deviations from atmospheric pressure within drug vials and syringes should be avoided.[1,2,9] The practice of using needles to 'vent' cytotoxic drug vials is not recommended because the risk of exposure is high. 'Venting' of cytotoxic drug vials can be carried out in one of several ways.

▼ Using a negative pressure procedure: The negative pressure procedure described by Wilson and Solimando[10] requires consistent, impeccable technique. Some operatives find it difficult to maintain and it may not always be possible with partially pressurized vials.

▼ Using a non-filtered air vent: Even though these equilibrate the pressure within the system they are not recommended because of the risk of escape of cytotoxic drug.

▼ Using a reconstitution device: A number of reconstitution devices are available, but not all are suitable for use with cytotoxic drugs. The devices usually have a short, fine plastic spike attached to a filter. Spikes can make large holes in rubber bungs, with the possibility of leakage of the solution from around the spike. In addition, there is a risk of producing a 'core' of rubber. Where devices with spikes are used for cytotoxic drug reconstitution they should be single use only and the spike should not constitute more than 50% of the surface area of the rubber bung of the vial. Reconstitution devices are useful for the repeated aspiration of measured volumes of diluent by syringe.

▼ Using a hydrophobic filter-needle unit: several types are available incorporating a 0.2 micron hydrophobic filter supplied as a reconstitution device or a unit which can be used separately. The latter type can be difficult to use with smaller vials as both the filter unit and the needle of the reconstituting syringe need to be accommodated in the rubber bung of the vial. Hydrophobic filter-needle units are relatively expensive but it is prudent to balance cost with increased safety to the individual.

INCIDENTAL ITEMS

1 Cleaning Equipment

All cleaning equipment should only be used in the designated cytotoxic reconstitution area. Any cloths, sponges or mop-heads can be used provided they are low-lint. Cloths, ideally, should be disposable. Where in-house sterilizing facilities are available it may be cheaper to buy unsterile cleaning equipment. If there are several areas to be cleaned, the use of colour coding might be applicable.

2 Trays

These can be used for many purposes, including collection of waste inside an isolator or VLFC, as a confined environment for cytotoxic drug reconstitution and for setting-up each preparation prior to reconstitution. They come in a variety of materials and sizes. It is important that they can be easily cleaned or sterilized depending on their use.

3 Absorbent Mats

These are used for lining working surfaces. Their use in VLFCs is not ideal because recirculation of air is hampered, but they may have a use in isolators. Their ease of disposal once contaminated is an advantage. Any absorbent material of suitable size can be used provided it can be sterilized for use within an aseptic area.

4 Tamper-evident Seals

The injection ports of infusion bags and the tops of infusion bottles should ideally be sealed after addition of a drug or reconstitution. This prevents the further addition of drugs and indicates any loss of integrity during storage and transport. A variety of caps and seals are commercially available.

5 Packaging

All cytotoxic preparations should be packed in leak-proof containers after preparation. Polythene tubing which can be heat sealed to give an air/water tight seal and which can be cut to enclose any size or shape of container is recommended. Grip top bags should be avoided as the seal is easily broken. Opaque polythene can be used for drugs requiring light protection. Polythene of gauge 200–250 g is suitable for most purposes; however 500 g polythene may be required for outer-packaging of items being transported to off-site centres.

Heat sealers are available from a number of sources. The sealer selected must create an adequate seal and must be durable enough to endure repeated use. Domestic heat sealers are not suitable for the grades of plastic recommended.

REFERENCES

1. Anon. (1983). Guidelines for the handling of cytotoxic drugs – working party report. *Pharm. J.* **230**, 230–231.
2. Anon. (1983). *The safe handling of cytotoxic drugs.* ASTMS, Health and Safety Office, Special Report.
3. Anon. (1987). *Sterile hypodermic syringes and needles, Part 1 Specification of sterile hypodermic syringes for single use. BS 5081.* British Standards Institute, London.
4. Anon. (1984). *Sterile hypodermic syringes for single use. ISO 7886.* (Available through the Standards Institute of the relevant country.)
5. Petersen, M.C. *et al.* (1981). Leaching of 2-(2-hydroxyethylmercapto) benzothiazole into contents of disposable syringes. *J. Pharm. Sci.* **70**, 1139–1143.
6. Reepmeyer, J.C. and Juhl, Y.H. (1983). Contamination of injectable solutions with 2-mercaptobenzothiazole leached from rubber closures. *J. Pharm. Sci.* **72**, 1302–1305.
7. Parkinson, R. *et al.* (1989). Stability of low-dose heparin in pre-filled syringes. *Brit. J. Pharm. Prac.* **11**, 34–36.
8. Forrest, S.C. (1984). Vepesid injection. *Pharm. J.* **232**, 88.
9. Anon. (1990). ASHP technical assistance bulletin on handling cytotoxic and hazardous drugs. *Am. J. Hosp. Pharm.* **47**, 1033–1049.
10. Wilson, J.P. and Solimando, D.A. (1981). Aseptic technique as a safety precaution in the preparation of antineoplastic agents. *Hosp. Pharm.* **16**, 575–581.

CHAPTER 5

Ambulatory Infusion Pumps for Cytotoxic Therapy

INTRODUCTION

Traditionally, cytotoxic chemotherapy has been administered in single or combined regimens which have been designed to maximize cell-kill whilst minimizing toxicity. However, in practice, these high dose, 'pulsed' regimens are not ideal because of the need to hospitalize the patients and the high incidence of side-effects which can delay further therapy.

Growing evidence has shown that continuous infusion of a low-dose of a cytotoxic drug achieves equivalent or higher tumour concentrations over a longer period than bolus, pulsed therapy.[1] The rationale for low-dose continuous infusion therapy is discussed in more detail in Chapter 10.

In response to the demand for this method of administration, there have been rapid advances in pump technology. A wide variety of ambulatory infusion pumps are now available, ranging in complexity from external syringe drivers to implantable, programmable pumps.

The pumps described are those available in the UK and the USA. A larger range of pumps is available worldwide and readers are directed to the literature available in their own country for details of other types of pump which have been used for the administration of cytotoxic chemotherapy.

SYRINGE PUMPS

Models: Braun Medical, Perfusor M (Figure 5.1); Graseby, MS16A (Figure 5.2) and MS26; Critikon, Syringe Minder 2

Syringe pumps are pocket-sized, usually battery-operated and are simple in design with only a few alarms, eg low battery, end of infusion and occlusion pressure. They use a range of syringes from 1 ml to 35 ml, although individual models may be limited to a narrower range.

The drug reservoir is a pre-filled syringe which is firmly clamped onto the pump. The pump is driven by a small battery-powered motor or, in the case of the Braun, Perfusor M, by a clockwork mechanism. A rotating lead screw (or drive shaft) moves the actuator (or drive nut) down the device at a constant rate, pushing the syringe plunger into the syringe barrel. The delivery rate of the drug is determined by the diameter of syringe and the speed at which the lead screw rotates.

Syringe pumps have been used successfully for self-administration of IV antibiotics[2] and cytotoxic agents.[3] They can be used with variable flow rates to a high level of accuracy (+/− 2% to 5%). Due to the pressure generated, the pump can be used for both intra-arterial and intravenous infusions. The syringe size is a limiting factor and, if larger volumes are required, it is necessary to replace the syringe reservoir several times.

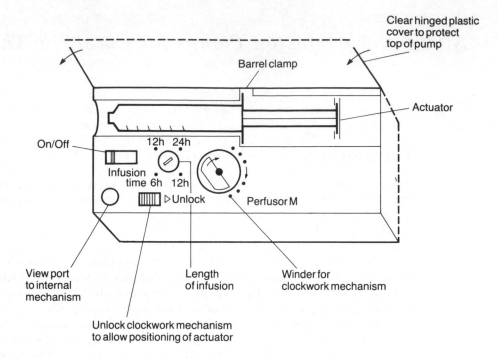

Figure 5.1: *Braun Medical Perfusor M Pump*

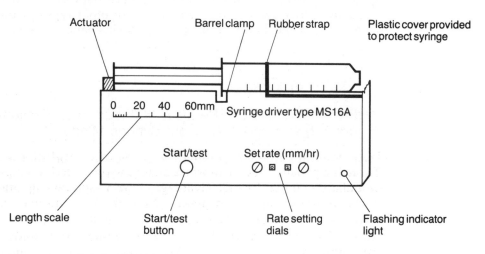

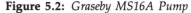

Figure 5.2: *Graseby MS16A Pump*

To set up the pumps, the administration line is primed either manually, before putting the syringe in the pump, or by a venting mechanism, if included in the pump. Priming should be carried out prior to rate setting in pumps that use the mm/hr or mm/day system, since at low infusion rates the dead volume of the tubing could alter the final infusion time by several hours. The syringe is placed into the pump and fixed in position. The actuator should be placed as close to the plunger as possible, so that there is little slack to take up in the lead screw when the pump is started. If the priming procedure or positioning of the actuator are not performed correctly, then, at low infusion rates, this could result in no drug being delivered for up to an hour and the patency of the venous access may be compromised.

The infusion rates are calculated in mm/hr for the Graseby, MS16A and Syringe Minder 2 pumps or mm/day for the Graseby, MS26 pump. Errors can occur when changing the pump setting if the patient or user does not understand the concept of mm/hr instead of ml/hr; or alternatively, confuses hours with days. The Syringe Minder 2 pump has preset rates of travel, 1, 2, 3, 4, 5, 6, 8, 10, 11, 12 mm/hr. The Graseby, MS16A and MS26 have continuously variable rates which are set as required. The Braun, Perfusor M has three preset rates of travel which deliver the contents of a 10 ml syringe in 6, 12 or 24 hr. Setting of infusion rates is straightforward for all those syringe drivers available in the UK. However, this simplicity also makes them easy to tamper with, which may be a disadvantage in some circumstances.

All of the pumps have a fixed occlusion pressure which causes the pump to alarm or stop. However, due to the need to overcome the build-up of pressure when infusing viscous fluids, the pressure at which the pump will alarm can be high. At low flow rates there is a considerable delay before the alarm is activated. This problem has been overcome in larger infusion pumps by positioning a pressure sensing device in the extension set rather than in the pump, but this feature is not yet available on the ambulatory pumps.

Patient education and training are required to ensure correct rate setting, mounting of syringe and priming of the set. They also need to be aware of the various alarms and how to deal with resulting malfunctions. Some knowledge is required of the mechanism of the syringe pumps. Checks must be kept on the batteries.

Despite their lack of sophistication, syringe drivers have several advantages as drug delivery systems. They are relatively cheap to purchase and the disposables associated with their use are cheap and readily available from several sources (excepting those devices dedicated to a certain brand of syringe). The simplicity of syringe drivers may make them less intimidating to patients and the necessity to change syringes frequently allows the patient to gain confidence rapidly in his or her mastery of the machine. The low weight and bulk of several of these devices is very popular with patients, who consider this a very important feature.[4] A further advantage of the syringe driver to the pharmacist is the large amount of published data on the stability of drugs in plastic syringes. There is a paucity of such information for the dedicated reservoirs of many other ambulatory pumps. The disadvantage of syringe drivers, apart from the susceptibility to tampering already alluded to, is the large number of syringes which have to be filled to provide a course of treatment, normally at least one per day. This can make them considerably more labour-intensive than pumps with larger drug reservoirs.

ELASTOMERIC PUMPS

Model: Baxter Infusor (Figure 5.3)

This is a novel delivery system which employs elastomer technology for drug delivery. The balloon, which acts as both drug reservoir and the pump, is made of an inert polyisoprene rubber material. This gives it elastic properties enabling the reservoir, once expanded, to contract back to its original shape and size.

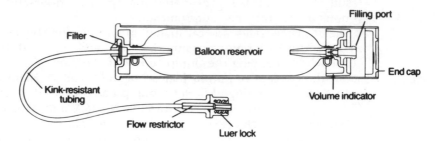

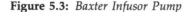

Figure 5.3: *Baxter Infusor Pump*

The operating principle of the pump is the Hagen-Poiseville Law[5] which states that flow through a tube is a function of pressure difference (P), radius of the lumen (r), length of the tube (l), and viscosity of the liquid (v).

The law is represented by the equation

$$F = \frac{P \times \pi r^4}{8 \times v \times l}$$

The variable function is viscosity, which will be affected by vehicle and temperature. The effects of the vehicle are known if glucose or 0.9% sodium chloride solution are used[6] and temperature fluctuations are kept to a minimum by wearing the Infusor close to the skin. High concentrations of drugs occasionally affect viscosity.

An increasing range of Infusors is being made available by Baxter. These infuse their contents over periods of up to 7 days.

Infusors are filled by connecting a luer-lock syringe, filled with drug solution, to the valve assembly in the Infusor, and forcing liquid into the elastomer reservoir. This requires significant force and can be tiring, especially if many Infusors are to be filled. Once filled, the microbore administration set primes automatically in about 15 minutes.

The patient removes the winged luer cap from the administration set and attaches the Infusor to the venous access device. The drug is delivered via a 10 µm filter at a constant rate, which depends upon the Infusor model and the diluent solution. The duration of infusion can be altered by adjusting the volume filled and dose rate can be altered by choice of Infusor model and by adjusting the volume filled or drug concentration. The Infusor can be used by the intra-arterial or intravenous route.

Infusors are intended for single use and are not designed to be refilled or resterilized for repeat use. Therefore, although there is no capital cost involved in the pump, since it cannot be reused, revenue costs are high. However, the ongoing introduction of Infusor models with longer discharge times may make them competitive with electromechanical pumps requiring dedicated disposables. Infusors are light-weight, small, comfortable in use and silent in operation. They are provided with a fabric holder which is pinned inside the patient's clothes.

The Infusor has been studied in 18 patients who received 52 treatment courses, representing 247 patient-days of treatment at home rather than in hospital. During this period there was no known failure to infuse and no reported flow rate or administration difficulties. There was one report of a leaking unit.[6]

The Infusor has been used to administer a number of drugs including morphine,[7] heparin,[8] cyclophosphamide, fluorouracil, doxorubicin, methotrexate, vincristine and vinblastine.

There are no published data on stability or compatibility of these injections in the devices. However, research has been conducted by Baxter Healthcare Ltd on the stability of a variety of drugs in Infusors; data are available from the company. Unfortunately, the parameters by which stability is considered to be satisfactory have not been fully described. This information should, therefore, be considered for guidance purposes only. It has been included in the relevant Drug Monographs.

The patient needs to be educated about storage, infusion rates, monitoring the infusion and care of his central line after completion of the infusion. The Infusor is popular with patients in comparison with more sophisticated pumps[1] because they do not have to be concerned with battery checks, setting of infusion rates or monitoring for mechanical malfunction of the pump. In addition, as the unit is disposable, they do not have equipment to return to the hospital at the end of treatment.

As well as constant rate Infusors, Baxter now market a variety of Infusors with additional flow controls which make them suitable for pulsatile or 'basal-bolus' drug delivery. Although primarily intended for antibiotic administration and patient-controlled analgesia, these devices are likely to be useful to those attempting to transfer more complex chemotherapy regimens from the hospital to the domiciliary setting.

PERISTALTIC PUMPS

Models: Pharmacia/Deltec, CADD-1 (Figure 5.4), CADD-PCA, CADD-PLUS

These pumps employ a motorized rotating drum powered by a battery, which rolls over a silicone tube. The drug reservoir is a 50 ml or 100 ml disposable bag enclosed in a rigid plastic shell. These pumps can also be used to deliver the contents of conventional collapsible infusion containers via a special administration set. They are more sophisticated than the other pumps discussed, since they are programmable and the infusion rate and drug dose can be varied. The CADD pumps have six alarms comprising internal malfunction, set up review, pump stopped, low residual volume in medication cassette, low battery and occlusion. There are a number of lock levels for varying patient involvement in the programming of the dose and rate of infusion. However, when used for chemotherapy, the patient is not normally involved in programming and the ability to 'lock' the pump memory against deliberate or accidental alteration is useful. Although these pumps are more sophisticated they aim to be user friendly, but still require a significant amount of training to ensure correct usage. With this in mind the company has prepared training programmes for operators. The pump is robust, but rather heavy and, with a 100 ml drug reservoir *in situ*, bulky (19.5 × 9 × 2.8 cm).

The manufacturers of the Pharmacia pump will provide information on the stability of various cytotoxic drugs in Pharmacia cassettes. This information, which is incorporated in the relevant Drug Monographs, was obtained from unpublished studies conducted at Apotekseolaget AB Central Laboratories and Apotekseolaget AB Karolinska Pharmacy, Stockholm, Sweden.

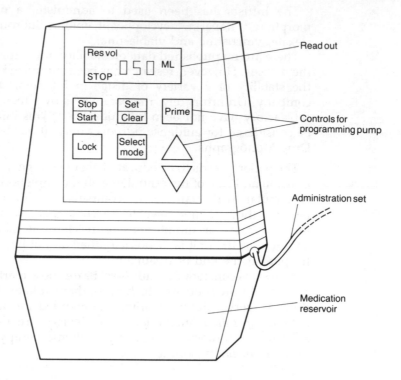

Figure 5.4: *Pharmacia/Deltec CADD-1 Pump*

As well as the CADD constant-rate pump, Pharmacia market two other pumps which differ only in their programming characteristics. The CADD-PCA delivers a continuous base drug infusion which may be boosted by the user activating a bolus control, whilst the CADD-PLUS (which is intended for antibiotic administration) can give pulsatile infusions. Both of these pumps are also capable of continuous, constant rate infusion and may be attractive to the user involved in providing a range of drug administration services, since they offer flexibility of application.

Model: Medfusion Inc., INFU-MED 300 (Figure 5.5)

The INFU-MED 300 is a linear peristaltic pump which delivers drug solutions from soft PVC reservoirs of 65, 150 or 250 ml via a silicone tubing administration set which is acted upon by the pump mechanism. Additionally, a special 'spike set' makes it possible to use the pump to infuse the contents of conventional collapsible infusion bags. The 65 ml drug reservoir will fit entirely within the pump's rigid plastic cover. Larger reservoirs are carried separately in the pump's fabric carrying pouch. Setting of the infusion rate is by means of an infusion rate setting dial. This is simple to operate, but also easily tampered with.

The INFU-MED 300 is simple to use, reasonably compact, and offers a comprehensive range of reservoir sizes, but is neither as small nor as lightweight as

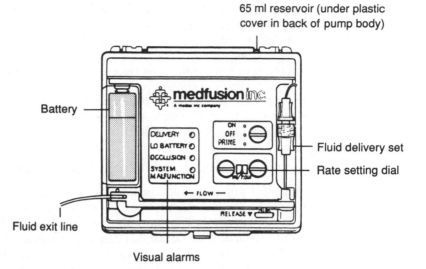

Figure 5.5: *Medfusion INFU-MED 300*

certain other devices and is, therefore, less popular with some patients. This pump is being superseded by the Walk Med pumps described below.

Models: Medfusion Inc., Walk Med 410c, Walk Med 420i/c, Walk Med 430pca, Walk Med 440pic

The Walk Med pumps share their pumping mechanisms and chassis construction with the INFU-MED 300 pump described above. However, flow control is achieved by programming the pump via an electronic keypad which can be locked in a similar way to that of the Pharmacia pump to prevent unauthorized tampering. Flow parameters are displayed on an LCD display.

The Walk Med 410c is the most basic pump for continuous, steady rate, drug infusion. The other three pumps in the range are all capable of fulfilling this task, and also function as devices for the delivery of patient controlled analgesia (430pca), intermittent drug infusion (420i/c) or both (440pic) and their flexibility may be attractive to the pharmacist involved in operating a range of services. No data are available yet on the stability of drugs in INFU-MED reservoirs, either from the distributors of the pump or from other published sources. This information will be required before the pump can be accepted for routine use.

IMPLANTABLE PUMP SYSTEMS

Implantable pump systems have been developed for drug delivery, offering the patient a more normal life-style, since there is no externalized portion of the system to be seen or to be managed. Additional advantages of the implantable pump system are a reduction in the potential for infections due to microbial contamination and improved patient compliance with therapy. These advantages are of particular benefit to the ambulatory patient receiving long-term therapy. The primary disadvantages of the implantable pump systems are the small volume capacity of the pump reservoirs, and the high cost of the pump and surgical implantation of the system.

Implanted in a subcutaneous pocket, the pump can easily be felt through the skin. The silicone injection septum is accessed through the skin using a special Huber-type needle for up to 1000 punctures, depending on needle size.

Two commercially available implanted pump systems are the Pfizer Infusaid Implantable Pump and the Medtronic SynchroMed Pump.

Model: Pfizer Infusaid Implantable Pump (Figure 5.6)

The Infusaid pump is made of titanium, is approximately 90 mm in diameter, 28 mm thick, weighs slightly more than 200 g, and has a reservoir capacity of approximately 50 ml. The operating mechanism of the pump utilizes a non-electronic metal bellows concept. The pump consists of two chambers, separated by flexible metal bellows, and is attached to a silicone rubber catheter placed into the delivery site. The outer chamber contains a fluorocarbon charging fluid, and the inner chamber serves as the drug reservoir. When the drug chamber is filled, the charging fluid is compressed. Expansion of the charging fluid exerts a vapour pressure which compresses the drug chamber, forcing drug from the reservoir through the flow restrictor and into the delivery catheter. Because there is no electromechanical component, the energy of the charging fluid is limitless, not requiring replenishment.

Flow rate is controlled by a restricted capillary tube which cannot be changed after implantation. Flow rate is affected by a number of variables, including fluid viscosity, patient temperature, and altitude. The Infusaid pump is supplied by the manufacturer with a specific capillary tube to deliver a specific drug at a specific flow rate for normal body temperature and at the geographical location of the patient. Increased temperatures, for example as experienced by a patient in a hot bath, will increase the flow rate of the pump by approximately 10 to 13% for each 1°C rise in temperature. Higher altitudes will also cause the pump to flow faster. An infusion pump calibrated for sea level will flow approximately 45% faster at an altitude of 2000 metres. After implantation, slight alterations in flow rate can be achieved by varying the concentration or viscosity of the fluid. Only one model of the Infusaid pump is commercially available, Model 400, although there is both a single catheter and a dual catheter version. The use of the sideport allows direct access to the catheter, bypassing the pump mechansm, for bolus doses, if required.

A programmable version of the Infusaid pump, Model 1000, is not yet commercially available, but is now in clinical trials. The pump uses telemetry via an external programmer to change delivery rates after implantation.

Model: Medtronic SynchroMed Pump (Figure 5.7)

This pump can be reprogrammed for delivery rate changes (0.1 to 18 ml/day) after implantation using an external programmer. Approximately 70 mm in diameter, 27 mm thick, and 200 g in weight, the pump has a usable capacity of 18 ml. The operating mechanism of the SynchroMed pump is a rotary peristaltic system that is powered by an internal lithium battery, improving delivery accuracy and eliminating the dependence on temperature, viscosity, and

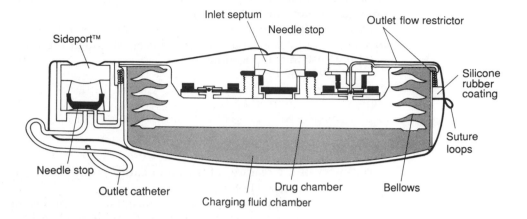

Figure 5.6: *Infusaid Model 400 implantable pump*

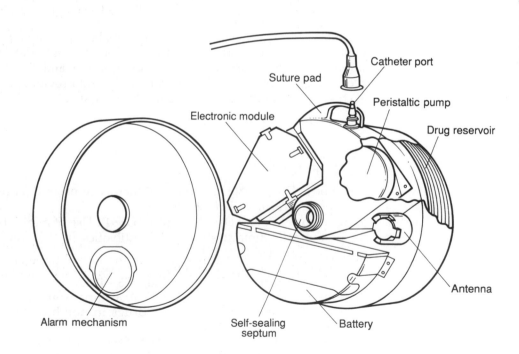

Figure 5.7: *SynchroMed implantable pump*

pressure characteristic of the Infusaid pump. The typical life of the battery is approximately three to four years at a flow rate of 0.5 ml/day. Two models of the pump are commercially available, Model 8611H and Model 8615. Model 8615 has a sideport access site to bypass the pumping mechanism for bolus doses.

The pump can be programmed to deliver continuous, intermittent and complex circadian administrations using the external programmer and a radio telemetry link via the programming wand.

The use of implantable pumps has been primarily restricted to regional deliveries, eg intra-arterial and intrathecal, although the pumps are also being used for systemic applications.[9–11]

CONCLUSION

A summary of the features of the ambulatory pumps discussed is contained in Table 5.1 (*see* pages 44–45).

Ambulatory pumps have made the concept of continuous infusion attainable, with all the concurrent benefits previously mentioned. All the pumps provide accurate dosing and are portable. Pumps differ in the number of features available, which may include flexible administration rates, variable reservoir sizes and range of alarms. The proposed use of the pump should be considered when selecting features required. With all the pumps, not only the capital cost of the pump, but also the cost of disposables that are required for each infusion are significant factors to be considered.

For successful home treatment with ambulatory pumps, the patient must feel confident and be proficient in the use of the unit. Patient education is an important part of any ambulatory programme and the level of knowledge required and staff time involved in training and providing a back-up service for each type of pump should be carefully evaluated.

REFERENCES

1. Moody, D.G. (1986). External ambulatory infusion devices and the oncology patient. *J. Pharm. Tech*. **2**, 160–165.
2. Johnston, J.B. and Davidson, M.R. (1984). Use of mini-infusor syringe pump for the self-administration of IV antibiotics in the home. *Natl. Intravenous Ther. Assoc. USA*. **7**, 381–383.
3. Adams, P.S. *et al.* (1987). Pharmaceutical aspects of home infusion therapy for cancer patients. *Pharm. J*. **238**, 476–478.
4. Summerhayes, M. *et al.* (1991). A comparison of two devices for the continuous infusion of cytotoxic drugs in non-hospitalized patients. *Int. J. Pharm. Pract*. **1**, 94–97.
5. Thomas, M. *et al.* (1985). Miniaturized continuous delivery systems for injectable solutions: individual patient control and physio-chemical properties. *Proc. of the Guild*, **19**, 3–37.
6. Akahoshi, M.P. *et al.* (1987). Safety and reliability of the Travenol Infusor in administering chemotherapy in the home. *J. Pharm. Tech*. **3**, 65–68.
7. Wermeling, D.P. *et al.* (1987). Evaluation of a disposable non-electric patient-controlled analgesia device for post-operative pain. *Clin. Phar*. **6**, 307–315.
8. Merrigan, D.M. *et al.* (1987). Continuous heparin infusion in the home-bound ambulatory patient using the Travenol Infusor. *Natl. Intravenous Ther. Assoc. USA*. **10**, 122–126.

9. Kwan, J.W. (1989). High technology IV infusion devices. *Am. J. Hosp. Pharm.* **46**, 320–335.
10. Kemeny, N. *et al.* (1987). Intrahepatic or systemic infusion of fluorodeoxy-uridine in patients with liver metastases from colorectal carcinoma. *Ann. Intern. Med.* **107**, 459–465.
11. von Roemeling, R. *et al.* (1988). Progressive metastatic renal cell carcinoma controlled by continuous 5-fluoro-2 deoxyuridine infusion. *J. Urol.* **139**, 259–262.

Table 5.1: *Summary of pumps described*

Make/Model	Range Infusion Time	Weight**	Dimensions***	Pump Mechanism	Reservoir	Battery	Flow Rate and	Accuracy	Alarm*
Graseby Medical									
MS16A	30 min to 60 h	275 g	16.5×2.3×5.3 cm	syringe pump electric	2 ml–35 ml syringe	9 V	0–99 mm/h variable	±5%	1,2,3
MS26	12 h to 60 days	275 g	16.5×2.3×5.3 cm	syringe pump electric	2 ml–35 ml syringe	9 V	0–99 mm/day	±5%	1,2,3
Braun Medical									
Perfusor M	6 to 24 h	450 g	17×7.5×3.5 cm	syringe pump clockwork	10 ml Braun Omnifix syringe	none	10 ml in 6–24 h fixed	±5%	none
Critikon									
Syringe Minder 2	4 to 50 h	270 g	11.7×5×1 cm	syringe pump electric	2 ml–20 ml syringe	9 V	1–12 mm/h fixed intervals	±3%	1,2,3
Pharmacia/Deltec									
CADD-1	1 h to 100 days	425 g	2.8×9×16 cm	peristaltic rotary programmable	50 ml/ 100 ml cassette	9 V	0–299 ml/day	theor. ±10% in studies ±3%	1,2,3, 4,5,6
CADD-PCA	1 h to 4 days	425 g	2.8×9×16 cm	peristaltic rotary programmable	50 ml/ 100 ml cassette	9 V	0–20 ml/h		1,2,3, 4,5,6
CADD-PLUS	1 h to 4 days	425 g	2.8×9×16 cm	peristaltic rotary programmable	50 ml/ 100 ml cassette	9 V	0–75 ml/h		1,2,3, 4,5,6
Baxter									
Single day Infusor	1 to 24 h	100 g	16.5×3 cm dia.	elastomeric pressure	60 ml	none	2 ml/h	±5%	none
Multi day Infusor	1 to 5 days	100 g	16.5×3 cm dia.	elastomeric pressure	60 ml	none	0.5 ml/h	±5%	none
Seven day Infusor	1 to 7 days	150 g	25×3 cm dia.	elastomeric pressure	90 ml	none	0.5 ml/h	±5%	none
Medfusion									
INFU-MED 300	1 h to 104 days	350 g	11.2×10.4×4.6 cm	linear peristaltic	65 ml/ 150 ml/ 250 ml collapsible reservoir	9 V	0.1–9.9 ml/h	±5%	2,3,4
WalkMed 410c	1 h to 104 days	360 g	11.2×10.2×4.6 cm	linear peristaltic programmable	65 ml/ 150 ml/ 250 ml collapsible reservoir	9 V	0.01–30 ml/h	±5%	2,3, 4,5
WalkMed 420i/c	1 h to 104 days	360 g	11.2×10.2×4.6 cm	linear peristaltic programmable	65 ml/ 150 ml/ 250 ml collapsible reservoir	9 V	0–9.9 ml/h	±5%	2,3, 4,5
WalkMed 430pca		360 g	11.2×10.2×4.6 cm	linear peristaltic programmable	65 ml/ 150 ml/ 250 ml collapsible reservoir	9 V		±5%	2,3, 4,5
WalkMed 440pic		360 g	11.2×10.2×4.6 cm	linear peristaltic programmable	65 ml/ 150 ml/ 250 ml collapsible reservoir	9 V		±5%	2,3, 4,5

Table 5.1: *Continued*

Make/Model	Range Infusion Time	Weight**	Dimensions***	Pump Mechanism	Reservoir	Battery	Flow Rate and Accuracy	Alarm*
Pfizer								
Infusaid 400	–	200 g	9×2.8 cm	non-electronic metal bellows concept	50 ml	none	flow rate affected by a number of variables	none
Medtronic								
SynchroMed 8611H	–	200 g	7×2.7 cm	rotary peristaltic system	18 ml	lithium	0.1–18 ml/day	none
SynchroMed 8615	–	200 g	7×2.7cm	rotary peristaltic system	18 ml	lithium	0.1–18 ml/day	none

*Alarms
1–end of travel/infusion, 2–low battery, 3–occlusion, 4–internal malfunction, 5–lower residual volume in medication cassette, 6–start-up review (power up)
**Includes batteries and smallest reservoir
***Includes smallest reservoir (empty) and protective cases for syringe pumps

CHAPTER 6

Health and Safety Aspects of Cytotoxic Services

INTRODUCTION

It is now well recognized that most anticancer drugs are potentially hazardous substances, since they are either mutagenic, teratogenic or carcinogenic. There is also substantial evidence to show that patients may develop secondary neoplasms as a result of treatment with cancer chemotherapeutic agents,[1-4] indicating the potential threat to the health of any persons exposed to this class of drugs. Such risks may be acceptable for patients with life-threatening diseases. It is clearly not acceptable to hospital personnel who are exposed to such chemicals in the workplace. There is now a large body of evidence to show that health care personnel involved in the preparation and manipulation of anticancer drugs can, if not adequately protected, absorb potentially harmful quantities of such compounds. Much of the evidence comes from epidemiological studies on such diverse groups as nurses, pharmacists and pharmacy technicians and has recently been extensively reviewed.[4-6] The potential dangers are, therefore, well established. Recent studies have, for example, shown the association between spontaneous abortions and malformations in the offspring of nurses with occupational exposure to cytotoxic agents.[7,8] Nurses handling these drugs have shown increased mutagenic activity in their urine when compared with unexposed personnel.[9-11] Similar patterns have also been reported in the serum of oncology nurses.[12-14] These and other studies indicate the potential high level of risk to staff working with anticancer drugs. A number of relevant safety measures have been introduced, many as a result of regulatory requirements, to protect health care personnel who prepare or administer cytotoxic drugs. Studies have now been reported highlighting the fact that such improvements can substantially reduce staff exposure levels. For example, improved care in handling has been shown to reduce mutagenic activity detected in nurses' urine.[6,15] Cooke et al.[16] reported that blood samples from pharmacy staff handling anticancer agents in purpose-designed cytotoxic units showed no greater evidence of mutagenicity than unexposed controls. In a comparative study, Kolmodin-Hedman et al.[17] showed that the provision of adequate safety precautions significantly reduced the mutagenic activity in the urine taken from staff working in oncology units and pharmacies. Ferguson et al.[18] reported that a group of pharmacists working in a fully protected environment preparing cytotoxic injections did not show evidence of drug absorption, although it was noted that an occasional individual did show evidence of exposure. Most recently, it has been confirmed that pharmacy staff preparing cytotoxics in a vertical laminar flow cabinet (biological safety cabinet Type 2b) with 30% recirculation and wearing gloves and arm protection, did not show any evidence of increased urine mutagenic activity.[19] It can be concluded that there is now sufficient evidence to indicate that staff working in pharmacies who prepare cytotoxic injections for administration, or nurses who work in oncology departments, either preparing drugs for administration or dealing with patients' urine or other contaminated fluids, are potentially at risk. This risk is sufficient to indicate, unequivocally, that all necessary measures should be adopted to protect these staff from occupational exposure. It is not possible to establish maximum safe exposure levels. Therefore, all recognized steps need to be taken to prevent, or at least reduce to a minimum, exposure to these hazardous substances in the workplace. As all approaches available are, by the nature of the problem, of an indirect form, many different aspects of service operation must be included to ensure adequate, state-of-the-art, staff protection. These should include the following:

▼ provision of adequate protective environments (suitable safety cabinet, isolators or hoods)
▼ regular staff monitoring by occupational health services
▼ effective written procedures and ongoing staff training
▼ regular application of service audits
▼ adequate procedures for dealing with spillages and disposal of all contaminated materials.

Another key question to be addressed by pharmacy managers is whether or not to rotate staff through this service and other departmental activities. A number of factors need to be considered in making such a judgement. The advantages of employing staff specifically to work in the cytotoxic service include assurance that a high level of expertise is established, that speed and efficiency of operation is optimized and such personnel can also fulfil training roles. The disadvantages are that the same staff are exposed to the hazards associated with cytotoxic drug handling over longer periods and it is more difficult to cover for staff absences. Finally, boredom from carrying out the same activities over long periods can lead to lowering of performance. If a rotational scheme is operated, this ensures that a maximum number of staff are trained and the levels of exposure to potentially harmful substances are reduced. However, it is likely that the overall level of competence is lower and a greater level of supervision and monitoring may be deemed necessary.

STAFF MONITORING

It is essential to maintain a system of health surveillance for staff directly involved in handling cytotoxic agents on a routine basis. This may comprise regular general health screening together with the use of specific biochemical and cytological tests to determine if an individual has been exposed to harmful levels of mutagenic substances.

1 Health Surveillance

Four data-gathering elements have been identified as contributing to a medical surveillance programme for staff working with cytotoxic drugs.[20] These are:

Medical history

The employee's medical and occupational history is rightly the prerogative of the occupational health department. Their staff have a key role to play in record keeping and counselling. The concept of an individual exposure record has been postulated as an attempt to quantify the drug 'burden' to which the individual has been exposed. A record of the length of time handling hazardous materials is logistically simpler to produce, and arguably more valid than a cumulative record of doses prepared. The scientific case for such records remains unproven and the problems of data interpretation are vast. Individual agents vary in their acute toxicity, particularly with regard to irritant effects, but differentiating between exposure to different drugs on an ongoing basis is unlikely to be possible.

Physical examinations

These should be routine pre-employment practice. For staff involved in cytotoxic drug handling, they should be repeated at regular intervals in order to identify symptoms which could be associated with acute exposure (for example, irritation of mucous membranes, dizziness, light-headedness[20]). Documentation of untoward events such as spills and accidents, together with estimations of potential exposure 'doses' should form a part of individual health surveillance records. One aim should be to determine whether abnormal findings or test results are associated with longer handling times.

Laboratory tests

Full blood and differential white cell counts are performed routinely in many centres. Such data gives little information except in the case of high exposure, and must be interpreted with care. Tests for changes in liver and renal function have also been advocated[20] in the light of the toxicity profiles of many cytotoxic drugs. There is also some evidence to link any such changes with adverse effects reported in health care workers handling cytotoxic drugs without adequate protection.[21]

Biological monitoring

The measurement of concentrations of specific cytotoxic agents in body fluids (for example in blood and urine) has been reported for certain drugs or their known metabolites.[22-24] The value of monitoring such levels is, however, limited, due to the increasing range of potential agents, and the likelihood that the extremely low concentrations of drug anticipated in an occupational exposure setting will be below the limits of sensitivity of assay procedures.

2 Health Surveillance in Practice

In practice, the cornerstone of an occupational health monitoring process is to give all new staff working with cytotoxic drugs a confidential interview, which is designed to review their medical history, and a physical examination. Simple laboratory tests, such as blood counts and differential white cell counts, together with urine and liver function tests, may also be performed to confirm their current state of good health. The interview should also be used as an opportunity for the staff member to discuss any fears they may have concerning work with such agents. This interview should be repeated at suitable intervals when the employee's exposure record can also be updated. Such interviews are usually recommended on an annual basis.

The exposure record is an essential part of staff surveillance programmes. It should include a record of times spent by each staff member working with cytotoxic agents, together with a specific record of involvement with accidental spillages or other occurrence which could increase that person's exposure. In addition, all incidences involving accidental exposure, such as gross spillages or needle-stick incidences, must be reported to the occupational health department. Following such incidents, blood testing and a physical examination should be undertaken to identify signs of acute toxicity to skin, mucous membranes, eyes etc. Records should be maintained centrally, ideally by occupational health or personnel departments. Computerization of these records allows for rapid data entry and recall, especially if linked to the pharmacy system used in the operation of the service. Exposure and incident records should be retained with the employee's personal record. A copy should be available on request to any employee who leaves the service or transfers to another hospital. If a local occupational health policy exists, this should be made available to general practitioners. Employees working for an authority without occupational health facilities should be advised to inform their general practitioner of the nature of their work. Many authorities now recommend that staff who are pregnant or contemplating pregnancy, or are breast-feeding, should be excluded from duties involving the preparation or administration of cytotoxic drugs. In addition to professional and technical staff, other grades may be involved in handling cytotoxic drugs. These can include porters, storekeepers etc. They need to be educated to an appropriate level in relation to their responsibilities, and provided with appropriate health screening and advice.

3 Cytogenetic Monitoring of Staff

The need to monitor staff for specific biological evidence of enhanced exposure to cytotoxic drugs is controversial. While such a system of staff surveillance offers, in theory, a sensitive means of monitoring the real biological risks to staff, in terms of indices of mutagenicity, test methods currently available do not appear to offer adequate assurance of their ability to identify the real risks.[3,5,6,20] Methods may be either insufficiently sensitive or poorly validated. The following tests are available and, in theory at least, offer a monitoring test for staff. These have been assessed in the context of hospital staff exposure to cytotoxic drugs by Ferguson et al.[18] and Kaijser et al.,[6] and for environmental exposure to mutagens and carcinogens by the International Commission for Protection against Environmental Mutagens and Carcinogens (ICPEMC).[5]

Test for urine mutagenicity

The Ames test is used as a routine method to measure mutagenic activity in urine. The test relies on the measurement of mutations in bacterial cells caused by carcinogenic agents. While relatively simple and cheap to perform, it lacks both sensitivity and specificity as a means of measuring staff exposure to cytotoxic agents in normal practice.[6] It is now considered unsuitable for staff monitoring.

Tests for cytogenetic changes

These tests are designed to identify biological changes which may have been caused by cellular exposure to mutagenic agents. They can be either chemical (eg carcinogens) or physical (eg ionizing radiation) agents. Biological markers are employed to detect either chromosomal aberrations or DNA interchange between chromatids.

Assay for chromosome aberrations

This method offers the most direct estimate of heritable changes, but is relatively insensitive and laborious to perform. Its main importance lies in the fact that it measures long-lasting effects and, therefore, provides an index of accumulative damage. In fact, if the test indicates that a particular individual does show an increase in chromosomal aberrations with time, this probably indicates that hazardous substances are being absorbed and urgent preventative measures are required.

Micronucleus assay

This method provides a more indirect method of detecting exposure to cytotoxic substances. It is less time consuming to perform than chromosomal aberration tests, and does not require the same high level of technical skill. It is, however, too variable to identify real differences in individuals[18] but it may be useful, when applied to sufficiently large groups of workers, to identify differences between populations or between working conditions. It may be improved by the use of the cytochalasin block method.[24]

Sister chromatid exchange (SCE)

This method detects reciprocal exchanges between chromatids. It is a sensitive method and detects changes that could be caused by very low levels of mutagenic compounds. However, it must be realized that SCE lesions are short lived and decline substantially within a few days. The test must be performed immediately after the sample has been collected. It will clearly have relevance to testing personnel while working with cytotoxic drugs. It has no retrospective value.

4 Should Blood Tests be Used to Monitor Staff?

Whether or not routine testing of staff for evidence of exposure to mutagenic substances should be conducted remains controversial. Many official guidelines suggest that currently these tests are not sensitive enough and not yet sufficiently validated to provide meaningful information concerning the levels of risk to which staff have been exposed.[5,6,20] However, Ferguson *et al.*[18] argue that a monitoring programme would provide a means of assessing if a relationship exists between consistent detection of abnormalities and occupational exposure to cytotoxic agents. Such testing may also provide a warning of equipment failure, poor technique practised by an individual, or inadequacies in protective clothing. The knowledge base relating to staff testing remains insufficient to offer firm guidance on the value of or the necessity for such testing. McDairmid[20] warns that, since it is not yet possible to interpret accurately the results of these various tests or link any single 'positive' result to occupational exposure, such a 'positive' result may provoke unjustifiable anxiety in individuals for whom its importance cannot be adequately explained.

In addition, it is not yet clear which test or tests would be of most value. Ferguson *et al.*[18] suggest that the SCE test is most relevant to testing personnel actively working in cytotoxic services. However, if tests are only performed as a routine on all staff, irrespective of their current duties, the chromosomal aberrations test is the only appropriate method. More recent comments, however, indicate that neither test alone is a reliable indicator of exposure to cytotoxic drugs, except possibly for very large exposures.[6] The prognostic value of these tests remains unproven.[20]

It has been suggested that the analysis of blood or urine for the presence of specific cytotoxic drugs or metabolites could be an alternative or additional valuable tool for monitoring staff exposure.[6] Both chromatographic and spectrophotometric methods have been investigated. A major methodological limitation with any current method is the poor sensitivity in relation to potential levels likely to be absorbed by staff working with cytotoxic drugs. In addition, there are no data available to determine or define threshold concentrations in blood or urine that relate to hazard for any of the drugs commonly handled. Until more epidemiological evidence is available, drug concentration monitoring of staff working with these agents is of no direct value as a tool in health surveillance.

CONTROL OF EXPOSURE

1 Regulations Controlling Exposure of Staff to Hazardous Substances

Many countries now have statutory controls concerning the protection of staff working with potentially hazardous substances. Specific examples include:

▼ UK–Control of Substances Hazardous to Health (COSHH) Regulations (1988)[25]
▼ USA–Federal Occupational Health and Safety Administration (OHSA).

Such regulations require employers to prevent or control exposure of their employees (or of visitors to their premises) to any substance potentially or actually hazardous to health.

2 The Working Environment

All aseptic preparative work involving the handling of cytotoxics must be conducted within a suitable safety cabinet or isolator. A detailed review of equipment options appears in Chapter 2, along with recommendations for quality control and monitoring of the environment. Adherence to strict quality assurance procedures ensures maximum operator protection and allows early detection of equipment failure.

Cabinets should ideally be situated within a dedicated area, with access restricted to authorized personnel only, to prevent the possible spread of contamination to other working areas.

Standard working practices prohibiting the consumption of food and drink in preparative areas will preclude the risk of ingestion of cytotoxic materials, as will strict adherence to cleanliness and hygiene procedures.

3 Handling Precautions

Exposure to cytotoxic materials may arise as a result of ingestion, inhalation, absorption through the skin or direct splashing, eg into the eye.

The safe handling of cytotoxic materials is dependent on attention to a number of factors. These are:

▼ appropriate protective clothing
▼ adequate containment facilities for the scale of the operation, properly maintained and monitored

▼ extensive training and regular assessment of technical competence
▼ clearly defined, written procedures for all stages of the operation from goods receipt to the disposal of cytotoxic waste.

A breakdown in any one of these areas will compromise safe working practice. It should be stressed that failure to perform in a safe and competent manner by a member of the team will create a potential risk, not only for that person, but also for the other staff working in the same unit.

In addition to professional and technical staff, other staff grades will be involved in cytotoxic drug handling, eg storekeepers, porters etc. They require education and training to an appropriate level in relation to their responsibilities.

Protective clothing

This is described in Chapter 3.

Equipment

In addition to the major containment equipment already described, there are a number of small disposable items which can make a significant contribution to safe handling practices. These are described in Chapter 4.

Training

Practical experience in basic aseptic technique is essential before staff are involved in cytotoxic manipulation. All staff who reconstitute cytotoxics should understand the theory behind their use in the treatment of cancer, and the risks associated with drug handling. Handling techniques should be taught and assessed using non-hazardous materials until the operator's technique has been validated. Particular attention should be paid to pressure equalization techniques. The following standard tests exist for such validation.

▼ A 1% quinine hydrochloride solution can be used in aseptic transfers. This will fluoresce under UV light, indicating spilt material and poor cleaning technique.
▼ The transfer of dye solutions such as amaranth or methylene blue between pressurized vials is a useful method of demonstrating aerosol formation.
▼ Recently published, although still experimental, work has explored more sophisticated techniques for identifying spilt materials and validating cleaning and inactivation procedures; these include direct fluorescence measurement[26,27] and the bioluminescent estimation of residual mutagenic activity.[28]

Handling guidelines for non-parenteral cytotoxics

Chemotherapy regimens frequently include oral cytotoxic preparations, and topical formulations containing cytotoxic drugs may occasionally be prescribed. Clinical staff are often unaware that these preparations pose a potential health hazard if handled carelessly.

Requests for extemporaneous preparation of medicines may arise whenever a dose regimen falls outside commercially provided dose forms. This is particularly true of paediatric doses. There may also be demands for liquid formulations if patients have difficulty in swallowing standard dosage forms.

The extemporaneous preparation of medicines containing cytotoxic drugs should be avoided wherever possible. If unavoidable, any manipulation of dosage forms, such as attempting to divide tablets must be restricted to a controlled environment within the pharmacy department. Such activities, which may cause release of drugs into the atmosphere, should be discouraged at ward level.

Recommendations for the preparation and dispensing of non-injectable cytotoxic drugs have recently been promulgated by the American Society of Hospital Pharmacists.[4]

All cytotoxic drugs dispensed for inpatient use should carry a warning label to alert nursing staff to the need for special handling precautions. Ward staff should be trained to examine all containers before opening and report signs of tablet/capsule deterioration to a pharmacist. Patients or their carers should be given appropriate advice on handling cytotoxic drugs.

Precautions in the pharmacy should include the following.

▼ Staff should wear gloves when handling products containing cytotoxics or equipment used to manipulate them.
▼ All counting of tablets/capsules must be undertaken using designated equipment. Automated tablet counting machines should not be used for cytotoxic preparations.
▼ Procedures should be developed to avoid the release of aerosolized powder or liquid into the working environment.
▼ Containment cabinets must have air flow characteristics which prevent the dispersal of powders. Fume cupboards with external ducting and fitted with a HEPA filter may be acceptable for small levels of activity (see Chapter 2).
▼ Isolators or cabinets used for aseptic preparation should not be employed for non-sterile work.
▼ Solutions of drugs are easier to handle than powders, and should be used whenever possible. If tablets need to be crushed, they should first be placed in a small sealable plastic bag.

Guidelines for the use of protective clothing, labelling, transport, disposal and dealing with spillages are the same as those used for parenteral cytotoxic preparations.

Spillage procedures

In the event of accidental spillage, personnel should be aware of clear written procedures for dealing promptly with the problem. Separate procedures may be required for:

▼ spillage within the cytotoxic reconstitution area
▼ spillage within the wider environs of the pharmacy department
▼ spillage within the ward/clinic areas of the hospital. This necessitates discussion with nursing, clinical and administrative staff, plus health and safety representatives.

General procedures for dealing with spillages are covered comprehensively by the latest ASHP technical assistance bulletin (TAB) on handling cytotoxic and hazardous drugs.[4]

In summary, the key elements are:

▼ adequate protective clothing for all individuals involved in the cleaning operation
▼ containment of the spillage as far as possible
▼ prompt action to remove the hazard

▼ adequate, clearly labelled containers for the disposal of waste associated with the clean-up operation
▼ the provision of emergency 'spill-kits' at appropriate locations
▼ documentation of all significant spillages; a report should be forwarded to the occupational health department if individuals have been exposed to risk, eg of skin absorption.

The novel techniques for monitoring the efficiency of spill cleaning procedures by visualization methods described above[26–28] may in the future enable a more quantitative approach to estimating exposure risk from spillage incidents.

Handling of waste from patients receiving cytotoxic drugs

The excreta from patients receiving cytotoxic chemotherapy may contain potentially hazardous amounts of cytotoxic drugs, or, in some cases, their active metabolites. These are mostly eliminated by renal or faecal excretion.[29–31]

The period over which staff handling patient waste are at risk depends on:

▼ the particular drug involved
▼ pharmacodynamic factors: dose, route of administration, duration of therapy, renal and/or hepatic function
▼ concomitant drug therapy, which may influence elimination rates.

Guidance on the potential hazard from patient excreta has been collated in Table 6.1, which summarizes the time over which additional protective measures are required for specific drugs.[30,31]

Table 6.1: *Details of drugs requiring extended precautionary periods for handling excreta after chemotherapy*[31]

Drug	Route	Duration (days) after completion of therapy for which precautions are necessary when handling:	
		Urine	Faeces
Bleomycin	inj.	3	?
Cisplatin	IV	7	?
Cyclophosphamide	any	3	5
Dactinomycin	IV	5	7
Daunorubicin	IV	2	7
Doxorubicin	IV	6	7
Epirubicin	IV	7	5
Etoposide	any	4	7
Melphalan	oral	2	7
Mercaptopurine	oral	3	?
Methotrexate	any	3	7
Mitoxantrone	IV	6	7
Thiotepa	inj.	3	?
Vinca alkaloids	IV	4	7

? : no information

As a general rule, the excreta from patients receiving cytotoxic drugs should be assumed to be hazardous for at least 48 hours after the completion of treatment.[31] Such patients should be clearly identified to ward staff.

Recommended precautions for staff/relatives caring for patients [29–31]

▼ Protective clothing, as described in Chapter 3, should be worn by staff dealing with blood or vomit from patients who have received cytotoxic drugs within the previous 48 hours, or longer if appropriate (*see* Table 6.1).

▼ All protective clothing should be treated as hazardous and disposed of accordingly.

▼ If contamination of skin, eyes or mucous membranes is suspected, the area should be rinsed thoroughly with large amounts of water and then washed with soap and water.

▼ Double sluicing of bedpans, vomit bowls and other items heavily contaminated with waste materials should be carried out. Disposable items are preferable, and should be treated as hazardous clinical waste and disposed of accordingly.

▼ Patients and staff should utilize different toilet facilities.

▼ Contaminated linen/uniforms may pose a threat to laundry staff. Lightly contaminated linen may be treated as 'infected waste' and dealt with by the normal laundry process. Heavily contaminated items may need to be incinerated. Soaking of linen in sodium hypochlorite solution has been recommended for drugs such as doxorubicin. [29]

4 Transport

Packaging and transport systems for cytotoxics must provide adequate physical, chemical and light protection during storage and transportation, be relatively impervious to the atmosphere, robust, and tamperproof, provide adequate protection to the handler, contain any leaked solution and allow easy identification of the contained drugs throughout.

All cytotoxic preparations should be packed in leak-proof containers after preparation. Polythene tubing which can be heat sealed to give an air/water tight seal and which can be cut to enclose any size or shape of container is recommended (*see* Chapter 4).

For transportation around the hospital, standard delivery containers may be utilized provided they fulfil the above criteria. Cytotoxics should not be transported in the same container as other drugs and the nature of the contained material should be clearly indicated on the outer container.

Transportation to other clinical settings outside the hospital may necessitate more stringent, possibly custom-designed packaging.

5 Disposal of Cytotoxic Drugs and Materials Contaminated with Them

Each institution should have a policy on the safe handling and disposal of cytotoxic drugs and materials contaminated with them. Clear and concise procedures for the collection, segregation and disposal of waste should be established; all staff involved, including non-pharmacy staff, should be trained in their use. Procedures should be updated at regular intervals and there should be a system of audit to ensure compliance with the procedures at all times.

Suitable containers, clearly labelled and reserved solely for cytotoxic waste, should be available in all areas where the drugs are handled. They should be brightly coloured with space to indicate the nature of the contents both during use and whilst awaiting disposal. 'Sharps' containers should be robust enough to contain any sharps and leaked solution. They should be constructed of plastic rather than lined cardboard with tightly fitting lids which can be sealed when the container is full. Absorbent material (paper or absorbent granules) should be placed in the bottom of the container to mop up any leaked solution. It is essential to carry out quality assurance on all disposal containers to check they are suitable for use and can be disposed of safely and in the appropriate manner.

Facilities for the storage of the cytotoxic waste awaiting destruction must safeguard the integrity of the packaging and not expose personnel to any risk. Waste should not be allowed to accumulate in either clinical or storage areas.

In the UK, prescription-only medicines are listed in Schedule 1 of the Control of Pollution (Special Waste) Regulations (1980)[32] as substances which are to be regarded as special waste. There is no specific reference to cytotoxics in these regulations, but their disposal will be subject to the general controls set out therein.

The risk associated with pharmaceutical waste which might enter the water cycle has been discussed in detail in a review by Richardson and Bowron.[33] They calculated that the major source of pharmaceutical chemicals as contaminants in potable water would be from domestic sources, including homes and hospitals, with only a marginal contribution to the load from industry. The authors concluded, from analytical and biodegradation data, that few drugs were likely to survive treatment in sewage works, river retention, reservoir retention and waterworks. Such drugs that did survive would be unlikely to pose a health risk at the concentrations likely to be found in water supplies. It can be concluded, therefore, that disposal to sewer may be used for small quantities of pharmaceuticals.

Disposal via the domestic sewerage system should not be used for large quantities of pharmaceutical waste. The Royal Pharmaceutical Society of Great Britain, in their guidelines, recommend pharmacists to use their professional judgement when deciding on the disposal of substances which may be particularly toxic, insidious or persistent.[34]

The relationship between hazard and the quantities of any particular cytotoxic substance requiring disposal is not generally addressed. However, in the USA, this issue is covered by regulations from the Environmental Protection Agency. These were recently summarized by Gallelli.[35] The relevant 'rules' are described as the '3%' and the 'mixture' rules. The former states that all empty containers that contain not more than 3% of cytotoxics by weight in relation to the total capacity of the container, need not be disposed of as hazardous waste. The 'mixture' rule states that if any amount of a listed waste is mixed with any other, the entire mixture is considered hazardous. This is to prevent the deliberate dilution of cytotoxic waste to avoid disposal regulations.

Many cytotoxics can be disposed of by chemical destruction. Details of recommended methods are summarized in Part 2 of this Handbook. Other important sources of information on chemical destruction of cytotoxics are recommended.[36,37]

The method recommended for disposal of cytotoxic drugs is incineration. Disposal into waste which might subsequently be tipped into a landfill site must not, under any circumstances, be used for cytotoxic drugs or materials contaminated with them. Several manufacturers recommend a temperature of 1000°C for the complete destruction of cytotoxic drugs.[38] Opinion differs as to the need for this, but until adequate research work has been carried out, this should be regarded as an ideal to be attained if possible. Perhaps of more importance than the actual temperature is the presence of an after-burner on the incinerator to be used. There is a possible risk of a solution containing a cytotoxic being aerosolized when passed into the incinerator. This may result in undegraded cytotoxic drug being emitted from the incinerator chimney. In the absence of a suitable incinerator, the services of a specialist waste disposal contractor should be employed.

A QUALITY AUDIT SCHEME FOR A CYTOTOXICS RECONSTITUTION SERVICE

The following audit scheme provides a systematic approach to examining the structure and process aspects of a cytotoxic reconstitution service. The main objectives of the audit process are as follows:

▼ to identify shortcomings and loopholes in the procedures and processes
▼ to determine whether those procedures are being followed and the processes are being carried out effectively by competent staff
▼ to determine whether the facilities, equipment and environment comply with relevant standards
▼ to monitor quality trends and assess the effectiveness of management action to remedy perceived deficiencies
▼ to motivate staff to provide a safe, efficient and cost-effective service.

The audit form (Table 6.2) incorporates a rating scale for level of compliance and also guidance on the means of assessment for each acceptance criterion. For some criteria, the assessment depends upon a process of peer review and it is, therefore, important that auditors have appropriate expertise.

This audit scheme is not proffered as a definitive statement applicable to all situations; it is intended to be a model which can be adapted to local circumstances. It should also be regarded as one of a number of quality assurance mechanisms that can be applied. It does not, for instance, attempt to address the outcomes of the patient's treatment.

1 Notes for Guidance when using Quality Audit Forms

Result ratings

1. Substantial compliance with Acceptance Criteria.
2. Significant compliance with Acceptance Criteria.
3. Partial compliance with Acceptance Criteria.
4. Minimal compliance with Acceptance Criteria.
5. Noncompliance with Acceptance Criteria.
NA Not applicable

Glossary of terms used in connection with the checks required for each criterion.

Assess	requires the auditor(s) to use their professional judgement in attributing a compliance rating.
Data	generally relates to validation studies and evidence taken from the literature.
Examine	generally relates to procedures and/or materials which need to be examined, for content and validity.
Observe	generally relates to activities which can be observed by auditor(s) and are representative of normal work practices. In some situations it may be appropriate to do this covertly.

Procedure	relates to written procedures which should be assessed for appropriateness and compliance with official guidelines (eg good manufacturing practice). They should have been recently appraised, signed and, where appropriate, countersigned (eg by quality control staff).	
Records	generally relates to requirements for documentary evidence. These should be inspected at the auditor(s) discretion.	
Test	applies to situations where the auditor(s) obtain their own evidence by test.	

Table 6.2: *Quality audit for cytotoxic reconstitutions*

HOSPITAL:		DATE:	CYTOTOXIC REGIMEN EXAMINED:		BATCH NO(S):
No.	Attribute	Acceptance Criteria	Check Req'd	Audit Result	Comments and Action to be Taken
001	Formulation acceptability	All formulations are stable (published or in-house evidence)	Data	1 2 3 4 5 NA	
002		All formulations are approved (with signature) by a pharmacist	Examine	1 2 3 4 5 NA	
003		Dose is for a single patient's requirements only	Procedure	1 2 3 4 5 NA	
005	Facilities	Facilities are adequate size for the activities undertaken	Assess	1 2 3 4 5 NA	
006		Facilities incorporate appropriate design features in terms of current GMP, ergonomics, work flow, ease of cleaning etc	Assess	1 2 3 4 5 NA	
007		Facilities include sufficient shelves, cupboards, benches etc for the activities undertaken	Assess	1 2 3 4 5 NA	
008		Walls, floors, ceilings, fixtures and fittings have acceptable finish and in good decorative order	Assess	1 2 3 4 5 NA	
	Environmental acceptability product protection	(A) Applicable to use of modified Class 2 (BS 5726) Microbiological Safety Cabinet			
009		Room used complies with (at least) Class J (unmanned) air (BS 5295) and tested within 3 months, and complies with European 'Orange Guide' Grades	Records	1 2 3 4 5 NA	
010		Safety cabinet complies with Class F (manned) air (BS 5295) and tested within 3 months	Records	1 2 3 4 5 NA	
011		The direction of the air-flow is inwards over the whole area of the work aperture (Smoke test confirmation)	Records/Test	1 2 3 4 5 NA	

Table 6.2: *Continued*

No.	Attribute	Acceptance Criteria	Check Req'd	Audit Result	Comments and Action to be Taken
012		The velocity of the down-flow air is in accordance with the requirements of BS 5726 (0.25–0.50 m/s)	Records	1 2 3 4 5 NA	
013		The mean air velocity through the working aperture by measurement of the exhaust velocity meets the requirements of BS 5726	Records	1 2 3 4 5 NA	
014		Safety cabinet and room comply with in-house standard for absence of micro-organisms and tested within one week	Records	1 2 3 4 5 NA	
015		Cleanroom garments/face mask/gloves used each session (see also 020)	Observe/ Procedure	1 2 3 4 5 NA	
016		Cleaning records comply with schedule	Records	1 2 3 4 5 NA	
017		Manometer readings show adequate differential pressure and are recorded daily	Records	1 2 3 4 5 NA	
	Environmental acceptability product protection	(B) Applicable to use of negative pressure isolator system			
018		Air complies with Class F air (BS 5295) within 2 minutes of opening and closing the transfer hatch and tested within 3 months	Records	1 2 3 4 5 NA	
019		Environment complies with in-house standard for absence of micro-organisms and tested within one week	Records	1 2 3 4 5 NA	
020		Cleaning records comply with schedule including sterilization of inside of cabinet when applicable	Records	1 2 3 4 5 NA	
021		The cabinet alarm system operates if the cabinet's seals are breached	Assess	1 2 3 4 5 NA	
022	Environmental acceptability operator protection	Safety cabinet complies with KI Discus test and tested within one year (not applicable for isolators)	Records	1 2 3 4 5 NA	
023		Systems prevent disturbance of air currents during use of cabinet, including opening/closing of door to room (not applicable for isolators)	Procedure/ Assess	1 2 3 4 5 NA	

Table 6.2: *Continued*

No.	Attribute	Acceptance Criteria	Check Req'd	Audit Result	Comments and Action to be Taken
024		Appropriate type of garments including gloves used by staff	Assess	1 2 3 4 5 NA	
025		The glove/sleeve system allows adequate dexterity in use and gloves are replaced as necessary (isolators only)	Assess	1 2 3 4 5 NA	
026		Luer-lock syringes and large-bore needles used during manipulations	Observe/ Procedure	1 2 3 4 5 NA	
027		Appropriate air-venting of vials occurs to prevent pressure differentials	Observe/ Procedure	1 2 3 4 5 NA	
028		Acceptable procedure for dealing with spillage in existence	Examine	1 2 3 4 5 NA	
029		Appropriate receptacles for contaminated liquids, 'sharps' and other consumables available	Assess	1 2 3 4 5 NA	
030		Appropriate procedure for disposal of contaminated waste available	Examine	1 2 3 4 5 NA	
031	Documentation (General)	Satisfactory standard operating procedures have been written for all items of equipment and signed and dated by the production pharmacist and independent quality control pharmacist	Examine	1 2 3 4 5 NA	
032		Worksheets for all different cytotoxic preparations have been written and signed and dated by the pharmacist and independent quality control pharmacist	Examine	1 2 3 4 5 NA	
033		Satisfactory procedures have been written, signed and dated on the following:			
		i) Changing and hand-washing prior to entry into preparation area (and is displayed)	Examine/ Observe	1 2 3 4 5 NA	
		ii) Laboratory cleaning and maintenance	Examine	1 2 3 4 5 NA	
		iii) Environmental and microbiological control	Examine	1 2 3 4 5 NA	
		iv) Other routine quality control testing	Examine	1 2 3 4 5 NA	
		v) Health and safety policy	Examine	1 2 3 4 5 NA	

Table 6.2: *Continued*

No.	Attribute	Acceptance Criteria	Check Req'd	Audit Result	Comments and Action to be Taken
034	Compounding	Documentary evidence of correct reconstitution	Records	1 2 3 4 5 NA	
035		Other documentary evidence completed and satisfactory	Records	1 2 3 4 5 NA	
036		Evidence to show that correct solutions incorporated into syringe/bag	Observe	1 2 3 4 5 NA	
037	Presentation	Label has acceptable legibility	Examine Sample	1 2 3 4 5 NA	
038		Label indicates route of injection	Examine Sample	1 2 3 4 5 NA	
039		Label bears unambiguous expression of ingredients/quantities	Examine Sample	1 2 3 4 5 NA	
040		Label shows correct expiry date/time	Examine Sample	1 2 3 4 5 NA	
041		Label shows correct storage conditions if other than room temperature	Examine Sample	1 2 3 4 5 NA	
042		Outer packaging is properly sealed and prevents contents leaking during transit	Examine Sample	1 2 3 4 5 NA	
043		Contents clear and free from visible particles	Examine Sample	1 2 3 4 5 NA	
044	Personnel	Appropriately trained and screened pharmacists/pharmacy technicians undertake the manipulations	Assess	1 2 3 4 5 NA	
045		All personnel are aware of and comply with the local policy on handling of cytotoxic materials	Assess	1 2 3 4 5 NA	
046		Staff perform satisfactory broth transfers every 6 months	Records	1 2 3 4 5 NA	
047	Effective use of resources	Notification of pharmacy by ward allows convenient scheduling	Assess	1 2 3 4 5 NA	
048		Most cost effective grade(s) of staff are used	Assess	1 2 3 4 5 NA	
049		Choice of units of ingredients minimizes wastage	Assess	1 2 3 4 5 NA	
050		The ingredients bear the nearest expiry date of stock	Examine	1 2 3 4 5 NA	
051		The wastage of disposables used is minimal	Observe	1 2 3 4 5 NA	

Table 6.2: *Continued*

No.	Attribute	Acceptance Criteria	Check Req'd	Audit Result	Comments and Action to be Taken
052	Storage/distribution and administration	Contents are suitably protected against heat/light etc	Examine	1 2 3 4 5 NA	
053		Syringes/bags are suitably protected for transport to ward	Examine	1 2 3 4 5 NA	
054		Bags can be delivered to ward by intended time of administration	Assess	1 2 3 4 5 NA	
055		Syringes/bags are appropriately stored on the ward if not to be used immediately and do not exceed their expiry date	Assess	1 2 3 4 5 NA	

NAME: JOB TITLE: SIGNATURE: DATE:

Auditor 1:

Auditor 2:

Auditor 3:

Other staff present:

Copies sent to:

Next Audit date:

REFERENCES

1. Sieber, S.M. and Adamson, R.H. (1975). Toxicity of antineoplastic agents in man: chromosomal aberrations, antifertility effects, congenital malformations and carcinogenic potential. *Adv. Cancer Res.* **22**, 57–155.
2. Boice, J.D. *et al.* (1983). Leukemia and preleukemia after adjuvant treatment of gastrointestinal cancer with semustine (methyl-CCNU). *N. Engl. J. Med.* **309**, 1079–1084.
3. Anon. (1986). OSHA work-practice guidelines for personnel dealing with cytotoxic (antineoplastic) drugs. *Am. J. Hosp. Pharm.* **43**, 1193–1204.
4. Anon. (1990). AHSP technical assistance bulletin on handling cytotoxic and hazardous drugs. *Am. J. Hosp. Pharm.* **47**, 1033–1049.
5. Carrano, A.V. and Natarajan, A.T. (1988). ICPEMC Publication No. 14: Considerations for population monitoring using cytogenetic techniques. *Mutation Res.* **204**, 379–406.
6. Kaijser, G.P. *et al.* (1990). The risks of handling cytotoxic drugs. 1. Methods of testing exposure. *Pharm. Weekbl. Sci. Ed.* **12**, 212–227.
7. Selevan, S.G. *et al.* (1985). A study of occupational exposure to antineoplastic drugs and fetal loss in nurses. *N. Engl. J. Med.* **313**, 1173–1178.
8. Hemminki, K. *et al.* (1985). Spontaneous abortions and malformations in the offspring of nurses exposed to anaesthetic gases, cytotoxic drugs and other potential hazards in hospitals, based on registered information of outcome. *J. Epidemiol. Community Health* **39**, 141–147.

9. Falck, K. (1982). Application of the bacterial urinary mutagenicity assay in detection of exposure to genotoxic chemicals. PhD dissertation, University of Helsinki, pp. 55.

10. Andersson, R.W. *et al.* (1982). Risks of handling injectable antineoplastic drugs. *Am. J. Hosp. Pharm.* **39**, 1881–1887.

11. Falck, K. *et al.* (1979). Mutagenicity in urine of nurses handling cytotoxic drugs. *The Lancet* **i**, 1250–1251.

12. Norppa, H. *et al.* (1980). Increased sister chromatid exchange frequencies in lymphocytes of nurses handling cytotoxic drugs. *Scand. J. Work Environ. Health* **6**, 299–303.

13. Sorsa, M. *et al.* (1982). Induction of sister chromatid exchanges (SCEs) among nurses handling cytotoxic drugs. *Banbury Proc.* Vol. 14. Cold Spring Harbor Laboratory, New York.

14. Waksvik, H. *et al.* (1981). Chromosome analyses of nurses handling cytotoxic drugs. *Cancer Treat. Rep.* **65**, 607–611.

15. Vainio, H. (1982). Mutagenicity in urine of workers occupationally exposed to mutagens and carcinogens. In Aito, A. *et al.* (Eds): *Biological monitoring and health surveillance of workers exposed to chemicals*. Hemisphere Publishing, Washington DC, 324–330.

16. Cooke, J. (1987). Environmental monitoring of personnel who handle cytotoxic drugs. *Pharm. J.* **239**, R2.

17. Kolmodin-Hedman, B. *et al.* (1983). Occupational handling of cytotoxic drugs. *Arch. Toxicol.* **54**, 25–33.

18. Ferguson, L.R. *et al.* (1988). The use within New Zealand of cytogenetic approaches to monitoring of hospital pharmacists for exposure to cytotoxic drugs: report of a pilot study in Auckland. *Aust. J. Hosp. Pharm.* **18**, 228–233.

19. Guinee, E.P. *et al.* (1991). Evaluation of genotoxic risk of handling cytostatic drugs in clinical pharmacy practice. *Pharm. Weekbl. Sci. Ed.* **13**, 78–82.

20. McDairmid, M.A. (1990). Medical surveillance for antineoplastic handlers. *Am. J. Hosp. Pharm.* **47**, 1061–1066.

21. Stellman, J.M. and Zoloth, S.R. (1986). Cancer chemotherapeutic agents as occupational hazards: A literature review. *Cancer Invest.* **4**, 127–135.

22. Venitt, S. *et al.* (1984). Monitoring exposure of nursing and pharmacy personnel to cytotoxic drugs: Urinary mutation assays and urinary platinum as markers of absorption. *The Lancet* **i**, 777.

23. Hirst, M. *et al.* (1984). Occupational exposure to cyclophosphamide. *The Lancet* **i**, 186–188.

24. Fenech, M. *et al.* (1986). Cytokinesis-block micronucleus method in human lymophocytes: Effect of *in vivo* aging and low-dose X-irradiation. *Mutation Res.* **161**, 193–198.

25. Anon. (1988). *The control of substances hazardous to health regulations*. HMSO, London.

26. Van Raalte, J. *et al.* (1990). Visible-light system for detecting doxorubicin contamination on skin and surfaces. *Am. J. Hosp. Pharm.* **47**, 1067–1074.

27. Dixon, T. (1990). Location of cytotoxic drug spillages using ultraviolet light. *Aust. J. Hosp. Pharm.* **20**, 469–470.

28. Wren, A.E. *et al.* (1991). A novel technique for the validation of cytotoxic decontamination procedures. *Int. Pharm.* **5**, 119.

29. Harris, J. and Dodds, L.J. (1985). Handling of waste from patients receiving cytotoxic drugs. *Pharm. J.* **235**, 289–291.

30. Anon. (1986). OHSA work-practice guidelines for personnel dealing with cytotoxic (antineoplastic) drugs. *Am. J. Hosp. Pharm.* **43**, 1193–1203.
31. Cass, Y. and Musgrave, C.F. (1992). Guidelines for the safe handling of excreta contaminated by cytotoxic agents. *Am. J. Hosp. Pharm.* **49**, 1957–1958.
32. Anon. (1980). *Joint circular from Department of Environment/Welsh Office, Control of Pollution (Special Waste) regulations.* HMSO, London.
33. Richardson, M.L. and Bowron, G.M. (1985). The fate of pharmaceutical chemicals in the aquatic environment. *J. Pharm. Pharmacol.* **37**, 1–12.
34. Appleby, G.E. (1988). Disposal of pharmaceutical waste. *Pharm. J.* **240**, 100.
35. Gallelli, J.F. (1988). Chemical destruction and disposal of antineoplastic drugs. In: *Proceedings of international symposium on oncology pharmacy practice*, Rotorua, New Zealand. New Zealand Hospital Pharmacists Association, Wellington, pp. 240–251.
36. Castegnaro, M. *et al.* (1985). *Laboratory decontamination and destruction of carcinogens in laboratory wastes.* International Agency for Research on Cancer, Scientific Publications No. 73, Oxford University Press, Fair Lane (NJ).
37. Armour, M.A. *et al.* (1986). *Potentially carcinogenic chemicals: information and disposal guide*, University of Alberta. Terochem Laboratories Ltd, Edmonton.
38. Garner, S. *et al.* (1988). Disposal of waste cytotoxics. *Pharm. J.* **241**, Hospital Supplement 32.

CHAPTER 7

Documentation

INTRODUCTION

Adequate and efficient documentation is an essential aspect of a pharmacy-operated cytotoxic service. The design of documentation is clearly of importance in ensuring the maintenance of safe procedures and good records of service operation. Furthermore, the use of pharmacy-based documentation, such as patient treatment records, is a vital support to the pharmacist's professional role in ensuring optimal patient care and minimizing the risks of adverse events associated with chemotherapy. The range of documents used, their design, reproduction and updating aspects will vary widely between hospitals. They will be governed by local circumstances such as the scale of operation, the grades of staff involved and the extent to which computers are used.

It may be considered that for some services, documents can be combined or contain superfluous information. However, in this text all those aspects that require consideration have been indicated. Local circumstances then dictate whether or not they are included in the user documentation.

Whether the storage and retrieval system devised is computerized or not, the basic needs of documentation remain the same.

DOCUMENTATION NEEDS

The various aspects of cytotoxics services requiring documents for safe, reliable and cost-effective operation are shown in Figure 7.1. The actual document needs have been summarized under each of the main categories depicted in the figure.

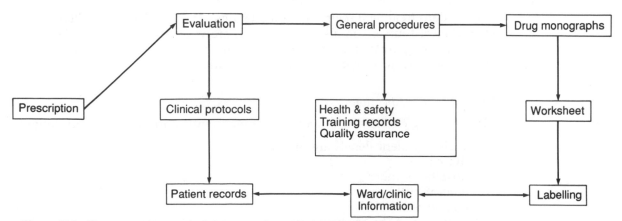

Figure 7.1: *Documentation required for cytotoxic services*

1 Prescriptions

There are several options regarding the ordering of chemotherapy.

▼ The patient's prescription may be sent to the pharmacy department.
▼ The patient's prescription may be transposed at ward or clinic level by the visiting pharmacist.
▼ A specially designed order form completed by the clinician may be supplied to the pharmacy. This may have a worksheet incorporated in its design.
▼ Visual display units or fax machines may be used with terminals at ward, clinic and pharmacy level.

Where a prescription is used, it must fulfil the minimum legal requirements of a prescription for any cytotoxic medicine.

Local hospital or state policy may deem additional information necessary (eg patient diagnosis, chemotherapy regimen being used in concise terms, patient details (surface area, height, weight), cycle or pulse number, etc.).

An appropriate design must adequately satisfy the requirements of medical, nursing and pharmacy staff, and a degree of compromise may need to be negotiated.

2 Evaluation

Clinical protocols and drug regimens

Chemotherapy regimens are divided mainly into two groups:

▼ protocols that are part of a formal clinical trial
▼ regimens which are based on experience and subject to the clinician's expertise and judgement, many of them being standard first-line treatments.

Clinical trial protocols are often complex and subject to randomization. For quick reference it may be appropriate to summarize the pharmaceutical aspects in a card or file system which details:

▼ schedules (induction, consolidation, maintenance, etc.)
▼ drug
▼ dose (/m² or /kg)
▼ how given (route, volume, equipment)
▼ timings (pulses, cycles, etc.)
▼ dosage reductions (when and how appropriate).

For standard treatment regimens, compilations of similar data from reference or from clinical sources can also be prepared. However, these are more likely to need updating frequently and hospital drug information units may be the appropriate means of gathering such information.

Prescription verification

The following checklist covers the key components of prescription verification:

▼ sufficient patient details are provided,
    full name
    hospital number
    date of birth
    diagnosis
▼ recognition of the regimen/protocol (reference source)

▼ the therapy prescribed is correct and complies with the reference source
▼ drug doses are calculated correctly against surface area/height/weight on prescription
▼ drug doses (single pulses within the cycle, stat doses, etc.) are time and date scheduled according to the protocol
▼ the form of administration: (route, diluent, volume, infusion rate) is acceptable and appropriate; for unlicensed drugs/routes of administration, a reference source should be provided by the prescriber, and the appropriate disclaimer documentation signed to accept liability
▼ patient record scrutiny will ensure that treatment progress through the protocol is appropriately timed; cycle delays, dose changes, protocol modifications, etc. should be documented within the pharmacy patient record.

Prescription checking

The checking process should be a separate stage between verification and final release of the product. A procedure based on a check-list such as the following should be implemented:

▼ the drug prepared is as stated on the label and as requested on the prescription
▼ the dose prepared is as stated on the label and as requested on the prescription
▼ diluents used are compatible with the drug
▼ infusion fluids are compatible with both drug and diluent used
▼ stability of the prepared drug is appropriate
▼ the storage conditions on the prepared drug label are appropriate
▼ the label details are correct
▼ all ingredients are batch number and expiry date checked and appropriate for use
▼ the intended route of administration is acceptable and appropriate (see above).

3 General Procedures

These should be clear, informative and comprehensive enough to cover all aspects of the pharmacy service. They should be readily accessible, comprehensible to all staff employed in the service and subject to regular review and updating.

Procedures covering personnel, education and training, staff monitoring, handling (suitable techniques and methods of evaluation) and waste disposal are of particular importance.

In each of these areas, definitive, concise standard operating procedures (SOPs) will form the basis of a training manual as well as providing a basis for routine audit of the service.

Education and training are essential components of a safe, high quality service. Documentational evidence in the form of a training record is required for all personnel involved in the provision of the service.

4 Drug Monographs

Drug monographs for commercially available injectable cytotoxic drugs are contained in Part 2 of this Handbook.

For unlicensed products, advice and further information should be sought from the supplier. Such information should be documented for reference and reviewed regularly.

5 Worksheets

A general worksheet may be used for all drugs or specific worksheets may be prepared for particular regimens. Prescription details can be transcribed on to the worksheet or the worksheet can be an integral part of the prescription.
Worksheets should include:

▼ name of the drug/s
▼ presentation (physical form, quantity, strength, etc.)
▼ reconstituting solutions/diluents (identification and quantities to be added)
▼ resultant solutions (quantity in volume)
▼ compatible infusion solutions (where appropriate)
▼ storage details
▼ stability
▼ labelling details or sample label
▼ pertinent 'special precautions' (eg carmustine vials should be inspected before use for signs of decomposition of the drug).

They should allow the following to be recorded:

▼ batch numbers of all ingredients used
▼ the number of containers used
▼ the quantities of solutions to be drawn up or removed
▼ label duplicate
▼ identification of personnel involved in the preparation stages (formulation, assembly of ingredients, reconstitution, etc.)
▼ identification of personnel involved in the checking procedures.

6 Labelling

Labels should comply with national regulations and should state the:

▼ intended route of administration (**particular attention must be paid to identifying clearly preparations intended for intrathecal or regional administration; these must be distinguished from the 'standard' intravenous preparations to reduce the potential for administrative error**)
▼ name of the drug
▼ quantity of the drug
▼ vehicle containing the drug (infusion solution as appropriate)
▼ final volume
▼ batch number allocated to the product
▼ expiry date
▼ storage conditions that ensure stability, etc.
▼ patient's name and location (ward, etc.)
▼ name and address of the cytotoxic dispensary.

Outer packs for transport should also clearly state details of the contained items and any possible handling hazards.

7 Information Documents for Ward/Clinic Staff

These should comprise the elements listed below. The detail required will depend on local circumstance.

General introduction detailing local policies

These may include:

▼ designated areas on ward/clinic for the preparation of cytotoxic agents
▼ personnel (ie groups of staff appropriate to undertake reconstitution/administration)
▼ protective garments that should be worn
▼ equipment that may be used
▼ extravasation policies
▼ disposal of waste.

Drug monographs

These will obviously be much less detailed than those required in pharmacy.

▼ Presentation.
▼ Reconstitution.
▼ Compatible solutions.
▼ Methods of administration.
▼ Special precautions (operator safety, extravasation, etc.).
▼ Stability.
▼ Accidental spillage (what to do in the event of).

Arrangements for the supply of cytotoxics from the pharmacy

▼ Procedure for the agreed method of service-operation at ward level (eg how and when to order).
▼ Communication access (personnel to contact, telephone numbers, etc.).
▼ Agreed presentations and possible alternatives for each drug.

CHAPTER 8

Education and Training

INTRODUCTION

All staff employed to handle cytotoxic materials should receive education and training appropriate to their level of involvement in the handling, preparation or administration of the drugs.

A training programme should include practical experience, one-to-one teaching, learning exercises which may be tested and information on health and safety. A more advanced programme will also include clinical and theoretical training.

The check-list on page 74–5 can be used as the starting point for a formal training programme.

THE TRAINING CHECK-LIST

This can be used as the starting point for a formal or informal training programme. Staff may use the list simply as a guide to the areas which should be covered, or a more extensive programme may be written around the headings in the check-list.

The aim of the check-list (see Table 8.1) is that staff acquire knowledge of and competence in aseptic procedures, cytotoxic reconstitution, local procedures, current awareness, active information, management and research and development. These are intended as broad guidelines for training. Local variations will exist depending upon circumstance.

The degree of training required in each section depends on the level of involvement of different groups of staff in the provision of chemotherapy. The staff groups are indicated at the top of each column.

Level 1 Full time and rotational technicians involved with the provision of a cytotoxic reconstitution service.

Level 2 Pre-registration pharmacists, junior/rotational pharmacists and senior pharmacists from other specialties.

Level 3 Senior pharmacists and technical staff managing a sterile preparation or cytotoxic reconstitution service.

The check-list attempts to differentiate between activities which comprise a fundamental part of the individual's job and those where information only is required. In the former, competence must be demonstrated against the standards defined by the manager of the unit. The latter may be covered by directed reading/open learning programmes. Smaller units may require external support to cover some areas.

Table 8.1: *Education and training check-list*

	Level 1	Level 2	Level 3
ASEPTIC TECHNIQUE			
What it is	A	A	A
Why it is needed	A	A	A
How it is achieved	A	A	A
Test for ensuring and maintaining it	A	A	A
How to realize it has failed	A	A	A
What to do when it fails	A	A	A
CYTOTOXIC RECONSTITUTION			
What are cytotoxics	A	A	A
Why are they a hazard	A	A	A
How aerosols are generated	A	A	A
How aerosols are prevented	A	A	A
Other possible routes of exposure/contamination	A	A	A
General reconstitution techniques	A	A	A
Special reconstitution techniques	A	A	A
Use of special equipment	A	A	A
Correct documentation	A	A	A
Expiry + storage	A	A	A
Tests for ensuring and maintaining good technique	A	A	A
LOCAL PROCEDURES			
For aseptic technique	A	A	A
For cytotoxic reconstitution	A	A	A
USE OF EQUIPMENT			
Special reconstitution devices	A	A	A
Special administration devices	I	I	I
Evaluation of new equipment	A	A	A
CLINICAL DATA/PHARMACEUTICAL DATA			
Clinical notes	I	A	A
Laboratory tests	I	A	A
Disease evaluation tests	I	I	A
Clinical/nursing procedures	I	I	A
Administration procedures	I	A	A
Practical pharmacokinetics	I	A	A
EVALUATION OF INFORMATION			
Publications	I	A	A
Protocols	I	I	A
Basic statistics	A	A	A
Drug representatives	I	A	A
Promotional material	I	I	A
Spoken communications	A	A	A
OBTAINING DRUG/CLINICAL INFORMATION			
In-house	A	A	A
Reading list	I	A	A
Library	I	A	A
Oral communications	A	A	A
On-line via Drug Information Centre	I	I	A

Key: A (activity)　　– trainee required to demonstrate competence in this area
　　　　I (information) – trainee requires information only

Table 8.1: *Continued*

	Level 1	Level 2	Level 3
DATA HANDLING			
Protocols	A	A	A
Documentation	A	A	A
Work-load statistics	A	I	A
Records	A	I	A
Clinical data	I	I	A
Adverse reaction reporting	I	I	A
Extravasation procedure	I	A	A
Mechanism of action	I	A	A
Overdose	I	A	A
Interactions with other drugs	I	A	A
Kinetics	I	I	A
Disposal	A	A	A
Legal and ethical considerations	A	A	A
HEALTH AND SAFETY REGULATIONS			
Nationally	A	I	A
Locally	A	A	A
Staff screening	A	I	A
Accident reporting	A	A	A
Accident procedure	A	A	A
HEALTH SERVICE BACKGROUND			
National framework for the provision of cytotoxic services	I	I	I
Current awareness	A	A	A
ACTIVE INFORMATION			
Bulletins	I	I	A
Seminars	I	I	A
Lectures	I	I	A
MANAGEMENT			
Education/training of appropriate pharmaceutical, nursing and medical staff	–	–	A
Monitoring of service quality	A	A	A
Work planning	A	A	A
Committee skills	–	–	I
Finance/budgeting	–	–	A
Interviewing	–	–	A
Guidelines for protocol submission preparation and evaluation	–	–	A
RESEARCH AND DEVELOPMENT			
Service development	–	–	A
Technique evaluation	–	–	A
Drug evaluation	–	–	A
Publication	–	–	A

Key: A (activity)   – trainee required to demonstrate competence in this area
      I (information) – trainee requires information only

CHAPTER 9

Extravasation

INTRODUCTION

Extravasation can be defined as the leakage into the subcutaneous tissue of a vesicant or irritant drug which is capable of causing pain, necrosis and/or sloughing of tissue. Tissue damage from extravasation can range from minor erythema to severe necrosis resulting in loss of function or loss of a limb. Its occurrence, and thus its treatment, must therefore be considered as a medical/oncological emergency which, although it does not have the critical time constraint of a myocardial infarction, should be dealt with within hours rather than days. Evidence exists to demonstrate that appropriately treated extravasation, dealt with within 24 hours, causes no further problem to the patient.[1–4]

It is a condition which is often underdiagnosed, undertreated and unreported. A large number of articles and reviews of extravasation have been published over the last ten years.[5–11] Their relevance is difficult to assess, as they often refer to isolated incidents that may have been treated in a haphazard way, without incorporating the knowledge which may be gleaned from a wider view of the literature. There are, however, several retrospective reviews and 'clinical trials' that go part of the way to offering evidence of the efficacy of various treatments.[12–15]

It must be borne in mind that some of the recommended antidotes could cause, and in animal models have caused, further tissue damage. This is especially likely if they are not used (with extreme care) by experienced persons. The use of sodium bicarbonate injection in anthracycline extravasation is an example.

RISK FACTORS ASSOCIATED WITH EXTRAVASATION

Many factors may increase the risk of extravasation occurring; these may be related to the patient, the injection technique or the drug.

1 The Patient

Extravasation injuries commonly occur in seriously ill patients and appear to be more prevalent in children, old people and patients requiring frequent venepunctures, such as those on chemotherapy. Patients unable to communicate pain produced by extravasated fluid are obviously more likely to develop tissue injury. These include neonates and young children, anaesthetized or comatose patients, and those undergoing cardiac resuscitation. Care should also be observed in patients with peripheral neuropathy whose peripheral sensation may be diminished and who are therefore unable to sense extravasation.

The state of the patient's venous system is an important risk factor. Fragile veins will increase the risk of extravasation. Elderly and debilitated patients are likely to have veins in poor condition. Patients with generalized vascular disease are more prone to extravasation, as are those with elevated venous pressure and those with obstructed venous drainage, after, for example, axillary surgery or radical mastectomy.

Severely ill patients frequently have reduced clotting factors and reduced platelet counts that consequently inhibit the formation of a firm haemostatic plug at the injection site, and increase the risk of leakage.

Venous spasm may lead to extravasation (see Recognition) and may be caused by a number of factors including change in body temperature, elevated blood pressure and psychological factors. Small vessel diameter will contribute to extravasation.

Patients who have had previous radiation therapy at the site of injection may develop severe local reactions from extravasated cytotoxic drugs. Cytotoxic drugs also have the potential to cause cutaneous abnormalities in areas that have been damaged previously by radiation, even if these areas are distant from the injection site. This is known as recall injury and has been noted in patients who have received doxorubicin.[16]

2 The Injection: Cannulation and Infusion Techniques

Many extravasation injuries are the result of inexperienced personnel performing venepuncture and administering vesicants. If a vein is punctured several times before an IV line is established, the stage is set for easier leakage. More extravasation injuries occur at night than during the day.

The type of cannula used can also affect the incidence of extravasation. It has been found that correctly positioned cannulae with steel needles extravasated drugs twice as often as those with plastic (Teflon) catheters.

The site of injection should be chosen to minimize damage if extravasation does occur. Sites near the joints of the arm and hand contain vital nerves and tendons and should be avoided.

Patients receiving drugs via infusion pumps should be observed closely because continued pumping of fluid after displacement of a cannula leads to mechanical compression of the tissues. This can have serious consequences, with the rise in extracellular hydrostatic pressure resulting in increased interstitial pressure, venous compression, arterial compromise and eventually tissue necrosis. Alarm devices for pumps which detect an increase in pressure are often insensitive and damage may occur before the alarm triggers. Extravasation alarms relying on decrease in skin temperature have been found to trigger when extravasation has not in fact occurred.

3 The Drugs

There are a number of risk factors which increase the prevalence of extravasation; these are listed below. These factors are useful predictive indices for clinical pharmacists when they are considering the risk represented by any IV infusion:

▼ ability to bind directly to DNA
▼ ability to cause direct cellular toxicity
▼ ability to cause local tissue ischaemia
▼ formulations with high osmolality

▼ formulation pH outside the range 5–9
▼ formulation likely to precipitate.

Table 9.1: *Classification of cytotoxic drugs according to their potential to cause serious necrosis when extravasated.*

Vesicants: Group 1	Irritants: Group 2	Non-vesicants: Group 3
Amsacrine	Aclarubicin	Asparaginase
Carmustine	Carboplatin	Azacytidine
Cisplatinum	Etoposide	Bleomycin
Dacarbazine	Methotrexate	Cyclophosphamide*
Dactinomycin	Mitozantrone	Cytarabine
Daunorubicin	Teniposide	Fluorouracil*
Doxorubicin		Ifosfamide*
Epirubicin		Melphalan
Idarubicin		Thiotepa*
Mitomycin		α Interferons
Mustine		Aldesleukin (IL-2)*
Plicamycin		
Streptozocin		
Vinblastine		
Vincristine		
Vindesine		

The classification of those drugs in group 3 marked with an asterisk is controversial. While being regarded by some as non-vesicant, others have argued that they represent an irritant hazard to subcutaneous tissues. These authors have further suggested that a simple/non-vesicant classification would be more helpful as this is less confusing with regard to the significance of the extravasation. It is the view of these authors that all extravasation is significant, but that the three-group classification can be helpful in individualizing the treatment.

Controversy about the classification of Aclarubicin suggests that extravasation should be treated as for Group 1 drugs.

PREVENTION OR MINIMIZATION OF THE PROBLEMS OF EXTRAVASATION

The position, size and age of the venepuncture site are the factors which have greatest bearing on the likelihood of problems occurring. However, if the following points are borne in mind, the likelihood of extravasation can be significantly reduced.

▼ For slow infusion of high risk drugs, a central line or drum catheter should be used.
▼ To ensure patency of a peripheral IV site, it is best to administer cytotoxics through a recently sited cannula. Site the cannula so it cannot become dislodged; use the forearm and avoid, if possible, sites near joints.

▼ Administer vesicants by slow IV push into the side arm port of a fast running IV infusion of compatible solution. The most vesicant drug should be administered first.

▼ Assess a peripheral site continually for signs of redness or swelling.

▼ Verify patency of the IV site prior to vesicant infusion and regularly throughout; if there are any doubts, stop and investigate. Resite the cannula if the patency of the cannulation is still not entirely satisfactory.

▼ Ask the patient to report any sensations of burning or pain at the infusion site. Some investigators suggest delaying the administration of antiemetics until after vesicant administration. The sedative and anti-inflammatory effects of antiemetics often mask the early warning signs of extravasation and may impede the patient's ability to report any sensation at the infusion site.

▼ Never hurry. Administer drugs slowly to allow the drug to be diluted by the carrier solution and to allow careful assessment of the IV site.

▼ Document carefully the rate of administration, location and condition of site, verification of patency, and patient's responses, on giving any potentially extravasable drugs.

If vein diameter or vein collapse are a problem, then the use of glyceryl trinitrate patches distal to the cannula may be helpful.[17-18]

RECOGNITION

The recognition of tissue extravasation, as opposed to venous irritation or local hypersensitivity, is based either on the patient's symptoms (pain, erythema or swelling at the injection site), a reduction in flow rate or lack of blood return. Early detection of extravasation is crucial. Administration should be halted and appropriate measures quickly implemented.

Extravasation should be suspected when:

▼ the patient complains of burning, stinging, pain or any acute change at the injection site. The patient is often the first person to become aware that something is wrong with their IV therapy, so instruct them at the beginning of treatment to inform staff of any acute change during the treatment. Explain the reason for this in a way which is not frightening but conveys the need for the patient's input and participation. Give reassurance that, if a leakage of drug should occur, it would probably not cause serious problems if the infusion is promptly stopped and the correct treatment instituted. Patients who are unable to communicate should be particularly closely observed

▼ induration, erythema, venous discolouration or swelling is observed at the site. (Discolouration alone may not indicate extravasation as doxorubicin, epirubicin and mitozantrone have been reported to produce this.)

▼ no blood return is obtained. The presence of blood return does not, however, negate the possibility of extravasation. The bevel of the needle can puncture the vein wall during venepuncture, allowing drug to escape into the tissues, whilst the lumen of the needle may still remain in the blood vessel and allow adequate blood return

▼ the flow rate is reduced. A reduced rate may not be observed when using an infusion pump, so close observation is necessary.

MANAGEMENT OF EXTRAVASATION

1 Policy for the Emergency Treatment of Extravasation

▼ It is vital to act promptly.
▼ There should be clear guidelines for prompt 'first aid' treatment.
▼ The 'extravasation kit' should remain simple to avoid confusion, but comprehensive enough to meet fully all reasonable needs. Comprehensive treatment and expert advice must be available as soon as possible.
▼ There should be clear, easy to follow instructions.
▼ The emergency treatment should aim to remove as soon as possible, as much as possible of the offending drug from the subcutaneous tissue.
▼ The emergency treatment should not cause further tissue damage or, in the event of misdiagnosis, cause damage where extravasation has not occurred.

2 The Basics of Treatment[19-29]

▼ ALWAYS aspirate then inject steroids IV, and subcutaneously (sc) and apply them topically
▼ THEN:
  EITHER spread and dilute using
    normal saline
    hyaluronidase
    warm continuous compression and elevation of the limb.
  OR localize and neutralize using
    antidote if available
    intermittent cold compression.

3 General Procedure for the Management of Extravasation

▼ Seek experienced assistance from someone more used to looking at extravasation.
▼ Stop the infusion, disconnect the drip but DO NOT REMOVE THE CANNULA.
▼ Mark the extravasated area with a pen.
▼ Aspirate the extravasated drug, trying also to draw some blood back from the cannula. This may be facilitated by sc injection of either 0.9% sodium chloride, to dilute the drug, or 1500 units of hyaluronidase in 2 ml water for injection. (Hyaluronidase should NEVER be used with vesicant drugs, unless as a specific antidote.)
▼ Remove the cannula.
▼ Give 100 mg hydrocortisone IV. This should be administered via a new cannula, resited remotely from the extravasation area.
▼ Give 100 mg hydrocortisone (2 ml) as 0.1–0.2 ml sc injections at about 6 to 8 points around the circumference of the extravasation site.
▼ Give sc injections of specific antidote where applicable.
▼ Apply 1% hydrocortisone cream to the area.
▼ Cover with sterile gauze and apply heat to disperse the extravasated drug or cool the area to localize the extravasation.
▼ Measure the area of the extravasation and document the treatment in the patient's notes. Complete a Green Card (*see* later). Photographing the area can be very helpful.

▼ Give antihistamine cover (terfenadine 60 mg, po, once only).
▼ Provide analgesia if required (indomethacin 25 mg tds, or dihydrocodeine have proved effective).

This general procedure can be refined, depending upon the type of extravasation provision it is required to make (*see* later). If this refinement is based on the 'group' classification of cytotoxics then the following general and specific procedures could be used.

4 General Procedure for the Management of Extravasation of a Non-vesicant Group 3 Drug

If a large volume has extravasated, aspirate as much fluid as possible. No further treatment should be required. Manage the situation symptomatically.

5 General Procedure for the Management of Extravasation of an Irritant Group 2 Drug

With the irritant group there exists the possibility of some local inflammation or necrosis, and/or some pain, particularly in sensitive individuals. Aspirate as much fluid as possible, give 100 mg hydrocortisone via the venflon, 100 mg sc hydrocortisone as 0.2 ml injections around the circumference of the affected area, apply topical hydrocortisone and cover area with an ice pack. There are no specific antidotes for these drugs.

6 Specific Procedures for the Management of Extravasation of a Vesicant Group 1 Drug

Dactinomycin	Infiltrate the affected area with 2–5 ml of 3% sodium thiosulphate.
Aclarubicin Daunorubicin Doxorubicin Epirubicin Idarubicin Mitomycin	Infiltrate the area with 2–5 ml of 2.1% sodium bicarbonate, leave for two minutes and aspirate off again. Paint dimethylsulphoxide (DMSO) topically to the extravasated area. This should be applied two-hourly, followed by hydrocortisone cream and 30 minutes of cold compression, for the first 24 hours. Treatment for the next 14 days should consist of topical application of DMSO at six-hourly intervals, alternating with six-hourly applications of topical hydrocortisone cream, a preparation thus being applied every three hours on an alternate basis. Contact with good skin should be avoided. If blistering occurs, the DMSO should be stopped and further advice sought.
Cisplatinum	Infiltrate the area with 2–5 ml of 3% sodium thiosulphate, aspirate back, then give 1500 units of hyaluronidase around the area and apply heat and compression.
Carmustine Plicamycin	Infiltrate the area with 2–5 ml of 2.1% sodium bicarbonate, leave for two minutes and aspirate off again.
Mustine	Infiltrate the area with 2–5 ml of 3% sodium thiosulphate. Introduce a further 100 mg of hydrocortisone to the infiltrated area. Apply cold compression intermittently for 12 hours.

Vincristine	Infiltrate the area with 1500 units of hyaluronidase. Apply
Vinblastine	heat and compression.
Vindesine	

Note that 2.1% sodium bicarbonate is not commercially available but can be produced when required at the scene, by a double dilution of 8.4% ampoules. However, 2.1% sodium bicarbonate still represents an extravasation hazard and should be used **with extreme care**. The 3% sodium thiosulphate is obtained by diluting 1.2 ml of the commercially available 50% sodium thiosulphate injection up to 20 ml with sterile water for injections.[30–35]

PROVISION OF AN EMERGENCY POLICY AND EXTRAVASATION KIT

Both the emergency treatment policy and extravasation kit should be simple and, therefore, easy to use without the risk of further damage; or complete and comprehensive but with the consequent necessity for expertise and care.

Whichever option is chosen for the local situation at ward or patient level, it will be necessary to hold the complete set of antidotes and hot and cold facilities at one or several locations within the hospital. Considering the following points may help in deciding the answer to the question, 'Is a "simple" or a "comprehensive" setup required?'

▼ Is it a department or ward routinely (ie more than 30% of the time) using potentially vesicant drugs?
▼ Are the staff particularly trained in the detection and treatment of extravasation?
▼ Does the treatment policy require a special antidote for any of these drugs?
▼ Are potentially hazardous treatments being carried out 24 hours a day?
▼ Is in- or out-patient treatment intended?

If the answer to the first four questions is 'yes', almost irrespective of the fifth, then a comprehensive setup is required.

Appendix 1 details the contents of a complete/comprehensive extravasation kit as used in the St Chad's Oncology Unit, Dudley Road Hospital, Birmingham, UK. The kit also contains details of the local emergency policy which are contained on two plastic covered cards within the box.

Appendix 2 details the contents of a simple extravasation kit which contains modified emergency cards giving 'first aid' treatment and directions indicating where full antidotes can be obtained.

DOCUMENTATION AND REPORTING OF EXTRAVASATION

It is important that a complete history of an extravasation event is documented, with diagrams and photographs, in the patient's notes. Observation and documentation of the injury should be on a daily basis for the first few days, extended then to weekly observation on a planned follow-up. (Figure 9.1 shows an ideal extravasation documentation slip.)

Extravasation Documentation Slip

Name: Date: Time: Location:

Drug sequence:

Needles size and type:

Technique:

Venepuncture site:

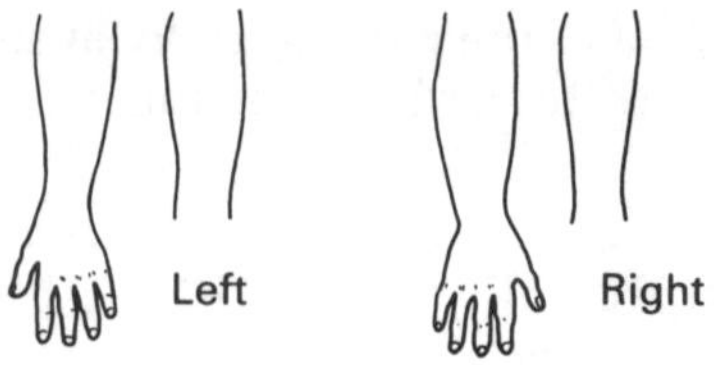

Approximate amount of extravasation:

Appearance:

Diameter of injured area:

Nursing management:

Patient's complaints and statements:

Signature:

Figure 9.1: *Extravasation documentation form*

In an attempt to collate and analyse data on extravasation events in a large number of patients, a 'Green Card' scheme for reporting extravasation incidences, their treatment and outcome is being co-ordinated through the St Chad's Unit, Dudley Road Hospital, Birmingham, UK.

1 Aims and Objectives of the Green Card Scheme

- To obtain accurate statistics on the number of incidents by extravasating drug and type of treatment.
- To collect data on treatment methods and antidotes being used for extravasation incidents.
- To obtain accurate information on the outcome of incidents.
- To feedback information on treatment and their effectiveness.

2 What do the Green Cards Ask For?

- Drug(s) involved.
- Circumstances of detection.
- Extent of the problem.
- Drugs used in the treatment.
- Procedure for treatment.
- Type of cannulation.
- Location and extent of the extravasation.

The green cards are intended to be user friendly. The information is strictly confidential and the reporting centre and patient remain anonymous.

The report cards are available from hospital pharmacy departments or oncology units in the UK or can be obtained direct from the Extravasation Report Co-ordinator, c/o St Chad's Unit, Dudley Road Hospital, Birmingham B18 7QH, UK.

An example of the Green Card is shown in Figure 9.2.

IN CONFIDENCE REGISTER OF EXTRAVASATION AND ITS TREATMENT FOR THE REPORTING OF EXTRAVASATION FROM ANY THERAPEUTIC COMPOUND

Patient   Male*/Female*   Age _____   Height (m) _____   Weight (kg) _____

Drug causing extravastion was _____   Dose _____

Infused in* _____   Added to last running drip of* _____ /Stat*

Given Cannula/Butterfly (please state size) _____ over _____ mins/hr

The above drug formed part of course No. _____ in the following regimen

Drug	Total Dose	Infusion Fluid/Stat	Time	Already Given	Not Yet Given
				Yes/No*	Yes/No*
				Yes/No*	Yes/No*
				Yes/No*	Yes/No*
				Yes/No*	Yes/No*

Other drugs being given concurrently (oral + IVs) _____

Were the drugs being administered via a pump or syringe driver? | YES | NO |

If YES please indicate model _____

Please indicate SITE and cannulation and area of extravasation with measurements on the diagrams below

Front   Back   Left or Right Arm*

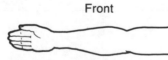 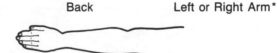

Other method of administration:

Central or long line*/Hickman line*/Portacath*/Drum catheter*

Other (please specify) _____

Location (please specify) _____

Details of extravasation treatment (Drug, Dose, Procedure)

_____

_____

Date of extravasation _____   Time of extravastion _____

Acute extravasation treatment started on _____ Stopped on _____

| This section is not compulsory. Contact name for further details (Dr, nurse, pharmacist)   Name _____   Tel.No. _____ |

Additional comments _____

_____

_____

* Please delete or fill in as appropriate

_____

FOLLOW UP REPORT ON THE OUTCOME OF PREVIOUSLY REPORTED EXTRAVASATION INCIDENCE

Please detach this portion of the Green Card

Please give details of any chronic pharmacological treatment _____

_____

_____

Outcome (please tick one)

Resolved following acute treatment ☐

Resolved using pharmacological treatment only ☐

Extravasation untreated and required skin grafting ☐

Patient lost to follow up ☐

If the extravasation injury ulcerated, was there any functional loss in the affected limb? | YES | NO |

If yes, please give details _____

_____

If surgery was performed please give brief details _____

_____

_____

Figure 9.2: *Example of a 'Green Card'*

REFERENCES

1. Hecker, J.F. (1990). Survival of intravenous chemotherapy infusion sites. *Br. J. Cancer* **62**, 660–662.
2. Bareford, D. (1985). Treatment of extravasation of vincristine with hydrocortisone and hyaluronidase. *Br. Med. J.* **291**, 1242.
3. Rudolph, R. (1978). Ulcers of the hand and wrist caused by doxorubicin hydrochloride. *Orthop. Rev.* **7**, 93–95.
4. Tsavaris, N.B., *et al.* (1990). Conservative approach to the treatment of chemotherapy-induced extravasation. *J. Dermatol. Surg. Oncol.* **16**, 519–522.
5. Ignoffo, R.J. and Friedman, M.A. (1980). Therapy of local toxicities caused by extravasation of cancer chemotherapeutic drugs. *Cancer Treat. Rev.* **7**, 17–27.
6. Banerjee, A. *et al.* (1987). Cancer chemotherapy agent-induced perivenous extravasation injuries. *Postgrad. Med. J.* **63**, 5–9.
7. Rudolph, R. and Larson, D.L. (1987). Etiology and treatment of chemotherapeutic agent extravasation injuries: A review. *J. Clin. Oncol.* **5**, 1116–1126.
8. Dorr, R.T. (1981). Extravasation of vesicant antineoplastics. *Ariz. Med.* **28**, 271–275.
9. Cullen, M.L. (1982). Current interventions for doxorubicin extravasations. *Oncol. Nurs. Forum* **9**, 52–53.
10. Linder, R.M. *et al.* (1983). Management of extensive doxorubicin hydrochloride extravasation injuries. *J. Hand Surg.* **8**, 32–38.
11. Cohen, M.H. (1979). Amelioration of adriamycin skin necrosis: An experimental study. *Cancer Treat. Rep.* **63**, 1003–1004.
12. Hart, L.L. and Middleton, R.K. eds. (1989). Treatment of doxorubicin extravasations. *D.I.C.P.* **23**, 386–387.
13. Larson, D.L. (1985). What is the appropriate management of tissue extravasation by antitumor agents? *Plast. Reconstr. Surg.* **75**, 397–405.
14. Coleman, J.J. *et al.* (1983). Treatment of adriamycin-induced skin ulcers: A prospective controlled study. *J. Surg. Oncol.* **22**, 129–135.
15. Olver, I.N. *et al.* (1988). A prospective study of topical dimethyl sulfoxide for treating anthracycline extravasation. *J. Clin. Oncol.* **6**, 1732–1735.
16. Donaldson, S.S. *et al.* (1974). Adriamycin activity: A recall phenomenon after radiation therapy. *Ann. Intern. Med.* **81**, 407–408.
17. Khawaja, H.T. *et al.* (1988). Effect of transdermal glyceryl trinitrate on the survival of peripheral intravenous infusions: A double-blind prospective clinical study. *Br. J. Surg.* **75**, 1212–1215.
18. Wright, A. *et al.* (1985). Use of transdermal glyceryl trinitrate to reduce failure of intravenous infusion due to phlebitis and extravasation. *The Lancet* **ii**, 1148–1150.
19. Olver, I.N. *et al.* (1988). A prospective trial of topical dimethyl sulphoxide (DMSO) for treating anthracycline extravasation. *Proc. ASCO* **7**, 279.
20. Svingen, B.A. *et al.* (1981). Protection by α-tocopherol and dimethyl-sulfoxide (DMSO) against adriamycin induced skin ulcers in the rat. *Res. Commun. Chem. Pathol. Pharmacol.* **32**, 189–192.
21. Zweig, J.I. and Kabakow, B. (1978). An apparently effective countermeasure for doxorubicin extravasation. *JAMA* **239**, 2116.
22. Dorr, R.T. *et al.* (1983). Cold protection from intradermal (ID) doxorubicin (Dox) ulceration in the mouse. Abstracts. *Proc. AACR* **24**, 255.

23. Cox, R.F. (1984). Managing skin damage induced by doxorubicin hydro-chloride and daunorubicin hydrochloride. *Am. J. Hosp. Pharm.* **41**, 2410–2414.
24. Zweig, J.I. *et al.* (1979). Rational effective medical treatment of skin ulcers due to adriamycin. *Cancer Treat. Rep.* **63**, 2101–2102.
25. Desai, M.H. and Teres, D. (1982). Prevention of doxorubicin-induced skin ulcers in the rat and pig with dimethylsulfoxide (DMSO). *Cancer Treat. Rep.* **66**, 1371–1374.
26. Crabbe, S.J. ed. (1990). *DMSO therapy for extravasation.* P&T. October, 1245–1248.
27. Dorr, R.T. *et al.* (1980). The limited role of corticosteroids in ameliorating experimental doxorubicin skin toxicity in the mouse. *Cancer Chemother. Pharmacol.* **5**, 17–20.
28. Dorr, R.T. and Alberts, D.S. (1981). Pharmacologic antidotes to experi-mental doxorubicin skin toxicity: A suggested role for beta-adrenergic compounds. *Cancer Treat. Rep.* **65**, 1001–1006.
29. Alberts, D.S. and Dorr, R.T. (1991). Case report: Topical DMSO for Mitomycin-C-induced skin ulceration. *Oncol. Nurs. Forum* **18**, 693–695.
30. Cox, K. *et al.* (1988). The management of cytotoxic drug extravasation: Guidelines drawn up by a working party for the Clinical Oncological Society of Australia. *Med. J. Aust.* **148**, 185–189.
31. Hirsh, J.D. and Conlon, P.F. (1983). Implementing guidelines for managing extravasation of antineoplastics. *Am. J. Hosp. Pharm.* **40**, 1516–1519.
32. Schneider, S.M. and Distelhorst, C.W. (1989). Chemotherapy-induced emergencies. *Semin. Oncol.* **16**, 572–578.
33. Harwood, K.V. and Aisner, J. (1984). Treatment of chemotherapy extravasa-tion: Current status. *Cancer Treat. Rep.* **68**, 939–945.
34. McNeece, J. and Lightly, J. (1986). *Cytotoxic extravasation manual.* Pharmacy Department, Leeds General Infirmary, Leeds.
35. Smith, R. (1985). Prevention and treatment of extravasation. *Br. J. Parent. Ther.* **6**, 114–118.

APPENDIX 1

Contents of a 'comprehensive' extravasation box:

▼ dimethylsulphoxide solution (50–100%)
▼ hyaluronidase 1500 units injection
▼ hydrocortisone 100 mg injection, and 1% cream
▼ sodium bicarbonate 8.4% injection*
▼ sodium chloride 0.9% injection
▼ sodium thiosulphate 50% injection*
▼ terfenadine 60 mg tablets
▼ water for injection (2 ml and 10 ml)
▼ selection of needles, syringes, alcohol wipes, cotton wool balls and sterile gauze
▼ directions to the nearest cold pack and heat pad.

* Overlabelled with directions for dilution.

Examples of the overlabels are shown below:

SODIUM BICARBONATE 8.4%
DO NOT USE UNDILUTED
5 ml of this solution should be added to 5 ml of water for injection and then 5 ml of this new solution added to a further 5 ml of water for injection. This will then give a 2.1% sodium bicarbonate solution.

SODIUM THIOSULPHATE 50%
DO NOT USE UNDILUTED
Dilute 1.2 ml of 50% sodium thiosulphate to 20 ml with water for injection. This will then give a 3% sodium thiosulphate solution.

APPENDIX 2

Contents of a 'simple' extravasation box:

▼ hyaluronidase 1500 units
▼ hydrocortisone 100 mg injection, and 1% cream
▼ sodium chloride 0.9% injection
▼ water for injections (2 ml)
▼ selection of needles, syringes, alcohol wipes, cotton wool balls and sterile gauze
▼ directions to the nearest cold pack and heat pad.

CHAPTER 10

Home-based Cytotoxic Chemotherapy

INTRODUCTION

1 Potential Benefits of Home Chemotherapy

Chemotherapy is a major weapon in the treatment of a wide variety of cancers and may be used either as a single modality or in combination with radiotherapy and/or surgery. Traditionally, patients requiring chemotherapy have been admitted into hospital as in-patients or as day-case patients to receive their medication. Day-case treatment often requires the patient to be hospitalized for two or three days either because of protracted treatment regimens or because a combination of severe side-effects and the remote geographical location of the patient's home from the hospital preclude discharge until the patient is well enough to travel. This approach to cancer chemotherapy results in the patient spending considerable time away from home, from the work-place and from their family.

Understandably, it is the desire of most patients to be able to remain at home and to live as normal a life-style as possible.[1] Demand for home-based treatment combined with developments in drug administration technology have resulted in the emergence of domiciliary chemotherapy programmes where the patient is able to receive parenteral chemotherapy in their own home. Home-based chemotherapy not only reduces the stress and inconvenience of attending hospital but also enables the patient to take an active role in his treatment.

Home chemotherapy enables the patient to enjoy greater independence, particularly if the chemotherapy is self-administered. The active involvement of patients in their treatment tends to encourage a more positive attitude to chemotherapy. Drug-related side-effects may be more readily tolerated if patients are able to remain at home with their families in familiar surroundings.

Families of cancer patients often experience a feeling of helplessness and inadequacy but home-based treatment provides an opportunity for families and close friends to give assistance and support with treatment. All of these factors can contribute to increased morale of patients and their families. Psychological studies[2] on both domiciliary and hospitalized patients receiving similar chemotherapy regimens have demonstrated improved quality of life and a greater sense of well-being in the home-based group of patients. Home treatment also reduces the exposure of immunocompromised cancer patients to hospital infections.[1]

From an economical perspective, a properly managed, home chemotherapy programme can reduce costs associated with hospitalization and increase treatment availability. In a randomized study of in-patient versus out-patient continuous infusion chemotherapy for patients with locally advanced head and neck cancer, Vokes *et al.*.[3] estimated a reduction in daily costs of $366 US per patient for domiciliary chemotherapy.

2 Potential Disadvantages and Limitations of Home Chemotherapy

In the home setting, professional assistance is not readily available to the patient. Acute drug-related toxicity, equipment failure, extravasation of the drug infusion and infection of the central venous catheter are difficulties which may cause patients severe distress. Acute toxicity can be minimized by using continuous ambulatory infusions for drug delivery and by pharmacodynamic individualization of drug dosage (*see* page 94). It is essential that patients are given thorough training on how to react in cases of equipment failure and that this is supported by written instructions and a 24-hour telephone number to enable home-based patients to contact a member of the oncology team. Most complications can be anticipated and dealing with them forms an integral part of the patient training programme. With experienced home care oncology teams, complications are rare and catheter infection rates of less than 1% are obtainable.[4]

It must also be accepted that some patients are not capable of maintaining their treatment at home. This may be because they are unable to understand basic instructions relating to their treatment or because of a physical disability (eg arthritis) that would prevent them from handling medication syringes and other equipment. In some cases support from family or friends may not be available and communications with the hospital-based oncology team may be difficult (eg the patient may not have access to a telephone). Some patients may prefer the security of a hospital and are unwilling to take on the responsibility of home-based treatment. Careful patient selection is essential and will exert a profound influence on the outcome of home chemotherapy.

The economics of home chemotherapy may not always be viewed in a favourable light, largely because health care financial systems are inflexible and geared to in-patient treatment. Although home chemotherapy may release hospital beds, costs will actually increase if these are subsequently occupied by other patients. At best, home-based treatment provides hospital managers with a choice: either they can reduce the number of oncology beds and save money or they can re-occupy the released beds with other patients (not necessarily cancer patients) and reduce waiting lists. In addition, savings made at ward level may be difficult to transfer to the budgets of those departments (eg pharmacy) where expenditure is increased as a result of home chemotherapy.

CLINICAL CONSIDERATIONS

1 Patient Selection

Careful patient selection is crucial to the success of a home chemotherapy programme. Before the option of domiciliary treatment is offered, the clinician must establish that the patient is well motivated, physically capable of managing their medication syringes, infusion pump or other equipment and that the patient is able to understand detailed instructions. Normally, patients should have a reasonable performance status (Karnofsky score of at least 60) and should be capable of enjoying a satisfactory quality of life during home treatment. Ideally, support should be available from family and friends who are able to adjust or disrupt their own routines in order to help care for the patient. The availability of transport to and from the oncology out-patient clinic must be considered and although it is possible to offer home chemotherapy to patients who live some distance from their hospital, access to a telephone is essential.

A wide range of cancers, including leukaemias (during remission) and solid tumours can be treated in the domiciliary setting. Patients with solid tumours of the breast, pancreas, colon, oesophagus and liver, often with metastatic disease, have been treated at a growing number of centres, both in the UK and abroad.[4-6] In many cases, home patients are being treated for recurrent disease following surgery or radiotherapy and the disease may be at an advanced stage. Patients in the late stages of disease or with fistulae, internal bleeding, ascites, systemic infection or severe nutritional deficiency are clearly not suitable for home treatment. Similarly, those patients who are unable to cope with the psychological and emotional stress associated with cancer should be offered the professional care available in the hospital or hospice system.

2 Dose Schedules

Bolus and short-term infusions

Although it is possible to administer home chemotherapy in traditional bolus or short-term infusion schedules, this approach is not always appropriate for domiciliary patients. In the hospital setting it is possible to control the acute toxicity (such as nausea and vomiting) associated with conventional chemotherapy. For domiciliary patients, such toxicity is more difficult to control and would be unacceptable, although this may become less of a problem in the future with the introduction of such symptomatic treatments as the $5HT_3$ antagonist antiemetics. Conventional bolus or short-term infusion schedules would normally be administered by a community nurse. Some patients may feel that this restricts their freedom and independence, negating the advantages of home treatment over hospital day-case treatment.

In cases where experience has shown that bolus chemotherapy is well tolerated, it may be possible to offer patients the option of self-medication by using a venous access device such as the Intraport shown in Figure 10.1. The catheter is inserted into a central vein (usually the subclavian vein) and the medication port is implanted subcutaneously, usually in the anterior chest wall, with the silastic septum located just beneath the skin. The septum is designed for multiple puncture and when not in use the patency of the system is maintained by flushing with dilute heparinized saline at monthly intervals.[7] Venous access devices provide a means of prolonged central venous access for cancer patients without frequent venepuncture and also for patients with difficult peripheral venous access as a result of obesity or emaciation. The safe administration of vesicant chemotherapy regimens is also made possible by these devices providing that the catheter is placed in a central vein.

The self-administration of small-volume subcutaneous injections may be appropriate for low-dose maintenance regimens providing that drug-related toxicity is minimal and the drug is non-vesicant. Home-care packs containing medication and the necessary syringes and needles are now available for this purpose. Devices used to aid the subcutaneous administration of insulin to diabetic patients may also be of benefit to leukaemia and cancer patients.

Prolonged continuous infusion

Attempts to improve the therapeutic index of antitumour drugs have focused on the replacement of traditional, rapid infusion schedules with prolonged continuous infusion regimens.[8] Recent developments with portable ambulatory infusion pumps have facilitated continuous infusion chemotherapy for domiciliary patients.

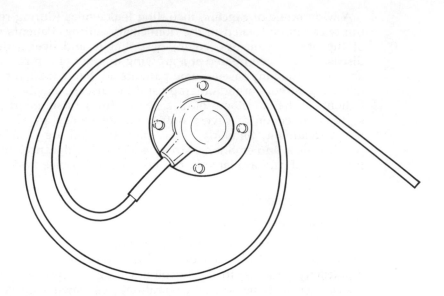

Figure 10.1: *Intraport Venous Access Port*

The rationale for continuous infusion chemotherapy is based on the pharmacokinetic characteristics of cytotoxic drugs and on the cytokinetic (growth cycle) profile of tumour cells.[8] Since many cytotoxic drugs have short plasma half-lives, continuous infusion regimens prolong the exposure of tumour cells to the drug. As tumour cells progress through the cell cycle, a greater proportion of the tumour cell population is exposed to the drug during the sensitive phase(s) of the cell cycle.

An additional advantage with continuous infusion regimens in home chemotherapy programmes is that adverse effects associated with peak plasma levels are reduced or eliminated. For example, doxorubicin is less cardiotoxic[9] and fluorouracil less myelosuppressive[10] in continuous infusion regimens. There is evidence that nausea and vomiting associated with bolus doses of cisplatinum are significantly reduced when infusional regimens are used.[11] However, other toxicities, such as mucositis and hand-foot syndrome in the case of fluorouracil,[12] may occur more readily with prolonged infusions.

Controlled studies[13,14] indicate that, on balance, drug-related adverse effects are reduced with infusional regimens and quality of life for the patient is improved.

LOGISTICAL CONSIDERATIONS

1 The Home Oncology Team

The success of home-based chemotherapy is dependent upon a team approach towards patient care. The team would typically include a consultant oncologist, oncology nurse and oncology pharmacist. If chemotherapy is to be administered as a continuous infusion using ambulatory pumps it will be necessary to include a surgeon in the team for the placement of central venous catheters or other venous access devices. If home-based patients are receiving ambulatory continuous infusion chemotherapy at least one member of the team (usually the pharmacist or nurse) should be available 24 hours a day to deal with any problems that may arise with infusion pumps or the central venous catheter.

The team should also be able to call upon the resources of other departments, such as microbiology and medical electronics (for the testing and calibration of infusion pumps). If home chemotherapy is to be based on nurse-administered bolus or short infusion schedules, the team should contain a fully trained oncology nurse. It is, of course, essential that the patient's general practitioner is informed of the treatment. If it becomes necessary to switch from chemotherapy to pain control, the venous access system used for chemotherapy can then be used for the infusion of opiates. In these cases, hospice nurses may become involved in the preparation and administration of opiate infusions.

2 Venous Access Devices

Central venous catheters have been widely used for many years to deliver chemotherapy and total parenteral nutrition. These devices provide a reliable system for the administration of prolonged continuous infusions and, when attached to a venous access port, may also be used to deliver concentrated bolus injections of cytotoxic drugs to a central vein. The Hickman[15] and the smaller internal diameter, Broviac[16] catheters are suitable for ambulatory use and give rise to very few complications. Central venous catheters are normally placed in the subclavian vein and are tunnelled subcutaneously for a few centimetres at the site of entry to provide a barrier against the ingress of micro-organisms. A Dacron cuff around the catheter just distal to the site of entry is used to hold the catheter in place. This cuff also helps to promote fibrosis of tissues at the site of catheter entry and this creates an additional barrier to micro-organisms. The site of catheter entry is further protected by an occlusive dressing which is changed at least fortnightly during visits to the oncology out-patient clinic.

Care should be taken not to infuse drug combinations which may exhibit physical incompatibility and form precipitate in the central venous catheter. Double and triple lumen catheters are available for the infusion of multiple drug regimens. Although the central venous catheter could be used to aspirate blood samples this practice may increase the risk of venous thrombosis and is not to be recommended. Venous thrombosis may occur at any time when the catheter is in place. Thrombosis usually occurs near the catheter tip and is characterized by venous distension in the neck, swelling of the arm and pain in the shoulder, arm or neck.[17] The catheter itself may become occluded and resistance to flow may prevent the correct function of relatively low-powered ambulatory infusion pumps. Thrombosis secondary to the placement of a central venous catheter is a clear indication for immediate catheter removal. Infusions of thrombolytic agents such as urokinase have been used in an attempt to salvage the catheter but the efficacy and safety of this approach is controversial.[17]

Infection at the site of catheter entry is another potential complication, although with good clinical practice and expert catheter placement the incidence of this complication can be reduced to below 1%.[4] Infections at the site of catheter entry usually present as an abscess or cellulitis where the catheter enters the skin. Blood cultures from the site of entry and from a remote peripheral site should be carried out to characterize the infecting micro-organism and to exclude systemic infection. Infections should be treated vigorously with systemic antibiotics, especially in febrile, neutropenic patients, who will require intravenous therapy. Infections involving the subcutaneous catheter tunnel usually necessitate removal of the catheter.

Instead of passing the central venous catheter out through the body for connection to an infusion pump, it may be connected to an implantable venous access port (Figure 10.1). These devices consist of a small-volume reservoir (usually 0.5 to 3 ml) and a silastic septum which is positioned subcutaneously. Venous access ports can be used to administer concentrated bolus injections which may prove vesicant to peripheral veins. Continuous infusions can also be administered via venous access ports by connecting the IV drug delivery tubing from the infusion pump to a 90° Huber needle. The Huber needle is then inserted through the skin into the septum of the venous access port where it can be left in position for at least two weeks.

Venous access ports are normally surgically implanted in the anterior chest wall. However, if the device is to be used for self-administration of bolus injections, it may be more convenient for the patient if the port is placed subcutaneously in the lower abdomen.

3 Ambulatory Infusion Pumps

A wide variety of ambulatory infusion pumps are now available, ranging in complexity from external syringe drivers to implantable, programmable pumps (*see* Chapter 5).

4 Patient Procedures

Although specific to the Home Oncology Programme, Exeter (HOPE)[4,18] the patient procedures described in this section represent a typical approach followed by other home oncology centres.

Suitable patients are introduced to the concept of home chemotherapy (and prolonged continuous infusion, if appropriate) by the consultant oncologist. If a patient decides to accept the option of home-based treatment he will then be referred to the oncology pharmacist for a more detailed explanation of the treatment. The patient is invited to view a video presentation, together with the oncology pharmacist, in which the consultant oncologist and oncology pharmacist discuss various aspects of home chemotherapy with previously treated patients and their relatives. The video is produced by the home oncology team and deals with specific issues of interest to the patient, including insertion of the central venous catheter, changing of medication reservoirs, management of the infusion pump or venous access port, and care of the dressing at the site of catheter entry. In the video presentation, previously treated patients discuss their treatment, their life-style and any difficulties they have encountered with the infusion pump. This often prompts the new patient to raise questions about the treatment and provides an opportunity for any anxieties or fears to be raised. The oncology pharmacist is required to take on the role of counsellor, a role that will be developed with each new patient as they attend the oncology out-patient clinic at fortnightly intervals.

The patient is then admitted to the oncology ward for a few days for insertion of the central venous catheter. This is an aseptic procedure and is carried out under local anaesthetic by an experienced anaesthetist. Prior to discharge from hospital, the patient is trained in the management of their treatment by the oncology pharmacist. The patient is taught how to operate the infusion pump, how to recognize and respond to any warning alarms the pump may have, how to store medication reservoirs and change these in the pump when necessary. Instruction is given in the safe disposal of cytotoxic waste and used medication reservoirs. Often potential problems can be anticipated and dealt with before they arise. For example, patients are often concerned by the presence of a small bubble of air in the infusion catheter. This is not clinically significant and the patient can be reassured before they even experience the problem themselves. Another problem that can occasionally occur is that the patient forgets to close the tap on the catheter before disconnecting the medication reservoir, resulting in venous blood flowing out through the catheter. Difficulties of this nature and the necessary action to take are always discussed with patients before they leave the hospital. The patient remains on the ward until the pharmacist is satisfied that they are fully competent. This usually takes 24 to 48 hours. In some cases it may be advisable to train patients' relatives in the relevant techniques so that they are able to offer constructive support to the patient. As a back-up to the training programme, patients also receive concise written instructions and are given telephone numbers which may be used to contact oncology nurses or the oncology pharmacist, 24 hours a day.

On discharge from the hospital, the patient is supplied with pre-filled syringes or a medication reservoir for ambulatory pump use, or with pre-filled syringes for bolus injection. Where drug stability permits, the patient is supplied with sufficient medication for 14 days treatment (or if the treatment schedule is based on a period of less than 14 days, sufficient medication to complete the course). During breaks in chemotherapy, to permit bone marrow recovery, heparinized saline is supplied to ensure that the subclavian catheter remains patent.

The patient is also given supplies of consumables to take home with him. These include spare batteries for infusion pumps, protective gloves, sterile wipes for absorbing any minor spillage and burn-bins for disposing of cytotoxic waste and used syringes/medication reservoirs.

Patients attend the oncology out-patient clinic once every two weeks where they are seen by the consultant oncologist who monitors the patient's clinical condition. The dressing at the site of catheter entry is changed by the oncology nurse and the oncology pharmacist is on hand to deal with any infusion pump-related problems or queries concerning adverse effects from the medication. During these fortnightly visits, patients collect further supplies of consumables from the out-patient clinic and further supplies of medication from the hospital pharmacy.

Many patients participating in home chemotherapy programmes will be entered into controlled clinical trials, usually of a phase II or phase III nature. Visits to the out-patient clinic provide the clinician with an opportunity to monitor the patient extensively and to determine the quality of life enjoyed by the patient during treatment. If pharmacokinetic studies also form part of the trial, it is preferable for blood samples to be taken by a visiting oncology nurse (or pharmacist trained in phlebotomy), rather than subject the patient to repeated hospital visits.

5 Commercial Services

For those hospitals where the pharmaceutical expertise or facilities are inadequate to provide all of the pharmaceutical elements of a home chemotherapy service, at least one commercial company (Unicare, a subsidiary of Baxter), which operates in the UK and USA is able to offer a supply service. The company will fill infusion devices and drug cassettes and deliver them direct to patients in their homes.

In the UK they will liaise with the patient's family practitioner to enable them to prescribe home chemotherapy, thereby transferring treatment costs from the hospital service into the community.

In the UK, at least, this is a novel service and several questions remain to be answered. Prominent amongst these are whether, under UK healthcare funding arrangements, general practitioners will be willing to take over expensive treatments initiated in hospitals, and whether hospital-based oncologists will be happy to devolve responsibility for the prescribing of complex and potentially toxic anticancer treatments to non-specialists who may, also, be unwilling to take on such a responsibility. There is also the question of whether the separation of supply and support functions will be considered satisfactory by those using the service.

PHARMACEUTICAL CONSIDERATIONS

1 Preparation of Medication for Home Chemotherapy Patients

The introduction of a home chemotherapy programme is likely to affect the work-load of the hospital pharmacy department in several areas. Consideration should be given to resource and funding implications before a home chemotherapy programme is implemented.

Unless the number of hospital-based oncology beds is reduced, the introduction of home chemotherapy may result in an increased patient throughput. This would be reflected by increased demands for the preparation of cytotoxic infusions and increased expenditure on the drugs budget. The preparation of pre-filled medication reservoirs for ambulatory infusion pumps will require additional staff training. The provision of several days or weeks supply of medication to home patients necessitates a marked deviation from the ideal practice of commencing drug administration within 24 hours of preparation. The issue of drug stability is addressed below but the microbiological aspects of long-term supply must also be considered. It cannot be assumed that cytotoxic infusions are bactericidal and it is, therefore, essential that all equipment associated with the aseptic preparation of medication for home patients is carefully monitored, and that all procedures are thoroughly validated.

2 Extended Role of the Oncology Pharmacist

As a member of the home chemotherapy team it is essential that the oncology pharmacist is prepared to accept new responsibilities in addition to the traditional functions of drug preparation and distribution. The hospital pharmacy department is an excellent centre for the co-ordination of the home chemotherapy programme.[1] The oncology pharmacist requires a detailed knowledge of infusion pumps, catheters and venous access ports to enable sound recommendations to be made on the type of ambulatory infusion system for each individual patient. The pharmacist should have a clear understanding of stability and compatibility issues so that clinicians can be made aware of both the possibilities and limitations of home chemotherapy regimens. As an educator, the pharmacist's role would include the preparation of training material, training patients, training other health care professionals and liaising with healthcare workers outside the hospital setting.

3 Drug Stability and Compatibility

For most cytotoxic drugs, some recommendations on drug stability and compatibility are available from the manufacturers and, in the UK, are published in the *Data Sheet Compendium*.[19] However, these recommendations are restricted to licensed regimens which are invariably bolus injections or short-term infusions. In the case of home chemotherapy it must be recognized that even pre-filled syringes for bolus medication may be stored in the patient's refrigerator for several weeks before use. Drug infusions delivered by ambulatory pumps are not only stored for long periods (up to 14 days) under refrigerated conditions before use but are also subjected to temperatures of 35–37°C in the pump reservoir which is worn under the patient's clothing. It is, therefore, essential to determine the physical and chemical stability of infusions used in home chemotherapy regimens under both storage (4–8°C) and 'in-use' (35–37°C) conditions. Exposure times will vary according to the type of infusion pump used. Pre-filled syringes used in the Graseby syringe driver contain 24 hours supply of medication and are changed daily by the patient. If it is proposed to give 14 days' supply of medication at a time, stability studies should be carried out under storage conditions (4–8°C) over 14 days and under in-use conditions (35–37°C) over 24 hours. In the case of infusion pumps with large volume cassettes or pouch-type medication reservoirs which contain sufficient infusion for five to 14 days treatment (depending on the regimen), drug stability under in-use conditions (35–37°C) should be determined over the treatment period. Since medication cassettes/pouches are normally connected to the infusion pump within 24 hours of preparation, stability studies under storage conditions (4–8°C) need only be continued over 24 hours. If, however, two pre-filled medication cassettes/pouches are supplied to give a total of 14 days treatment, drug stability would be determined over seven days under both storage and in-use conditions. It is advisable to monitor the temperature of each patient's own refrigerator to ensure that medication is stored at the correct temperature.

In view of the limited information available on the pharmacology and toxicology of degradation products arising from cytotoxic drugs, only fully validated stability-indicating assay methods should be used in chemical stability studies. All stability investigations should be carried out on infusions in the type of syringe or medication reservoir to be used clinically. Weight changes of infusions should be monitored during storage, particularly at 37°C, since moisture loss from medication reservoirs can mask a reduction in drug assay arising from degradation.[20] Chemical stability data for some cytotoxic drug infusions in a variety of pump reservoirs are presented in the appropriate drug monographs. Before a new type of medication reservoir or catheter is used for the first time, the level of extractives released from the plastic into the infusion should be determined. Plasticizer levels (as diethylhexylphthalate) extracted into infusions from medication reservoirs are low with typical concentrations of less than 1 µg/ml.[21] Care should be taken when using concentrated infusions of cytotoxic drugs formulated in co-solvent solutions (eg etoposide) since these can react with certain plastics causing hair-line cracks.[22]

THE PHARMACIST'S ROLE IN FUTURE DEVELOPMENTS

Most hospital pharmacists who have worked with a home oncology team have found the experience both rewarding and challenging. Both practice and research aspects of home-based oncology have required pharmacists to develop and use their scientific, clinical and counselling skills at the highest level. Future developments in home oncology treatment will also require a significant pharmaceutical input. Recent chronobiological studies[23,24] have suggested that administration of chemotherapy in accordance with circadian rhythms may reduce drug-related toxicity and improve the outcome of treatment. Dose calculations based on pharmacodynamic parameters[25] may also help in the control of adverse effects. Both approaches offer considerable potential for home chemotherapy treatment, where avoidance of severe drug toxicity is essential. These new developments require the modification and control of drug delivery systems and will clearly be dependent upon the availability of pharmaceutical expertise.

REFERENCES

1. Bacovsky, R.A. (1988). *Home parenteral chemotherapy programs*. Proceedings of 1st international symposium on oncology pharmacy practice. New Zealand Hospital Pharmacists' Association, 294–300.
2. Payne, S. (1989). *Quality of life in women with advanced breast cancer*. PhD Thesis, Department of Psychology, University of Exeter.
3. Vokes, E.E. *et al.* (1989). A randomized study of in-patient versus out-patient continuous infusion chemotherapy for patients with locally advanced head and neck cancer. *Cancer*, **63**, 30–36.
4. Sewell, G.J. *et al.* (1989). Home-based cancer therapy by continuous infusion. *Pharm. J.* **243**, 139–141.
5. Ausman, R.K. *et al.* (1982). Long-term, ambulatory, continuous intravenous infusion of 5-fluorouracil for the treatment of metastatic adenocarcinoma in the liver. *Wisc. Med. J.* **81**, 25–28.
6. Lokich, J.J. *et al.* (1982). The delivery of cancer chemotherapy by constant venous infusion: ambulatory management of venous access and portable pump. *Cancer* **50** (12), 2731–2735.
7. Finley, R.S. (1988). Ambulatory infusion pumps and venous access devices. Proceedings of 1st international symposium on oncology pharmacy practice. New Zealand Hospital Pharmacists' Association, 279–293.
8. Lokich, J.J. (1987). Introduction to the concept and practice of infusion chemotherapy. In: Lokich, J.J. (ed.). *Cancer chemotherapy by infusion*, Precept Press Inc., Chicago, 3–11.
9. Legha, S.S. *et al.* (1982). Reduction of doxorubicin cardiotoxicity by prolonged continuous intravenous infusion. *Ann. Int. Med.* **96**, 133–139.
10. Seifert, P. *et al.* (1975). Comparison of continuously infused 5-fluorouracil with bolus injection in treatment of patients with colorectal adenocarcinoma. *Cancer* **36**, 123–128.
11. Thigpen, J.T. (1989). A randomized comparison of a rapid versus prolonged (24 hr) infusion of cisplatin therapy of squamous cell carcinoma of the uterine cervix: A gynecologic oncology study. *Gyn. Onc.* **32**, 198–202.
12. Mortimer, J. and Anderson, I. (1989). Managing the toxicities unique to high-dose leukovorin (CF) and fluorouracil (FU). *Proc. Amer. Soc. Clin. Onc.* **8**, 98.

13. Lokich, J.J. *et al.* (1989). Prospective randomized comparison of continuous infusion fluorouracil with a conventional bolus schedule in metastatic colorectal carcinoma; a mid-Atlantic oncology program study. *J. Clin. Onc.* **7**, 425–432.

14. Coates, A. *et al.* (1987). Improving the quality of life during chemotherapy for advanced breast cancer. A comparison of intermittent and continuous treatment strategies. *New Eng. J. Med.* **317**, 1490–1495.

15. Hickman, R.O. *et al.* (1979) A modified right atrial catheter for access to the venous system in marrow transplant recipients. *Surg. Gynecol. Obstet.* **148**, 871–875.

16. Broviac, J.W. *et al.* (1973). A silicone rubber atrial catheter for prolonged parenteral alimentation. *Surg. Gynecol. Obstet.* **136**, 602–606.

17. Moor, C.L. (1987). Nursing management of infusion catheters. In: Lokich, J.J. (Ed.). *Cancer chemotherapy by infusion*, Precept Press Inc., Chicago, 64–74.

18. Sewell, G.J. *et al.* (1987). HOPE for cancer. *J. Dist. Nur.* April, 4–6.

19. Anon. (1989). *ABPI Data Sheet Compendium, 1989–90.* Datapharm Publications Ltd, London.

20. Sewell, G.J. *et al.* (1987). The stability of carboplatin in ambulatory continuous infusion regimes. *J. Clin. Pharm.* **12**, 427–432.

21. Sewell, G.J. (1988). *Cancer chemotherapy by infusion, drug stability and compatibility considerations.* Proceedings of 1st international symposium on oncology pharmacy practice. New Zealand Hospital Pharmacists' Association, 253–278.

22. Schwinghammer, T.L. and Reilly, M. (1988). Cracking of ABS plastic devices used to infuse undiluted etoposide injection (letter). *Am. J. Hosp. Pharm.* **45**, 1277.

23. Hrushesky, W.J.M. (1983). The clinical application of chronobiology to oncology. *Am. J. Ant.* **168**, 519–542.

24. Von Roemling, R. and Hrushesky, W.J.M. (1989). Circadian patterning of continuous floxuridine infusion reduces toxicity and allows higher dose intensity in patients with widespread cancer. *J. Clin. Onc.* **7**, 1710–1719.

25. Belani, C.P. *et al.* (1989). A novel pharmacodynamically-based approach to dose optimization of carboplatin when used in combination with etoposide. *J. Clin. Onc.* **7**, 1896–1902.

CHAPTER 11

Monitoring and Treatment of Adverse Effects in Cancer Chemotherapy

INTRODUCTION

Despite significant efforts over the last ten years to develop antineoplastic compounds with fewer adverse effects, the toxicity of cancer chemotherapy remains one of the main obstacles to its effective use. Most of the currently available drugs have been selected on the basis of their activity against proliferating cells. Unfortunately this cytotoxic activity is not highly selective and does not discriminate between malignant cells and normal cells undergoing rapid division. As a result, cytotoxic drugs probably have the narrowest therapeutic index of any class of drug in common use.

The adverse effects occurring most frequently with this group of drugs in the days and weeks immediately following treatment include suppression of bone marrow activity, anorexia, nausea and vomiting, mucositis and alopecia. Patients will require supportive care, both in the hospital and in the community, to help overcome these problems. Organ toxicities, such as pulmonary toxicity, neurotoxicity and cardiotoxicity, are more drug specific and, unlike most of the acute adverse effects, may not be reversible. Long-term effects may not be apparent until months or years following treatment. These problems include infertility due to suppression of ovarian or testicular function and occasionally the induction of a secondary malignancy in patients who have previously been successfully treated. In addition, cytotoxic drugs can give rise to a whole spectrum of rare, unpredictable or idiosyncratic reactions. The use of cytotoxic drugs in combination, in an attempt to increase their activity, adds to the toxicity of treatment, despite efforts being made to combine agents with different dose limiting toxicities.

Reductions in dose or delays in treatment as a result of toxicity may compromise the success of potentially curative therapy, but, for the majority of patients, chemotherapy is given to palliate the disease and sometimes to prolong life. This has a considerable bearing on the degree of toxicity which is considered 'acceptable' by the patient.

Managing the toxicity of chemotherapy involves a number of approaches. Treatment must be individually tailored for each patient and appropriate measures taken to avoid or minimize predictable toxicity. Adverse effects which do arise in spite of these measures must be treated and accurately documented. To effectively contribute to patient care the pharmacist must have a detailed knowledge of the drugs prescribed and must be able to anticipate potential adverse effects, in order to monitor prescribing and to advise on appropriate supportive therapy.

INDIVIDUALIZING THERAPY

Although each cytotoxic drug varies in its particular spectrum of toxicity, some general precautions can be taken to minimize the risk of predictable adverse effects occurring. Appropriate investigations must be carried out before treatment commences to ensure that the patient is fit for chemotherapy; in particular their haematological, renal and hepatic functions should be investigated. In general, patients with a white cell count below 3000/mm^3 or a platelet count below 100 000/mm^3 should not be given myelosuppressive cytotoxics.

Unlike most classes of drug, where a standard dose range can be safely recommended for the majority of patients, the dose of cytotoxic drugs must be individually calculated for each patient on the basis of their weight or, more commonly, on body surface area. Doses may then require further adjustment in the presence of renal or hepatic impairment to ensure that delayed excretion does not result in increased toxicity.

Methotrexate serum concentrations are measured following high dose therapy to help determine the dose and duration of folinic acid necessary for adequate rescue. The concept of individualizing treatment based on serum drug concentrations is being explored with other agents, largely to optimize the efficacy of treatment.

MANAGEMENT OF ADVERSE EFFECTS

Significant progress has been made in reducing the mortality and morbidity of cancer chemotherapy through the improved management of adverse effects. Ondansetron and granisetron, the 5HT$_3$ receptor antagonists, have been significant additions to the armoury of available antiemetics. Reduced mortality in the febrile neutropenic patient has been achieved by the prompt use of combinations of antibiotics, usually an aminoglycoside and an anti-pseudomonal penicillin, to provide broad spectrum cover. The availability of new antifungal and antiviral agents has also been invaluable. Despite these advances, successful treatment of chemotherapy-related toxicity is expensive, involves prolonged hospitalization and a reduction in patients' quality of life. Thus, patient management must focus on the **prevention** of toxicity.

1 Extravasation

Extravasation of many cytotoxic drugs can have disastrous consequences. The long-term outcome may be permanent tissue damage, despite the best efforts made to rescue the situation. In the absence of adequate treatment, the approach to this problem relies heavily on safe techniques for administration of cytotoxic drugs (*see* Chapter 9).

2 Nausea and Vomiting

Occasionally cytotoxic regimens or single agents such as vincristine or fluorouracil, do not require antiemetic drugs to be given routinely, but, for any cytotoxic causing severe or moderate emesis, antiemetics should always be prescribed prophylactically and not used on an 'as required basis' after vomiting has started. Although the availability of new, effective antiemetics and better use of existing agents has improved the control of acute nausea and vomiting, delayed emesis remains a significant problem, particularly for patients who have received cisplatin. Antiemetics should be taken regularly by all patients following treatment with cisplatin. Dexamethasone is probably the most effective available agent at the present time for delayed emesis and should be the basis of therapy, but further work is required in this area. More detailed information can be found by referring to the reference list at the end of the chapter.

3 Infection

A number of measures can be taken to minimize the risk of infection developing. Good oral hygiene is important as the mouth is a major source of infection, particularly in neutropenic patients. Patients should be instructed to brush their teeth regularly with a soft toothbrush and use regular antiseptic mouthwashes following tooth brushing and after every meal. Prophylactic antifungal therapy may also be appropriate.

Focal sepsis is a particular problem with IV catheter sites and is more prevalent with the increased use of central venous catheters. Ideally lines should only be handled by trained staff, using strict aseptic techniques and following agreed procedures for handling.

The haematopoietic growth factors G-CSF and GM-CSF shorten the duration of neutropenia following chemotherapy, thus reducing the incidence of infection. They are also being exploited to allow increased intensity of treatment where bone marrow suppression is the dose limiting toxicity, in the hope of improving response rates and survival.

4 Alopecia

In an effort to avoid alopecia, scalp cooling techniques have been developed using ice caps and more sophisticated refrigeration systems. The procedure itself is unpleasant and can only be used with agents with a short elimination half-life such as doxorubicin with a half-life of 30 minutes. The results of studies carried out over the last 15 years remain equivocal. Hair loss may be avoided when single agent doxorubicin is used, but is less effective when doxorubicin is used in combination with other drugs capable of causing alopecia or is used at doses above 40 mg/m^2. In the absence of reliable methods of avoiding alopecia, patients should be prepared for hair loss and given practical advice on coping with this, for example when to expect loss of hair, how rapidly this will occur and advice on obtaining a wig.

MONITORING TOXICITY

Safe administration of chemotherapy relies on clear and accurate documentation of all treatment given. The total cumulative dose administered should be recorded for drugs such as doxorubicin where this is critical. Both the response to and the toxicity of therapy should be carefully documented. A detailed assessment of response is normally carried out after a pre-determined number of treatment cycles, and toxicity is generally assessed following every cycle. The occurrence of toxicity may result in a dose reduction, delay or some other modification to treatment on subsequent cycles. A number of international rating scales are available for rating the predictable, acute reactions arising from chemotherapy, including that of the World Health Organization (WHO) and National Cancer Institute (NCI). Standardizing the assessment of treatment related toxicity in this way allows comparison to be made between published reports of clinical trials. One example is shown in Figure 11.1.

Figure 11.1: *An example of the classification for patient toxicity and response used in a monitoring chart*

	Toxicity Grade (based on WHO ratings)				
	0	1	2	3	4
Alopecia	No change	Minimal hair loss	Moderate, patchy alopecia	Complete alopecia but reversible	Non-reversible alopecia
Nausea/ vomiting	None	Nausea	Transient vomiting	Vomiting requiring treatment	Intractable vomiting
Diarrhoea	None	Transient <2 days	Tolerable but >2 days	Intolerable requiring therapy	Haemorrhagic dehydration
Oral	No charge	Soreness Erythema	Erythema, ulcers: can eat solids	Ulcers: requires liquid diet	Alimentation not possible
Neurotoxicity	None	Parasthesiae, and/or decreased tendon reflexes	Severe parasthesiae and/or mild weakness	Intolerable parasthesiae and/or marked motor loss	Paralysis
Skin	No change	Erythema	Dry desquamation, vesiculation, pruritus	Moist desquamation, ulceration	Exfoliative dermatitis: necrosis requiring surgical intervention
Performance status	Capable of normal activity No restrictions	Incapable of strenuous activity Capable of light work Ambulatory	Ambulatory Capable of all self-care Unable to work Up and about >50% waking hours	Limited self-care Confined to bed/chair >50% waking hours	Completely disabled No self-care Totally confined to bed/chair

Source: Birmingham Oncology Treatment Chart, St Chad's Unit, Dudley Road Hospital, Birmingham.

CLINICAL MONITORING

Prescriptions for cancer chemotherapy are often complex, involving combinations of both parenteral and oral cytotoxic drugs, intravenous fluids and other supportive therapies. To effectively monitor and check prescribing the pharmacist must recognize and anticipate a whole range of potential problems. Table 11.1 presents a framework for monitoring the prescribing of cytotoxic drugs to help ensure that the treatment received by patients is optimal.

Table 11.1: *A check-list for prescription monitoring in cancer chemotherapy*

Patient details
　diagnosis
　age
　weight, height, body surface area
　haematological function
　renal function
　liver function
　underlying disease
　allergy
　previous treatment
　previous reaction to treatment, ie toxicity from previous cycles requiring dose
　　modification of subsequent cycles
　total exposure to drugs with cumulative toxicity, eg doxorubicin

Protocol
　is treatment prescribed according to established regimen or clinical trial protocol?
　is drug name clear and unambiguous?
　dose
　timing, scheduling number of days therapy
　have all drugs in regimen been prescribed?
　recommended dose modifications for organ dysfunction or previous toxicity
　stop date indicated for oral therapy

Administration
　appropriate route of administration
　suitable venous access
　appropriate infusion fluid and dilution
　appropriate rate of administration
　appropriate scheduling, with regard to time of day, day of week

Interactions
　with other prescribed therapy
　pharmaceutical interactions with concurrent IV therapy, or infusion fluids

Supportive care
　ensure appropriate adjuvant therapy prescribed, eg:
　　antiemetics
　　mouth care
　　eye care
　　hydration
　　allopurinol
　　prophylactic antibiotics/antifungals/antivirals
　　growth factors
　　antidotes; folinic acid, mesna

The following drug tables highlight the main acute toxicities of specific cytotoxic drugs which can occur in the initial weeks following treatment. They do **not** include all documented adverse effects of the drugs but attempt to provide a guide to clinical monitoring of chemotherapy. For example, allergic or hyper-sensitivity reactions have occurred with many cytotoxic drugs. For more comprehensive information the reader should refer to original reference sources. A rating scale has been used to indicate the incidence and severity of adverse effects (Table 11.2), however, these effects may be dependent on the dose and method of administration and will also be influenced by patient factors such as the presence of any pre-existing disease. In addition, the toxicity of treatment will be compounded if these agents are used in combination.

Table 11.2: *Toxicity rating scale and abbreviations used in the following tables*

+	occasional or mild
+ +	common or moderately severe
+ + +	invariable or dose limiting
FBC	full blood count
ECG	electrocardiogram
LFT	liver function tests
WBC	white blood cell
SIADH	syndrome of inappropriate anti-diuretic hormone secretion
CNS	central nervous system

CHEMOTHERAPEUTIC AGENTS

Aclarubicin

	Toxicity Grading	Comment	Clinical Monitoring/ Intervention
Gastrointestinal tract			
Nausea/vomiting	+ +	Severe at doses greater than 120 mg/m^2	Prophylactic antiemetics
Other	+ + +	Mucositis Oral ulceration Diarrhoea	Good mouth care
Haematological			
Myelosuppression	+ + +	WBC nadir days 14–21, recovery days 21–28 Thrombocytopenia nadir days 7–14, recovery days 14–28	Pre-treatment FBC
Cutaneous			
Alopecia	+	–	–
Tissue necrosis (on extravasation)	Group 1/2	–	–
Cardiovascular	+ + +	Acute cardiotoxicity Congestive heart failure	ECG monitoring Caution in patients with impaired cardiac function or previously treated with anthracyclines
Pulmonary	–	–	–
CNS	–	–	–
Renal/bladder	–	–	–
Hepatic	+ +	–	Monitor liver function and consider dose reduction in presence of hepatic impairment

Amsacrine

	Toxicity Grading	Comment	Clinical Monitoring/ Intervention
Gastrointestinal tract			
Nausea/vomiting	+ +	–	Prophylactic antiemetics
Other	+ +	Mucositis	Prophylactic mouth care
Haematological			
Myelosuppression	+ + +	Prolonged Nadir days 10–16 Recovery days 21–25	Pre-treatment FBC
Cutaneous			
Alopecia	+ +	–	–
Tissue necrosis (on extravasation)	Group 1	–	–
Other	–	Irritant to intact skin	–
Cardiovascular	+ +	Rare, but potentially serious, ventricular arrhythmias and congestive heart failure	Pre-treatment ECG Caution in patients previously treated with anthracyclines Avoid in hypokalaemia
Pulmonary	–	–	–
CNS	–	–	–
Renal/bladder	–	–	–
Hepatic	–	Cholestasis	Monitor liver function and consider reduction in presence of hepatic impairment

Asparaginase

	Toxicity Grading	Comment	Clinical Monitoring/ Intervention
Gastrointestinal tract			
Nausea/vomiting	+	Usually acute in onset and short lived	–
Haematological			
Myelosuppression	+	Nadir day 14 Recovery day 21	Pre-treatment FBC
Coagulation	+	Depressed clotting factors	Monitor prothrombin time
Cutaneous			
Alopecia	–	–	–
Tissue necrosis (on extravasation)	Group 3	–	–
Cardiovascular	–	–	–
CNS	+ +	Encephalopathy	Monitor renal status
Renal/bladder	+	Mild decrease in renal function	Monitor renal function
Hepatic	+ + +	Liver enzyme abnormalities common Severe hepatotoxicity rare	Consider dose reduction in hepatic impairment
Other		Hypersensitivity	Consider intradermal test dose of 50 IU in 0.1–0.2 ml Observe for 3 hours Facilities for management of anaphylaxis should be available
	+ + +	Pyrexia and rigors	
	+	Hyperglycaemia	Monitor urine glucose
	+	Pancreatitis	Monitor amylase

Bleomycin

	Toxicity Grading	Comment	Clinical Monitoring/ Intervention
Gastrointestinal tract			
Nausea/vomiting	+	Onset 3–6 hours	–
	+	Mucositis	
Haematological			
Myelosuppression	–	Uncommon	–
Cutaneous			
Alopecia	–	–	–
Tissue necrosis (on extravasation)	Group 3	–	–
Other	+ +	Hyperpigmentation of mucous membranes, skin and nails	–
Cardiovascular	–	–	–
Pulmonary	+ + +	Pneumonitis Fibrosis Post-operative respiratory failure	Monitor pulmonary function Regular chest X-rays Avoid cumulative doses greater than 500 IU Treatment with cortico-steroids may be considered
CNS	–	–	Caution in patients underdoing surgery following treatment with bleomycin
Renal/bladder	+ +	–	Monitor renal function Consider dose reduction in renal impairment
Hepatic	–	–	–
Other	+ +	Fever	Prophylactic paracetamol or concomitant hydrocortisone

Carboplatin

	Toxicity Grading	Comment	Clinical Monitoring/ Intervention
Gastrointestinal tract			
Nausea/vomiting	+ +	Onset 2–6 hours Duration 6–12 hours	Prophylactic antiemetics
Haematological			
Myelosuppression	+ + +	Mainly thrombo-cytopenia Nadir days 10–21 Recovery days 28–35	Pre-treatment FBC
Cutaneous			
Alopecia	+	Rare	–
Tissue necrosis (on extravasation)	Group 2	–	–
Cardiovascular	–	–	–
Pulmonary	–	–	–
CNS	+	Peripheral neuropathies Ototoxicity	–
Renal/bladder	+ +	Nephrotoxicity mainly at high doses	Hydration with high doses Monitor renal function Consider dose modification on basis of renal function
Hepatic	–	–	–
Other	+	Electrolyte disturbance	Monitor biochemistry Supplement as required

Carmustine (BCNU)

	Toxicity Grading	Comment	Clinical Monitoring/ Intervention
Gastrointestinal tract			
Nausea/vomiting	+ +	Dose related Onset 2–4 hours Duration 4–6 hours	Prophylactic antiemetics
Haematological			
Myelosuppression	+ +WBC + + +platelets	Delayed Nadir 4–6 weeks	Pre-treatment FBC Treatment interval >6 weeks
Cutaneous			
Alopecia	+	Rare	–
Tissue necrosis (on extravasation)	Group 1	–	–
Cardiovascular	–	–	–
Pulmonary	–	Acute pulmonary infiltrate and/or fibrosis Also delayed onset pulmonary toxicity	–
CNS	+	Rare	–
Renal/bladder	–	–	–
Hepatic	–	Reversible elevation of LFTs	–
Other	+ +	Pain on injection	Administer slowly by infusion

Cisplatin

	Toxicity Grading	Comment	Clinical Monitoring/ Intervention
Gastrointestinal tract			
Nausea/vomiting	+ + +	Onset 1–2 hours Duration 12–48 hours	Prophylactic antiemetics
Other	+ +	Diarrhoea Sudden onset	Anti-diarrhoeal prophylaxis for future cycles
Haematological			
Myelosuppression	+	Nadir days 14–23 Recovery days 21–35	
Cutaneous			
Alopecia	–	–	–
Tissue necrosis (on extravasation)	Group 1	–	–
Cardiovascular	–	–	–
Pulmonary	–	–	–
CNS	+ + +	Peripheral neuropathy Ototoxicity	Regular neurological examinations Audiometry
Renal/bladder	+ + +	Renal toxicity	Adequate pre- and post-treatment hydration, to maintain diuresis Mannitol may be given Monitor renal function prior to each cycle and adjust dose accordingly
Hepatic	–	–	–
Other		Electrolyte imbalance:	Rarely symptomatic
	+ + +	hypomagnesaemia	Monitor and
	+ +	hypocalcaemia	supplement as
	+	hypersensitivity	appropriate

Cyclophosphamide

	Toxicity Grading	Comment	Clinical Monitoring/ Intervention
Gastrointestinal tract			
Nausea/vomiting	+ +	Onset 4–12 hours Duration 4–10 hours	Prophylactic antiemetics
	+ +	Mucositis	
Haematological			
Myelosuppression	+ + +	Nadir days 10–14 Recovery days 21–28	Pre-treatment FBC
Cutaneous			
Alopecia	+ + +	Complete with IV therapy Partial with oral therapy	–
Tissue necrosis (on extravasation)	Group 3	–	–
Cardiovascular	+	Cardiac toxicity reported with high doses	–
Pulmonary	+	Interstitial pneumonitis Pulmonary fibrosis	–
CNS	–	–	–
Renal/bladder	+ + +	Haemorrhagic cystitis Tubular damage	Less problematic than ifosfamide Ensure adequate hydration Consider mesna at doses greater than 1.5 g/m^2 Monitor renal function
Hepatic	–	–	–
Others	+	SIADH	

Cytarabine

	Toxicity Grading	Comment	Clinical Monitoring/ Intervention
Gastrointestinal tract			
Nausea/vomiting	+ +	Dose related Onset 6–12 hours Duration 3–8 hours	Prophylactic antiemetics
Other	+ +	Mucositis Diarrhoea	Prophylactic mouthcare
Haematological			
Myelosuppression	+ + +	Nadir days 14–18 Recovery days 21–28 Thrombocytopenia Rapid recovery	Pre-treatment FBC
Cutaneous			
Alopecia	+	+	–
Tissue necrosis (on extravasation)	Group 3	–	–
Cardiovascular	–	–	–
Pulmonary	+ +	Respiratory distress Pulmonary oedema	–
CNS	+ +	Toxicity at high dose, including dysarthria, ataxia	May be alleviated by pyridoxine
Renal/bladder	–	–	Reduce dose in renal impairment
Hepatic	+	Rare hepatic dysfunction	Monitor liver function and modify dose as necessary
Other	+ +	Ocular toxicity: including conjunctivitis, and photophobia	Prophylactic steroid eye drops with high dose therapy
		'Cytarabine syndrome': fever, myalgia, bone pain, conjunctivitis, chest pain, malaise	Corticosteroids

Dacarbazine

	Toxicity Grading	Comment	Clinical Monitoring/ Intervention
Gastrointestinal tract			
Nausea/vomiting	+ + +	Onset 1–3 hours Duration 1–12 hours	Prophylactic antiemetics
Haematological			
Myelosuppression	+ +	Nadir days 10–14 Recovery days 21–28	Pre-treatment FBC
Cutaneous			
Alopecia	+	Rare	–
Tissue necrosis (on extravasation)	Group 1	–	–
Cardiovascular	–	–	–
Pulmonary	–	–	–
CNS	–	–	–
Renal/bladder	–	–	–
Hepatic	+	Rare hepatotoxicity	–
Other	+	Rare flu-like syndrome, myalgia, fever, malaise starting within 7 days of treatment	

Dactinomycin

	Toxicity Grading	Comment	Clinical Monitoring/ Intervention
Gastrointestinal tract			
Nausea/vomiting	+ +	Onset 2–6 hours	Prophylactic antiemetics
	+ +	Mucositis	Prophylactic mouthcare
Haematological			
Myelosuppression	+ +	Nadir days 10–14 Recovery days 21–28	Pre-treatment FBC
Cutaneous			
Alopecia	+	–	–
Tissue necrosis (on extravasation)	Group 1	–	–
Cardiovascular	–	–	–
Pulmonary	–	–	–
CNS	–	–	–
Renal/bladder	–	–	–
Hepatic	–	–	Monitor liver function Consider dose reduction in hepatic impairment

Daunorubicin

	Toxicity Grading	Comment	Clinical Monitoring/ Intervention
Gastrointestinal tract			
Nausea/vomiting	+ +	Onset 2–6 hours	Prophylactic antiemetics
	+ +	Mucositis	Prophylactic mouthcare
Haematological			
Myelosuppression	+ + +	Nadir days 9–14 Recovery days 21–28	Pre-treatment FBC
Cutaneous			
Alopecia	+ +	–	–
Tissue necrosis (on extravasation)	Group 1	–	–
Cardiovascular	+ + +	Cardiomyopathy	Monitor cardiac function Maximum cumulative dose 600 mg/m^2
Pulmonary	–	–	–
CNS	–	–	–
Renal/bladder	–	–	–
Hepatic	–	–	Monitor hepatic function Consider dose reduction for hepatic impairment

Doxorubicin

	Toxicity Grading	Comment	Clinical Monitoring/ Intervention
Gastrointestinal tract			
Nausea/vomiting	+ +	Onset 4–6 hours Duration 6 hours	Prophylactic antiemetics
Other	+ + +	Mucositis	Prophylactic mouthcare
Haematological			
Myelosuppression	+ + +	Nadir days 10–14 Recovery days 21–28	Pre-treatment FBC
Cutaneous			
Alopecia	+ + +	–	–
Tissue necrosis (on extravasation)	Group 1	–	–
Cardiovascular	+ + +	Dose limiting toxicity Cardiomyopathy arrhythmias	ECG monitoring Caution in patients with impaired cardiac function or previously treated with anthracyclines Maximum cumulative dose 450–550 mg/m^2
Pulmonary	–	–	–
CNS	–	–	–
Renal/bladder	–	–	–
Hepatic	+ +	Increased bilirubin Rare hepatocellular necrosis	Monitor hepatic function and modify dose as required
Other	–	Hyperpigmentation of skin, mucous membranes, nails	–

Epirubicin

	Toxicity Grading	Comment	Clinical Monitoring/ Intervention
Gastrointestinal tract			
Nausea/vomiting	+ +	Onset 4–6 hours Duration 6 hours	Prophylactic antiemetics
Other	+ + +	Mucositis	Prophylactic mouthcare
Haematological			
Myelosuppression	+ + +	Nadir days 10–14 Recovery days 21–28	Pre-treatment FBC
Cutaneous			
Alopecia	+ + +	–	–
Tissue necrosis (on extravasation)	Group 1	–	–
Cardiovascular	+ + +	Dose limiting toxicity Cardiomyopathy arrhythmias	ECG monitoring Caution in patients with impaired cardiac function or previously treated with anthracyclines Maximum cumulative dose 950 mg/m^2
Pulmonary	–	–	–
CNS	–	–	–
Renal/bladder	–	–	–
Hepatic	+ +	Increased bilirubin Rare hepatocellular necrosis	Monitor hepatic function and modify dose as required
Other	–	Hyperpigmentation of skin, mucous membranes, nails	–

Etoposide

	Toxicity Grading	Comment	Clinical Monitoring/ Intervention
Gastrointestinal tract			
Nausea/vomiting	+ +	Onset 3–8 hours Duration 12 hours	Prophylactic antiemetics
Other	+ +	Mucositis	Prophylactic mouthcare
Haematological			
Myelosuppression	+ + +	Nadir days 14–16 Recovery days 21–28	Pre-treatment FBC
Cutaneous			
Alopecia	+ +	–	–
Tissue necrosis (on extravasation)	Group 2	–	–
Cardiovascular	+	Hypotension on rapid infusion	Administer over 1 hour
Pulmonary	–	–	–
CNS	–	–	–
Renal/bladder	–	–	Monitor renal function Consider dose modification in patients with renal impairment
Hepatic	–	–	Monitor liver function Consider dose modification in patients with hepatic impairment

Fluorouracil

	Toxicity Grading	Comment	Clinical Monitoring/ Intervention
Gastrointestinal tract			
Nausea/vomiting	+	Onset 3–6 hours Dose limiting	Prophylactic antiemetics
Other	+ + +	Diarrhoea	Treatment may need to be stopped
		Stomatitis	Possible benefit from sucralfate or prophylactic allopurinol suspension
Haematological			
Myelosuppression	+	Nadir day 14 Recovery days 21–25	Schedule dependent
Cutaneous			
Alopecia	+	–	–
Tissue necrosis (on extravasation)	Group 3	5FU 'burns' can cause problems with venous access	–
Cardiovascular	+ +	Rare vascular toxicity including angina/ cardiac spasm Myocardial infarction	Monitor cardiac function Caution in patients with cardiac disease
Pulmonary	–	–	–
CNS	+	Rare CNS dysfunction, ataxia, confusion, headaches	–
Renal/bladder	–	–	–
Hepatic	–	–	–

Idarubicin

	Toxicity Grading	Comment	Clinical Monitoring/ Intervention
Gastrointestinal tract			
Nausea/vomiting	+ +	–	Prophylactic antiemetics
Other	+ +	Mucositis	Prophylactic mouthcare
Haematological			
Myelosuppression	+ + +	–	Pre-treatment FBC
Cutaneous			
Alopecia	+ + +	–	–
Tissue necrosis (on extravasation)	Group 1	–	–
Cardiovascular	+ + +	Cardiomyopathy	Monitor cardiac function Caution in patients with cardiac disease or previously treated with anthracyclines
Pulmonary	–	–	–
CNS	–	–	–
Renal/bladder	–	–	Monitor renal function Consider dose reduction for renal impairment
Hepatic	–	–	Monitor hepatic function Consider dose reduction for hepatic impairment

Ifosfamide

	Toxicity Grading	Comment	Clinical Monitoring/ Intervention
Gastrointestinal tract			
Nausea/vomiting	+ + +	Onset 1–2 hours Duration 12–24 hours	Prophylactic antiemetics
Haematological			
Myelosuppression	+ + +	Nadir days 5–10 Recovery days 14–21	Pre-treatment FBC
Cutaneous			
Alopecia	+ + +	Usually complete Onset 1–3 weeks	–
Tissue necrosis (on extravasation)	Group 3	–	–
Cardiovascular	–	–	–
Pulmonary	–	–	–
CNS	+ + +	Encephalopathy Neurotoxicity Confusion/lethargy	Assess risk factors: renal function, albumin, presence or absence of pelvic disease
Renal/bladder	+ + +	Haemorrhagic cystitis Urothelial toxicity Tubular damage	Prophylactic mesna required Ensure adequate hydration Monitor renal function Consider dose reduction in presence of renal impairment
Hepatic	–	–	–

Melphalan

	Toxicity Grading	Comment	Clinical Monitoring/ Intervention
Gastrointestinal tract			
Nausea/vomiting	+ +	Onset 6–12 hours	Prophylactic antiemetics
Haematological			
Myelosuppression	+ +	Delayed Nadir days 10–18 Recovery 6–7 weeks	Pre-treatment FBC
Cutaneous			
Alopecia	–	Uncommon	–
Tissue necrosis (on extravasation)	Group 3	–	–
Cardiovascular	–	–	–
Pulmonary	+	Rare pulmonary fibrosis	–
CNS	–	–	–
Renal/bladder	–	–	Monitor renal function Consider dose reduction for renal impairment
Hepatic	–	–	–

Methotrexate

	Toxicity Grading	Comment	Clinical Monitoring/ Intervention
Gastrointestinal tract			
Nausea/vomiting	+ +	Dose related	Prophylactic antiemetics with doses >100 mg/m^2
Other	+ + +	Stomatitis	Ensure folinic acid rescue starts at 24 hours post-chemotherapy with doses >100 mg/m^2
Haematological			
Myelosuppression	+ +	Dose related Nadir day 10 Recovery day 21	Pre-treatment FBC
Cutaneous			
Alopecia	–	–	–
Tissue necrosis (on extravasation)	Group 2	–	–
Cardiovascular	–	–	–
Pulmonary	–	–	–
CNS	–	–	–
Renal/bladder	+ + +	Electrolyte disturbance Tubular damage and destruction	Monitor renal function Maintain diuresis Maintain urinary pH at >7.5 With doses >1 g/m^2 monitor methotrexate plasma concentration and adjust folinic acid dose accordingly
Hepatic	–	–	–
Other	–	Conjunctivitis Sore, itching eyes	Symptomatic treatment with hypromellose 0.3% eyedrops

Mitomycin

	Toxicity Grading	Comment	Clinical Monitoring/ Intervention
Gastrointestinal tract			
Nausea/vomiting	+	Onset 1–4 hours	Prophylactic antiemetics
Haematological			
Myelosuppression	+ +	Nadir 3–4 weeks Recovery 6–8 weeks	Pre-treatment FBC
Cutaneous			
Alopecia	–	–	–
Tissue necrosis (on extravasation)	Group 1	–	–
Cardiovascular	–	–	–
Pulmonary	+	Pulmonary fibrosis	–
CNS	–	–	–
Renal/bladder	–	Renal toxicity	Monitor renal function
Hepatic	–	–	–

Mitozantrone

	Toxicity Grading	Comment	Clinical Monitoring/ Intervention
Gastrointestinal tract			
Nausea/vomiting	+	–	Prophylactic antiemetics
	+	Mucositis	
Haematological			
Myelosuppression	+	Nadir day 14 Recovery day 21	Pre-treatment FBC
Cutaneous			
Alopecia	+ +	–	–
Tissue necrosis (on extravasation)	Group 2	–	–
Cardiovascular	+ +	Cardiomyopathy	Monitor cardiac function if cumulative dose >160 mg/m^2, in presence of cardiac disease or previous anthracycline therapy
Pulmonary	–	–	–
CNS	–	–	–
Renal/bladder	–	–	–
Hepatic	+	+	Particular problem in patients with bilirubins >35–40 Monitor hepatic function

Mustine

	Toxicity Grading	Comment	Clinical Monitoring/ Intervention
Gastrointestinal tract			
Nausea/vomiting	+ + +	Onset 0.5–2 hours	Prophylactic antiemetics
Haematological			
Myelosuppression	+ + +	Nadir days 9–14 Recovery days 16–28	Pre-treatment FBC
Cutaneous			
Alopecia	+ +	–	–
Tissue necrosis (on extravasation)	Group 1	–	–
Cardiovascular	–	–	–
Pulmonary	–	Rarely pulmonary fibrosis	–
CNS	–	–	–
Renal/bladder	–	–	–
Hepatic	–	–	–

Plicamycin

	Toxicity Grading	Comment	Clinical Monitoring/ Intervention
Gastrointestinal tract			
Nausea/vomiting	+ +	Onset 4–6 hours Duration 12–24 hours	Prophylactic antiemetics
Haematological			
Myelosuppression	+ +	Mainly thrombocytopenia Nadir day 14 Recovery day 21	Pre-treatment FBC
Other	+	Coagulopathy	Monitor coagulation
Cutaneous			
Alopecia	–	Uncommon	–
Tissue necrosis (on extravasation)	Group 1	–	–
Cardiovascular	–	–	–
Pulmonary	–	–	–
CNS	–	–	–
Renal/bladder	–	Nephrotoxic	Monitor renal function Consider dose reduction for renal impairment
Hepatic	–	Hepatotoxic	Monitor hepatic function Consider dose reduction for hepatic impairment
Other	–	Hypocalcaemia	Monitor calcium level

Thiotepa

	Toxicity Grading	Comment	Clinical Monitoring/ Intervention
Gastrointestinal tract			
Nausea/vomiting	+	–	Antiemetics as required
Haematological			
Myelosuppression	+ +WBC + + +platelets	Nadir day 14 Recovery 4 weeks	Pre-treatment FBC
Cutaneous			
Alopecia	–	Rare	–
Tissue necrosis (on extravasation)	Group 3	–	–
Cardiovascular	–	–	–
Pulmonary	–	–	–
CNS	–	–	–
Renal/bladder	–	–	–
Hepatic	–	–	–

Vinblastine

	Toxicity Grading	Comment	Clinical Monitoring/ Intervention
Gastrointestinal tract			
Nausea/vomiting	+	Onset 4–8 hours	Antiemetics as required
Other	+ +	Constipation	Consider prophylactic laxatives
	+	Stomatitis	Prophylactic mouthcare
Haematological			
Myelosuppression	+ +	Nadir day 10 Recovery days 14–21	Pre-treatment FBC
Cutaneous			
Alopecia	+	–	–
Tissue necrosis (on extravasation)	Group 1	–	–
Cardiovascular	–	–	–
Pulmonary	–	–	–
CNS	+ +	Neuropathy	–
Renal/bladder	–	–	–
Hepatic	–	–	Monitor hepatic function Consider dose reduction for hepatic impairment
Other	+	SIADH	–

Vincristine

	Toxicity Grading	Comment	Clinical Monitoring/ Intervention
Gastrointestinal tract			
Nausea/vomiting	+	Onset 4–8 hours	Antiemetics as required
Other	+ +	Constipation	Consider prophylactic laxatives ·
	+	Stomatitis	Prophylactic mouthcare
Haematological			
Myelosuppression	+	Nadir day 10 Recovery day 21	Pre-treatment FBC
Cutaneous			
Alopecia	+	–	–
Tissue necrosis (on extravasation)	Group 1	–	–
Cardiovascular	–	–	–
Pulmonary	–	–	–
CNS	+ + +	Neuropathy	–
Renal/bladder	–	–	–
Hepatic	–	–	Monitor hepatic function Consider dose reduction for hepatic/biliary impairment
Other	–	SIADH	–

Vindesine

	Toxicity Grading	Comment	Clinical Monitoring/Intervention
Gastrointestinal tract			
Nausea/vomiting	+	Onset 4–8 hours	Antiemetics as required
Other	+	Constipation	Consider prophylactic laxatives
Haematological			
Myelosuppression	+ +	Nadir days 3–5 Recovery days 7–10	Pre-treatment FBC
Cutaneous			
Alopecia	+ +	–	–
Tissue necrosis (on extravasation)	Group 1	–	–
Cardiovascular	–	–	–
Pulmonary	–	–	–
CNS	+ +	Neuropathy	–
Renal/bladder	–	–	–
Hepatic	–	–	Monitor hepatic function Consider dose reduction for hepatic/biliary impairment
Other	–	–	–

CYTOKINES

Filgrastim

	Toxicity Grading	Comment	Clinical Monitoring/ Intervention
Gastrointestinal tract			
Nausea/vomiting	–	–	–
Haematological			
Myelostimulation	+ +	–	If leukocyte count exceeds $50 \times 10^9/l$ discontinue therapy
Cutaneous			
Alopecia	–	–	–
Tissue necrosis (on extravasation)	Group 3	–	–
Cardiovascular	+	Transient hypotension	–
Pulmonary	–	–	–
CNS	–	–	–
Renal/bladder	+	Mild to moderate dysuria	–
Hepatic	–	–	–
Other	+ +	Musculoskeletal pain	Standard analgesics
	+ +	Elevation of lactate dehydrogenase, alkaline phosphatase, uric acid, δ glutamyl transpeptidase: reversible, dose dependent	Monitor levels

α Interferon

	Toxicity Grading	Comment	Clinical Monitoring/ Intervention
Gastrointestinal tract			
Nausea/vomiting	+	Usually accompanied by diarrhoea	–
Other	+ +	Anorexia	Regular monitoring of patient's weight
Haematological			
Myelosuppression	+ +	Nadir day 14 Recovery day 21	Pre-treatment FBC Monitor with regular FBCs
Cutaneous			
Alopecia	+	Mild to moderate	–
Tissue necrosis (on extravasation)	Group 3	–	–
Cardiovascular	+	Dose related transient hypotension, arrhythmias, palpitations	Monitor cardiac function in at-risk patients
Pulmonary	–	–	–
CNS	+ +	Depression, confusion, dizziness, vertigo At high doses: convulsions, coma, paraesthesia, neuropathy	–
Renal/bladder	–	–	–
Hepatic	–	–	–
Other	–	'Flu'-like symptoms: fever, chills, headaches, malaise	Administer injection in the evening Prophylactic paracetamol
		Pain/reaction at injection site	Rotate site of injection
		Elevated serum glucose levels	

Aldesleukin (IL-2)

	Toxicity Grading	Comment	Clinical Monitoring/ Intervention
Gastrointestinal tract			
Nausea/vomiting	+ +	–	Prophylactic antiemetics
Other	+ +	Diarrhoea Mucositis	Anti-diarrhoeals
Haematological			
Myelosuppression	+	Anaemia Thrombocytopenia	Pre-treatment FBC
Cutaneous			
Alopecia	–	–	–
Tissue necrosis (on extravasation)	Group 3	–	–
Other	+ +	Erythematous rash	Prophylactic Antihistamine
		Skin desquamation	Water based lotion
Cardiovascular	+ + +	Hypotension/arrhythmias Peripheral and pulmonary oedema Weight gain/dyspnoea	Monitor throughout treatment
Pulmonary		Capillary leak syndrome	
CNS	+ +	Confusion Disorientation	–
Renal/bladder	+ + +	Nephrotoxic creatinine	Monitor renal function
Hepatic	+ +	Liver enzymes disturbance	Monitor hepatic function
Other	+ +	'Flu'-like symptoms: fever, chills, malaise, nasal congestion	Prophylactic paracetamol

SOURCES OF INFORMATION

ABPI Data Sheet Compendium 1991–92. (1991). Datapharm Publications, London.

Borison, H.L. and McCarthy, L.E. (1983). Neuropharmacology of chemotherapy induced emesis. *Drugs* **25(Suppl.1)**, 8–17.

Cain, M. and Tenni, P. (1992). *Drug therapy in cancer: a practical guide for health professionals*. Society of Hospital Pharmacists of Australia.

Chabner, B.A. and Myers, C.E. (1989). Clinical pharmacology of cancer chemotherapy. In: DeVita, V.T. *et al.* (eds) *Cancer: principles and practice of oncology*, 3rd edition. Lippincott, New York, 356.

Dollery, C. editor. (1991). *Therapeutic drugs*. Churchill Livingstone, Edinburgh.

Fahey, M. *et al.* (1984). Prescription monitoring and the oncology patient. *Pharm. J.* **233**, 483–485.

Middleton, J. *et al.* (1985). Failure of scalp hypothermia to prevent hair loss when cyclophosphamide is added to doxorubicin and vincristine. *Cancer Treat. Rep.* **69**, 373–375.

Perry, M.C. and Yarbro, J.W. (1984). *Toxicity of chemotherapy*. Grune & Stratton, Orlando.

Priestman, T.J. (1989). *Cancer chemotherapy: an introduction*, 3rd edition. Springer-Verlag.

Reynold, J.E.F., editor (1982). *The extra pharmacopoeia*, 29th edition. Pharmaceutical Press, London.

Souhami, R. and Tobias, J. (1986). *Cancer and its management*. Blackwell Scientific, Oxford.

Stanley, A.P. (1992). Management of symptoms associated with cancer treatment. (I). *Pharm. J.* **249**, 50–53.

Stanley, A.P. (1992). Management of symptoms associated with cancer treatment. (II). *Pharm. J.* **249**, 90–92.

Tierney, A.J. (1987). Preventing chemotherapy induced alopecia in cancer patients: Is scalp cooling worthwhile? *J. Adv. Nurs.* **12**, 303–310.

Triozzi, A. and Laszlo, J. (1987). Optimum management of nausea and vomiting in cancer chemotherapy. *Drugs* **34**, 136–149.

WHO handbook for reporting results of cancer treatment. (1989). WHO, Geneva.

PART TWO: Drug Monographs:
Compendium of Intravenous Drugs
in Cancer Chemotherapy

Storage of Cytotoxic Drugs After Reconstitution or Repackaging: A Statement Regarding Extended Shelf-life

Many parenteral cytotoxics require reconstitution. In a centralized service, cytotoxic injections will normally be drawn up into a syringe or into an infusion container ready for administration. Manufacturers are currently required by licensing authorities to indicate on the Data Sheet and package insert that reconstituted drugs, with or without preservative, should be stored in a refrigerator (unless dictated by the chemical nature of the drug) and must be used within a specified period, usually not more than 24 hours. This is to ensure that, although the drug may be stable, any micro-organisms introduced during the reconstitution procedures (assumed to be on the ward) will have insufficient opportunity to multiply and reach hazardous numbers before the injection is administered.

This recommendation or directive, therefore, will not usually relate to considerations of chemical stability. Consequently, provided that any manipulations undertaken to prepare the drug for administration are carried out under aseptic conditions, ensuring that an adequate level of sterility assurance is maintained, the shelf-life of such reconstituted or repackaged injections can be extended at the discretion of the responsible hospital pharmacist.

It is essential that good aseptic techniques are employed and adequate quality assurance programmes maintained. The shelf-life of such injectables can then be governed by chemical stability considerations together with local practice and procedures. This allows far greater flexibility and opportunities for greater efficiency in operating centralized cytotoxic services.

Guidance in each Monograph regarding storage after reconstitution assumes that subsequent manipulations are undertaken under appropriate aseptic conditions. The Monographs have been prepared from reviews of the literature, guidance from the respective manufacturer and the author's own studies and experience. However, responsibility for the final preparation must rest with the pharmacist responsible for the cytotoxic services.

Drug Monographs: Compendium of Intravenous Drugs in Cancer Chemotherapy

These Monographs describe injectable cytotoxics and biologicals used in cancer chemotherapy. Information has, wherever possible, been referenced to specific sources of information. Data and information from the particular manufacturer may originate from a variety of sources, including UK Data Sheets, package inserts and personal communications, held on file by the author of each Monograph. Since the content of Data Sheets changes frequently, the reader is referred to the current product Data Sheet for the latest information. A glossary of drug names and product titles used in different countries is included for reference purposes.

Each Monograph has a common structure for ease of reference and uniformity. The purpose of each section is described below. The major aim in producing the Monographs is to provide the user with all the available information for each injection concerning stability in the context of a cytotoxic service operated by a pharmacy department.

1 General Details

Under the heading Approved names, the first name(s) refers to INNM titles, followed by alternatives in common use.

As well as nomenclature, this section includes manufacturers and suppliers in the UK. Details for other countries are included in the Glossary (page 305).

2 Chemistry

A summary of the chemical properties of the drug relevant to the injection form (structure, solubility, etc.).

3 Stability Profile

A summary of the chemical stability of each drug is given, including chemical and physical parameters that influence stability after reconstitution and repackaging. Degradation pathways, when known, are included as background information. Important practical aspects, including container compatibility, and reported incompatibilities with other drugs are noted. Although useful for reference purposes, much of the data relates to short-term physical compatibility of admixtures in the laboratory, and is not necessarily applicable to the clinical setting. A summary of the stability of the reconstituted injection completes this section.

4 Clinical Use

A brief summary of dosage regimens commonly used is included for guidance purposes only.

5 Preparation of Injection

Details of how the injection is prepared for bolus injection and infusion, as relevant, are included, together with handling precautions and details concerning treatment of extravasation. With regard to injections prepared for different routes of administration, the pharmacist responsible for these services should ensure that everything possible is done to distinguish **intrathecal** injections, in particular, from those intended for other routes.

6 Destruction of Drug or Contaminated Articles

The recommended methods of inactivating each cytotoxic drug are summarized under the headings Incineration, Chemical, and Contact with skin. The incineration conditions indicate the minimum temperatures recommended, usually by the manufacturer. *See* Chapter 6 for more details concerning safe handling.

NOTE: While the authors of each Monograph have taken every care to provide accurate and complete information, as far as it is possible to do so, the authors or publishers cannot accept any liability for the information therein.

ACLARUBICIN

1 General Details

Approved name: Aclarubicin.

Proprietary name: Aclacin.

Manufacturer or supplier: Lundbeck Ltd.

Presentation and formulation details: Sterile, pyrogen-free, yellow or orange-yellow, freeze-dried powder in vials containing aclarubicin hydrochloride equivalent to 20 mg aclarubicin.[1]

Storage and shelf-life of unopened container: Three years, protected from sunlight. Store at room temperature.[1]

2 Chemistry

Type: Aclarubicin is a cytotoxic antibiotic of the anthracycline group (Class II).

Molecular structure: A trisaccharide (containing L-cinerulose, 2-deoxy-1-fucose, and L-rhodosamine), linked through a glycosidic bond to the C7 of a tetracyclic aglycone, aklavinone.[2]

Molecular weight: 848.34.

Formula: $C_{42}H_{53}NO_{15}HCl$

Solubility: Aclarubicin is very soluble in methanol and chloroform, freely soluble in water, acetone and ethyl acetate, sparingly soluble in benzene and toluene, and almost insoluble in ethyl ether and R-hexane. The solubility of aclarubicin is pH-dependent. In buffered solution at pH 6 solubility is approximately 400 mg/ml, whereas at pH 7.4 it is only 0.05 mg/ml.[3]

3 Stability Profile

Physical and chemical stability

The manufacturer states that the reconstituted solution is stable for 24 hours, below 4°C, when protected from light, or 6 hours at room temperature.[1] A review of the literature suggests that aclarubicin may be stable for longer periods.[4,5] However, very few data have been published. In addition, Krämer and Wenchel[4] quote 'in-house data', the full details of which have not been published. For these reasons further studies are needed to assess the long-term stability of aclarubicin.

The stability of aclarubicin in aqueous solution depends on a number of factors, the most important of which are pH, temperature, and the type of solvent used for reconstitution. Aclarubicin is also light sensitive and may adsorb onto glass and certain plastics, in the same way as other anthracyclines.

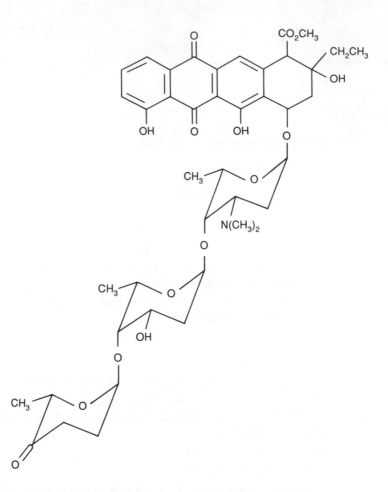

Effect of pH: Aclarubicin is most stable at pH 5–6. At pH values greater than 7 the hydrochloride is insoluble and/or very slightly soluble degradation products are formed.[6] Aclarubicin is not stable at pH values less than 4.[3]

Poochikian *et al.*[5] studied the stability of aclarubicin (128 μg/ml) in glass at ambient temperature (21°C) in 5% glucose (pH 4.5), 0.9% sodium chloride (pH 6.2), lactated Ringer solution (pH 6.3) and Normosol-R (pH 7.4). Results showed that aclarubicin was more stable in 0.9% sodium chloride ($t_{90\%}$ = 108 hours) than in 5% glucose ($t_{90\%}$ = 88 hours), lactated Ringer's ($t_{90\%}$ = 72 hours), or Normosol-R ($t_{90\%}$ = 32 hours). These data indicate that the stability of aclarubicin is highly dependent on the pH of the medium.

In acidic solution, the rate of degradation of the anthracyclines is strongly dependent on structural modifications in the amino sugar moiety and unaffected by structural modifications in the aglycone portion of the molecule.[7] As aclarubicin contains a trisaccharide, its rate of degradation is likely to be different to doxorubicin, daunorubicin and epirubicin which all contain monosaccharides. However, there are no published data available to confirm this hypothesis. Acidic hydrolysis of aclarubicin is expected to result in cleavage of the glycosidic bond to yield a water-insoluble aglycone, aklavinone, and water-soluble amino sugar residues.

In alkaline solution, the rate of degradation of the anthracyclines is affected by structural modifications in the aglycone portion of the molecule and unaffected by structural modifications in the amino sugar moiety.[8] As aclarubicin possesses a unique aglycone, aklavinone, its stability in alkaline media cannot be predicted from existing data for other anthracyclines. In addition, its poor solubility in alkaline solution may preclude stability determination under these conditions.

Effect of light: Data on the photodegradation of doxorubicin, daunorubicin and epirubicin have been published[9,10] but there are no data available for aclarubicin. The rates of photodegradation of doxorubicin, daunorubicin and epirubicin have been reported to be similar and may be substantial at concentrations less than 100 μg/ml if solutions are exposed to light for sufficient time.[10] The manufacturers of aclarubicin warn that exposure of very dilute solutions to light promotes degradation. At higher concentrations, such as those used for cancer chemotherapy (at least 500 μg/ml), no special precautions are necessary to protect freshly prepared solutions of doxorubicin, daunorubicin and epirubicin from light.[10] The manufacturers of aclarubicin suggest that all solutions are protected from light.[1]

Effect of temperature: At ambient temperature (21°C) Poochikian *et al.*[5] observed that aclarubicin was chemically stable (less than 10% degradation) in 5% glucose, 0.9% sodium chloride, lactated Ringer's and Normosol-R for at least 48 hours. At 5°C, aclarubicin (2 mg/ml) has also been stated to be stable in 0.9% sodium chloride, water for injections and 5% glucose, for at least 14 days when protected from light.[6]

Container compatibility: Aclarubicin appears to be compatible with polypropylene, PVC, EVA and glass.[4-6] Doxorubicin, daunorubicin and epirubicin adsorb onto glass but not onto siliconized glass or polypropylene.[11] Therefore, aclarubicin may behave in a similar manner. In clinical practice, when aclarubicin is used at concentrations of approximately 500 μg/ml, adsorptive losses during storage and delivery are expected to be negligible.

Compatibility with other drugs: The manufacturer recommends that no other drugs are mixed with aclarubicin.[1]

Stability in clinical practice

Aclarubicin (2 mg/ml) appears to be chemically stable for at least 24 hours, and possibly 14 days, in 0.9% sodium chloride, water for injections and 5% glucose at 5°C, when protected from light.[6] However, the manufacturer recommends that if 5% glucose is used to dilute aclarubicin its pH should be between 5 and 6.[1]

4 Clinical Use

Main indications: Remission induction in patients with acute non-lymphocytic leukaemia (ANLL) who are resistant or refractory to first line chemotherapy. Aclarubicin may be used in combination regimens with other cytotoxic agents when the dosage may need to be reduced.[1]

Dosage and administration: Dosage is usually calculated on the basis of body surface area. The manufacturer gives the following recommendations:

▼ In adults, including the elderly, the usual initial dosage is 175 to 300 mg/m^2 over three to seven consecutive days, for example, 80 to 100 mg/m^2 daily for three days or 25 mg/m² daily for seven days.[1] Maintenance dosage should be treatments of 25 mg/m² to 100 mg/m² given as a single infusion every three to four weeks.[1]

▼ In children, experience suggests that aclarubicin is well tolerated at the standard dosage level.[1]

The dosage schedules should, however, take into account the haematological status of the patient and the dosages of other cytotoxic drugs when used in combination. Aclarubicin should be used with caution in patients with impaired hepatic, renal or cardiac function. The total cumulative dose administered should be decided according to the cardiological status of the patient. Most patients have received a maximum of not more than 400 mg/m², however, larger dosages in some patients have been used without ill consequence.[1]

5 Preparation of Injection

Reconstitution: The contents of the 20 mg vial should be reconstituted with 10 ml of water for injections or 0.9% sodium chloride. After addition of the diluent and gentle shaking the contents of the vial will dissolve to produce a solution of 2 mg/ml.[1] To prepare an intravenous infusion, the required volume of reconstituted solution should be diluted with 200–500 ml of 0.9% sodium chloride or, if necessary, 5% glucose (with a pH value between 5 and 6). The final concentration should be between 0.2 and 0.5 mg/ml.[1]

Bolus administration: In Phase I–II trials, aclarubicin has been administered by bolus injection.[12–14] However, it is currently recommended that aclarubicin is administered by intravenous infusion over 30–60 minutes.[1]

Intravenous infusion: In Phase I–II trials aclarubicin has been given by short-term infusion using various schedules: 20 mg daily for 7–14 days,[15] 0.33 to 0.70 mg/kg daily for 7–20 days[16] and 60 mg/m² daily for five days.[17] In another study, short-term infusion (10–30 mg/m² daily for 10–30 days) was compared with bolus injection, 15 mg/m² daily, for ten days.[18]

Extravasation: Irritant. (May cause inflammation and induration on extravasation, but is unlikely to cause tissue necrosis [19–22] (*see* Chapter 9).)

6 Destruction of Drug or Contaminated Articles

Incineration: 1000°C.[1]

Chemical: 10% sodium hypochlorite (1% available chlorine)/24 hours.[6]

Contact with skin: Wash well with water, or soap and water. If the eyes are contaminated, immediate irrigation with 0.9% sodium chloride should be carried out.[1]

References

1. *ABPI Data Sheet Compendium 1991–92.* (1991). Datapharm Publications Ltd, London, pp. 843–844.
2. Lundbeck Ltd. Personal communication.
3. *Aclacin – product monograph.* Lundbeck Ltd, Luton, UK.
4. Krämer, I. and Wenchel, H.M. (1991). Viability of micro-organisms in antineoplastic drug solutions. *Eur. J. Hosp. Pharm.* **1**, 14–19.

5. Poochikian, G.K. *et al.* (1981) Stability of anthracycline antitumor agents in four infusion fluids. *Am. J. Hosp. Pharm.* **38**, 483–486.

6. *Pharmaceutical expert report (GDy/UHM).* (1988). Lundbeck Ltd, Copenhagen, Denmark, 19–21.

7. Beijnen, J.H. *et al.* (1985). Aspects of the chemical stability of daunorubicin and seven other anthracyclines in acidic solution. *Pharm. Weekbl. (Sci.)* **7**, 109–116.

8. Beijnen, J.H. *et al.* (1986). Aspects of the degradation kinetics of doxorubicin in aqueous solution. *Int. J. Pharm.* **32**, 123–131.

9. Tavoloni, N. *et al.* (1980). Photolytic degradation of adriamycin. *J. Pharm. Pharmacol.* **32**, 860–862.

10. Wood, M.J. *et al.* (1990). Photodegradation of doxorubicin, daunorubicin and epirubicin measured by high-performance liquid chromatography. *J. Clin. Pharm. Ther.* **15**, 291–300.

11. Bosanquet, A.G. (1986). Stability of solutions of antineoplastic agents during preparation and storage for *in vitro* assays. II. Assay methods, adriamycin and the other antitumour antibiotics. *Cancer Chemother. Pharmacol.* **17**, 1–10.

12. Machover, D. *et al.* (1984). Phase I–II study of aclarubicin for treatment of acute myeloid leukaemia. *Cancer Treat. Rep.* **68**, 881–886.

13. Mitrou, P.S. *et al.* (1985). Aclarubicin (aclacinomycin A) in the treatment of relapsing acute leukaemias. *Eur. J. Cancer Clin. Oncol.* **21**, 919–923.

14. Mitrou, P.S. (1987). Aclarubicin in single agent and combined chemotherapy of acute myeloid leukaemias. *Eur. J. Haematol.* **38 (suppl. 47)**, 59–65.

15. Takahashi, I. *et al.* (1980). Treatment of refractory acute leukaemia with aclacinomycin A. *Acta Med. Okayama* **34**, 349–354.

16. Suzuki, H. *et al.* (1980). Phase I and preliminary Phase II studies on aclacinomycin A in patients with acute leukaemia. *Jpn. J. Clin. Oncol.* **10**, 111–117.

17. Rowe, J.M. *et al.* (1988). Aclacinomycin A and etoposide (VP-16-213): An effective regimen in previously treated patients with refractory acute myelogenous leukaemia. *Blood* **71**, 992–996.

18. Maral, C. *et al.* (1983) Aclacinomycin A: Present status of experimental and clinical studies. *Drugs Exptl. Clin. Res.* **IX**, 375–382.

19. Warrell, R.P. *et al.* (1982). Phase I–II evaluation of a new anthracycline antibiotic, aclacinomycin A, in adults with refractory leukaemia. *Cancer Treat. Rep.* **66**, 1619–1623.

20. Majima, H. (1980). Preliminary clinical study of aclacinomycin A. In *Recent Results in Cancer Research* (Carter, S.K. and Sakurai, Y. eds). **70**, 75–81.

21. Spehn, J. *et al.* (1983). Aclacinomycin A in thyroid cancer. *Proc. 13th Int. Congr. Chemotherapy, Vienna* 211/63–211/66.

22. Bedikian, A.Y. *et al.* (1983). Phase II evaluation of aclacinomycin A (ACM-A, NSC208734) in patients with metastatic colorectal cancer. *Am. J. Clin. Oncol.* **6**, 187–190.

Prepared by M.J. Wood

AMSACRINE

1 General Details

Approved names: Amsacrine, AMSA, m-AMSA.

Proprietary name: Amsidine Concentrate for Infusion.

Manufacturer or supplier: Parke-Davis Research Laboratories Ltd.

Presentation and formulation details: Orange/red solution of amsacrine in 2 ml ampoules containing 1.5 ml injection, 50 mg/ml amsacrine (75 mg/vial). The diluent vial contains 13.5 ml of 0.0353 M/L lactic acid solution. Amsacrine is dissolved in anhydrous N,N-dimethylacetamide (DMA). The diluent vial contains lactic acid in order to form the lactate salt of amsacrine when the drug is added to the diluent, under the acid conditions prevailing. The presence of DMA also prevents the formation of gelatinous material normally seen in aqueous amsacrine lactate solutions.

Storage and shelf-life of unopened container: Three years at ambient temperature not exceeding 25°C, protected from light.

2 Chemistry

Type: Acridine-like DNA intercalating agent.

Molecular structure: 4'-(Acridine-9-ylamino)methanesulphon-*m*-anisidine.

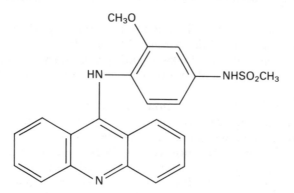

Molecular weight: 393.5.

Solubility: in water = 0.3 mg/ml
          DMA = 100 mg/ml.

3 Stability Profile

Physical and chemical stability

Amsacrine is relatively stable in an aqueous vehicle, provided reconstitution takes place in the presence of lactate ions, and pH remains acid. It is stable for 48 hours after dilution in 5% glucose.[1] As the drug is incompatible with chloride or sulphate ions, saline must be avoided as a diluent. The hydrochloride salt of amsacrine is poorly water soluble.

Degradation pathways: 9(10H)-acridone, 9-chloroacridine and 4-aminomethanesulphon-m-amsidine are formed as degradation products.

Physical stability is not significantly affected by normal temperature ranges. The drug is light-sensitive. After dilution in 5% glucose at a final concentration of 150 μg/ml, amsacrine is stable during exposure to diffuse daylight or fluorescent light over a 48 hour period.[1] Since amsacrine solutions are relatively insoluble in water, DMA is included in the drug diluent to prevent precipitation when the drug is reconstituted.

It has been reported that DMA may increase extraction of components of rubber or certain plastic material.[2] Consequently, it is recommended that only glass syringes should be employed to transfer the drug concentrate to the diluent vial and from vial to infusion. However, this study examined only leaching from PVC infusion containers and administration sets. Most plastic syringes are composed of polypropylene barrels with rubber plungers so this study is not relevent. The company points out that studies using the amsacrine/DMA solution in polypropylene syringes were not conclusive in demonstrating elution of these substances; however, contamination with such chemicals may affect the stability and toxicity profile of amsacrine and glass syringes should be used for the initial steps in the preparation of the infusion. Once diluted in 500 ml 5% glucose, however, DMA is sufficiently dilute not to interact with plastic infusion containers, sets or lines.[3] One other problem that can arise is the effect of DMA on the physical performance characteristics of syringes. Experience indicates that amsacrine concentrate does not affect the physical performance of polypropylene syringes.

Compatibility information: No further information available.

Stability in clinical practice

The reconstituted drug is stable in the diluent provided for 48 hours at room temperature and ambient lighting. It should be protected from exposure to strong daylight. Amsacrine is also stable after dilution in 5% glucose for 8 hours,[4] although there is evidence to indicate that such solutions are stable for 48 hours.[5]

Amsacrine must not be diluted in saline infusions.[4] Amsacrine diluted in 5% glucose at a concentration of 150 μg/ml is not degraded during exposure to diffuse daylight or fluorescent light over a 48-hour period.[3] It was also reported that amsacrine was not absorbed by PVC or polybutadiene-containing administration sets.[3]

4 Clinical Use

Type of cytotoxic: Inhibitor of DNA.

Main indications: Acute leukaemia.

Dosage: Induction of remission – 90 mg/m²/day for five days. In patients with impaired hepatic or renal function, reduce the dose by 20–30% (60–75 mg/m²/day). Maintenance – 150 mg/m² as a single dose or 50 mg/m²/day for 3 days.

5 Preparation of Injection

Dilution: Transfer 1.5 ml of amsacrine solution in DMA (in the ampoule) to the diluent vial, preferably using a glass syringe. The resulting solution contains 5 mg/ml amsacrine.

Bolus administration: Not recommended.

Intravenous infusion: Add required volume of diluted amsacrine to 500 ml 5% glucose infusion. Infuse over 60 to 90 minutes. Problems of phlebitis are more likely with higher concentrations and the data sheet recommends dilution of 75 mg amsacrine in 500 ml 5% glucose solution.[4]

Extravasation: Very damaging; no known antidote. Apply ice-pack to affected area (*see* Chapter 9).

6 Destruction of Drug or Contaminated Articles

Incineration: >260°C.

Chemical: 10% sodium hypochlorite/24 hours (not recommended by the manufacturer).

Contact with skin: wash with soap and water.

References

1. D'Arcy, P.F. (1983). Reactions and interactions in handling anticancer drugs. *Drug Intell. Clin. Pharm.* **17**, 532–538.
2. Vishnuvajjala, R.B. and Cradock, J.C. (1984). Compatibility of plastic infusion devices with diluted N-Methyl-Formamide and N,N-dimethyl-acetamide. *Am. J. Hosp. Pharm.* **41**, 1160–1163.
3. Cartwright-Shamoon, J.M. *et al.* (1988). Examination of sorption and photo-degradation of amsacrine in intravenous burette administration sets. *Int. J. Pharm.* **42**, 41–46.
4. *ABPI Data Sheet Compendium 1991–92.* (1991). Datapharm Publications Ltd, London, pp. 1100–1101.
5. Trissel,L.A. (1992). *Handbook on injectable drugs,* 7th edn. American Society of Hospital Pharmacists, Bethesda, USA.

Prepared by M.C. Allwood

ASPARAGINASE

1 General Details

Approved names: Crisantaspase, Erwinia L-asparaginase.

Proprietary name: Erwinase.

Manufacturer or supplier: Porton Products Ltd.

Presentation and formulation details: White, freeze-dried powder in 2 ml rubber-capped vials containing 10 000 IU asparaginase. Each pack contains 20 vials.

Inactive ingredients: Glucose 5.0 mg, sodium chloride 0.6 mg. 1 IU Crisantaspase releases 1 μmol ammonia/minute from L-asparagine.

Storage and shelf-life of unopened container: Three years at 2 to 8°C.[1]

2 Chemistry

Type: Bacterial enzyme protein from *Erwinia chrysanthemi*.

Molecular weight: 130,000.

Activity: 700 U/mg.

Solubility in water: Highly soluble.[2]

3 Stability Profile

Physical and chemical stability

Stable in solution for at least 20 days at 37°C. Denaturation of the protein and loss of enzyme activity occur outside physiological pH range (6–7.5).[3]

Degradation pathways: No information available.

Physical: Polymerization of the reconstituted enzyme solution occurs after 15 minutes. Gelatinous fibres are produced. Enzyme activity is retained. Polymerization is accelerated by contact with the rubber closure of the vial.[3]

Container compatibility: Stable in glass containers and glass or polypropylene syringes,[4] avoid contact with rubber. No data on stability in plastic syringes, but most syringes contain a rubber plunger.

Compatibility with other drugs: The manufacturer recommends that asparaginase should not be mixed with other drugs.

Stability in clinical practice

Solutions should be administered as soon as possible after reconstitution since gelatinous fibres form after 15 minutes. The effect, however, is not progressive and does not affect the potency of the solution. Sterile solutions transferred to glass syringes retain potency for at least 20 days at 37°C.[4]

4 Clinical Use

Type of cytotoxic: Therapeutic enzyme – not a true cytotoxic agent.

Main indications: Used in combination with other agents in treatment of acute lymphatic leukaemia and some other neoplastic conditions.

Dosage: 200 IU/kg body-weight (5,000–6,000 IU/m² body-surface area) by intramuscular injection three times per week for nine doses.[3] Also refer to current MRC protocols.

5 Preparation of Injection

Reconstitution: The contents of the vial should be reconstituted with 1 to 2 ml of 0.9% sodium chloride injection and dissolved with gentle mixing to avoid contact with the rubber stopper.

Administration: The intramuscular route is preferred as it is associated with less risk of anaphylaxis. The solution may also be given by subcutaneous injection. Intravenous injection or infusion is rarely indicated but may be used if necessary.

Intravenous infusion: Administration by infusion is not usually necessary. Asparaginase is stable for at least seven days in solution in 0.9% sodium chloride and 5% glucose.[2] Enzyme activity may be adversely affected if the pH of the solution is outside the normal physiological range.[3]

Extravasation: Administration is usually by intramuscular or subcutaneous injection. No harmful local effects will result from extravasation of solutions given intravenously.

6 Destruction of Drug or Contaminated Articles

Incineration: 800°C.

Chemical: Strong acids or alkalis will denature the protein.

Contact with skin: Wash with water.

References

1. *ABPI Data Sheet Compendium 1991–92.* (1991). Datapharm Publications Ltd, London, p. 1164–6.
2. Wade, H.E. (1986). *Development of Erwinase (Erwinia Asparaginase).* Lecture to symposium: Erwinia Asparaginase in the treatment of leukaemia. Frankfurt, Germany, 21 November 1986.
3. Porton Products Ltd. (1988). Data on file.
4. Porton Products Ltd. (1991). Data on file.

Prepared by J.M. Oakes

BLEOMYCIN

1 General Details

Approved name: Bleomycin, bleomycin sulphate.

Proprietary name: Bleomycin Lundbeck Injection.

Manufacturer or supplier: Lundbeck Ltd.

Presentation and formulation details: Cream-coloured freeze-dried plug of bleomycin sulphate equivalent to 15 IU bleomycin in a clear glass ampoule. Contains no excipients.

Storage and shelf-life of unopened container: Store at room temperature and protect from light.[1] Shelf-life is 3 years.

2 Chemistry

Type: Anti-tumour antibiotic.

Molecular structure: Glycopeptide. The drug consists of at least 10 components, the main ones being bleomycin A_2 and bleomycin B_2.[2]

Solubility in water: Very soluble.

3 Stability Profile

Physical and chemical stability

Bleomycin is reported to be stable at room temperature in 0.9% sodium chloride, protected from light for 28 days (data on file at company). Equally stable at 2 to 8°C.[2,3] Less stable in 5% glucose.

Degradation pathways: No information available.

Physical: Stable in pH range 4–10.[4] Light may cause bleomycin to break down.[1]

Container compatibility: Early studies suggested that bleomycin binds to PVC containers.[5,6] Recent work indicates that sorption does not occur, but adducts are formed in 5% glucose.[7] The stability of bleomycin in the following systems has been investigated by the manufacturer:

▼ 0.9% saline in an infusion bag (bleomycin 15 IU/100 ml)
▼ 5% glucose in an infusion bag (bleomycin 15 IU/100 ml)
▼ 0.9% saline in polypropylene syringes (bleomycin 60 IU/100 ml).

The stability of bleomycin A_2 and B_2 was evaluated after 28 days storage at room temperature in the dark. Bleomycin was found to be relatively stable in 0.9% sodium chloride with only 4% loss in infusion bags and 6% loss in plastic syringes. In contrast, a 54% loss occurred from the glucose solution in the infusion bag. It can be concluded that bleomycin is relatively stable in PVC containers and plastic syringes provided that the diluent is 0.9% saline.

Compatibility with other drugs: Bleomycin is reported to be compatible at an infusion 'Y' site with tobramycin, gentamicin, potassium chloride, fluorouracil, heparin sodium, vincristine, vinblastine, hydrocortisone sodium phosphate and phenytoin;[4,8] incompatible with ascorbic acid, hydrogen peroxide, any agents containing sulphydryl groups, amino acids, riboflavin, penicillins, methotrexate, mitomycin, dexamethasone, frusemide, aminophylline and diazepam.[4]

Stability in clinical practice

The solution, after reconstitution in 0.9% sodium chloride, is stable for at least seven days, protected from light and stored in the refrigerator. After further dilution in 0.9% sodium chloride, in PVC containers, it is similarly stable. Drug diluted in 5% glucose or glucose/saline appears to be unstable and such diluents should be avoided.

4 Clinical Use

Type of cytotoxic: Anti-tumour antibiotic.

Main indications: Squamous cell carcinoma. Hodgkin's disease and lymphomas, testicular teratoma, and malignant effusions of serous cavities.

Dosage: As single agent 15 to 30 IU twice or three times weekly up to a total of 100–500 IU, dependent on age and condition of patient; lower doses in combination therapy. For malignant effusions, use 60 IU in 100 ml 0.9% sodium chloride.

5 Preparation of Injection

Dilution: Dissolve dose in up to 5 ml water for injection or 0.9% sodium chloride. (1% lignocaine may be used if pain occurs at injection site. IM use only.)

Bolus administration: Inject slowly or via fast-running drip.

Intravenous infusion: Dilute in up to 200 ml 0.9% sodium chloride and administer slowly.

Extravasation: Non-irritant.

6 Destruction of Drug or Contaminated Articles

Incineration: 1000°C.

Chemical: 10% hypochlorite/24 hours.

Contact with skin: Wash with soap and water.

References

1. Douglas, K.T. (1983). Photoactivity of bleomycin. *Biomed. Pharmacother.* **37**, 191–193.
2. McEvoy, G.K. (ed.) (1985). *American Hospital Formulary service drug information.* American Society of Hospital Pharmacists, Bethesda, Maryland, USA.
3. Anon. (1981). *Outline guide for the use of cancer chemotherapeutic agents.* MD Anderson Hospital and Tumor Institute, University of Texas Cancer Center, Houston, Texas.
4. Dorr, R.T. *et al.* (1982). Bleomycin compatibility with selected intravenous medications. *J. Med.* **13**, 121–130.
5. Benvenuto, J.A. *et al.* (1981). Stability and compatibility of antitumor agents in glass and plastic containers. *Am. J. Hosp. Pharm.* **38**, 1914–1918.
6. Adams, J. *et al.* (1982). Instability of bleomycin in plastic containers. *Am. J. Hosp. Pharm.* **39**, 1636.
7. Koberda, M. *et al.* (1990). Stability of bleomycin sulphate reconstitued in 5% dextrose or 0.9% sodium chloride injection stored in glass vials or PVC containers. *Am. J. Hosp. Pharm.* **47**, 2528–2529.
8. Salamone, F.R. and Muller, R.J. (1990). Intravenous admixture compatibility of cancer chemotherapeutic agents. *Hosp. Pharm.* **25**, 567–570.

Prepared by R.J. Needle

CARBOPLATIN

1 General Details

Approved names: Carboplatin, JM8.

Proprietary names: Paraplatin.

Manufacturer or supplier: Bristol-Myers Squibb Pharmaceuticals Ltd.

Presentation and formulation details: Vials containing 50, 150 and 450 mg carboplatin, as a 10 mg/ml solution in water for injection.

Storage and shelf-life of unopened container: 18 months at room temperature.[1]

2 Chemistry

Type: Platinum-containing complex.

Molecular structure: Cis-diammine (1,1-Cyclobutanedicarboxylato) platinum.

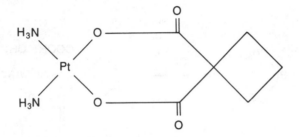

Molecular weight: 371.24.

Solubility in water: 18.6 mg/ml.[2]

3 Stability Profile

Physical and chemical stability

Carboplatin is relatively stable in aqueous solutions. Degradation is accelerated by chloride and hydroxyl ions.[3] The $t_{95\%}$ values for carboplatin in 0.9% sodium chloride and water for injections at 25°C are 52.7 and 29.2 hours respectively.[3]

Degradation pathways: Carboplatin degrades by two simultaneous pathways summarized in Figure 1[3,4] and described as follows:

▼ hydrolytic reactions which give 'activated' platinum species, including cisplatin
▼ nucleophilic substitution with chloride or other nucleophiles resulting in the replacement of the cyclobutanecarboxylate ligands with chloride.

One degradation product is cisplatin.

Degradation obeys pseudo first order kinetics.[3] The overall rate of reaction can be simplified in the following reaction:

$$K_{obs} = K_1 + K_2 (Cl^-)$$

where K_{obs} = observed degradation constant
K_1 = hydrolytic rate constant
K_2 = chloride-dependent nucleophilic substitution rate constant.

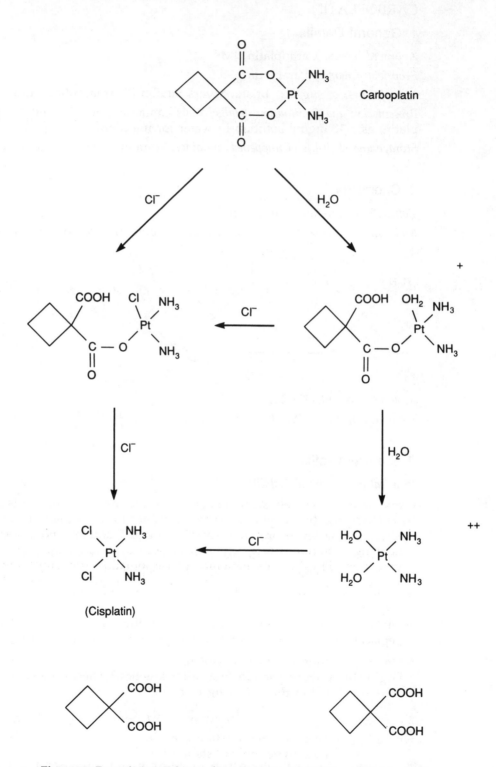

Figure 1: *Degradation pathways for carboplatin in chloride-containing solutions*

Values of K_1 and K_2 at 25°C were 9.74×10^{-4}/h and 3.14×10^{-3}/h, respectively.[3] Apparent first-order kinetics is obeyed.

The range of degradation products (some are intermediates) possibly include:

▼ monosubstitution with Cl^-
▼ disubstitution with Cl^- (cisplatin)
▼ monosubstitution with water
▼ substitution with water and chloride ions.

The aquated 'intermediates' are likely to be the most toxic (but also the species with most anti-tumour activity). They can form various dimers, trimers and other oligomers in their own right.

Effect of pH: Carboplatin is relatively stable within the range pH 4–6.5.[3] Degradation rate constants increase rapidly above pH 6.5.[3] The $t_{95\%}$ values for carboplatin at pH 7.0 stored at 4°C in the absence and presence of chloride ions (equivalent to 0.9% sodium chloride) are 737 and 559 hours respectively.[3]

Effect of temperature: The stability of carboplatin at various temperatures in different vehicles is summarized in Table 1.[3,5]

Table 1: *The effect of temperature on the stability of carboplatin in different infusions*

Temp. (°C)	Conc. (mg/ml)	$t_{95\%}$ (hours) in:		
		0.9% Sodium Chloride	Water for Injections	5% Glucose
4	3.7	24.0	32.0	40
21	3.7	22.0	32.0	44
25	1.0	29.2	52.7	–
37	3.7	9.0	14.0	16

Certain frozen solutions may also be stable.[6]

Effect of light: Carboplatin is not especially light-sensitive.

Container compatibility: Carboplatin is compatible with PVC infusion containers[4] and plastic syringes.[5,7]

Compatibility with other drugs: Mixing of carboplatin with any drug solution containing chloride ions (eg hydrochloride salts) leads to accelerated degradation. Physical compatibility of carboplatin with etoposide has been reported although no details are provided of concentration or conditions.[8]

Stability in clinical practice

If diluted in water for injections or 5% glucose as directed, carboplatin is stable for at least eight hours at room temperature or 24 hours stored in the refrigerator.[1] Cheung *et al.*[4] have reported that carboplatin, 0.1 or 1 mg/ml, in 5% glucose, 0.9% sodium chloride or a range of other infusions, is stable for 24 hours at 25°C. It has also been reported that carboplatin, 1 mg/ml, in 0.9% sodium chloride, is stable for 24 hours at 5°C, with less than 1% degradation.[9] Carboplatin, 10 mg/ml, stored in plastic syringes is stable for at least five days at 4°C with no loss recorded over that period.[7]

The stability of carboplatin in ambulatory pumps has been reported. Sewell *et al.*[7] reported that carboplatin, 10 mg/ml, in plastic syringes showed 3.1%

degradation after storage for 24 hours at 37°C. In a later study, carboplatin, 1 mg/ml, diluted in water for injections, stored in the reservoir of the Parker Micropump, was stable for 14 days at either 4°C or 37°C.[10]

4 Clinical Use

Main indications: First and second line therapy of advanced ovarian carcinoma of epithelial origin and small cell carcinoma of the lung. Carboplatin is also used in treating testicular and bladder tumours in combination with other cytotoxic drugs.

Dosage and administration: Carboplatin is administered intravenously. Recommended dosage in previously untreated adult patients with normal kidney function is 400 mg/m² as a single IV dose administered by short-term (15–30 minutes) infusion.

The following formula may be used to calculate the dose of carboplatin:

$$Dose = AUC \times (GFR + 25)$$

where AUC = desired area under the plasma concentration curve, the value depending on individual chemotherapy protocols; it may vary from 2 to 12.[11] GFR = glomerular filtration rate. Therapy should not be repeated until four weeks after the previous carboplatin course. Reduction of initial dosage by 20–25% is recommended for those patients with risk factors, such as myelosuppressive treatment. Carboplatin should not be used in patients with severe pre-existing renal impairment (creatinine clearance at or below 20 ml/minute).

5 Preparation of Injection

Bolus administration: Solution may be administered by slow intravenous injection (over 15–30 minutes) using an infusion pump.

Intravenous infusion: Dilute the injection (10 mg/ml) to as low as 500 µg/ml (1 : 20) in 5% glucose or 0.9% sodium chloride.[1]

Extravasation: Mildly irritant (*see* Chapter 9).

6 Destruction of Drug or Contaminated Articles

Incineration: 1000°C.

Chemical: Dilute in large volumes of water; allow to stand for 48 hours.

Contact with skin: Wash with water.

References

1. *ABPI Data Sheet Compendium 1991–92.* (1991). Datapharm Publications Ltd, London, pp. 263–265.
2. Harrap, K.R. (1986). Paraplatin preclinical development. In *Abstracts of a symposium on paraplatin*, Imperial College, London, 1986, pp. 3–7. Bristol Myers Oncology.
3. Allsop, M.A. *et al.* (1991). The degradation of carboplatin in aqueous solutions containing chloride or other selected nucleophiles. *Int. J. Pharm.* **69**, 197–210.
4. Cheung, Y. *et al.* (1987). Stability of cisplatin, iproplatin, carboplatin and tetraplatin in commonly used infusion solutions. *Am. J. Hosp. Pharm.* **44**, 124–130.

5. Institute of Cancer Research, London. (1988). Personal communication.
6. Bosanquet, A.G. (1989). Stability of solutions of antineoplastic agents during preparation and storage for *in vitro* assays. *Cancer Chemother. Pharmacol.* **23**, 197–207.
7. Sewell, G.J. *et al.* (1987). The stability of carboplatin in ambulatory continuous infusion regimens. *J. Clin. Pharm. Therap.* **12**, 427–432.
8. Salamone, F.R. and Muller, R.J. (1990). Intravenous admixture compatibility of cancer chemotherapeutic agents. *Hosp. Pharm.* **25**, 567–570.
9. Perrone, R.K. *et al.* (1989). Extent of cisplatin formation in carboplatin admixtures. *Am. J. Hosp. Pharm.* **46**, 258–259.
10. Northcott, M. *et al.* (1991). The stability of carboplatin, diamorphine, 5-fluorouracil and mitozantrone infusions in an ambulatory pump under storage and prolonged in-use conditions. *J. Clin. Pharm. Therap.* **16**, 123–129.
11. Calvert, A.H. *et al.* (1989). Carboplatin dosage: prospective evaluation of a simple formulation based on renal function. *J. Clin. Oncol.* **7**, 1748–1756.

Prepared by T. Root and D. Kan

CARMUSTINE

1 General Details

Approved names: Carmustine, BCNU.

Proprietary names: Bicnu.

Manufacturer or supplier: Bristol-Myers Squibb Pharmaceuticals Ltd.

Presentation and formulation details: White freeze-dried flaky powder in 30 ml capacity vial, containing 100 mg carmustine, with diluent vial containing 3 ml absolute alcohol.

Storage and shelf-life of unopened container: Three years at 2 to 8°C, protect from light.

2 Chemistry

Type: nitrosourea.

Molecular structure: N,N'-bis(2-chloroethyl)-1-nitrosourea.

$$CICH_2CH_2N - \overset{\overset{\displaystyle NO}{|}}{C} - NHCH_2CH_2Cl$$
$$\quad\quad\quad\quad \overset{\overset{\displaystyle O}{\parallel}}{}$$

Molecular weight: 214.04.

Melting point: 27°C (Merck Index quotes 30–32°C).

Solubility: 4 mg/ml in water; 150 mg/ml in 95% ethanol.

3 Stability Profile

Physical and chemical stability

Carmustine is relatively unstable after reconstitution. Its stability depends on a number of factors. The most important chemical factor is pH.

Degradation pathways (in aqueous solution):[1] BCNU degrades to:

2 chloroethylamine hydrochloride + acetaldehyde + nitrogen + carbon dioxide.
$(Cl.CH_2\ CH_2\ NH_3\ HCl\ +\ CH_3CHO\ +\ N_2\ +\ CO_2)$.

Carmustine has a very low melting point (27°C according to the manufacturer,[2] although another source quotes 30–32°C)[3]. The drug, if melted, liquifies to become an oily film in the base of the vial. The physical change may also be associated with decomposition and such vials must be discarded. There is slow decomposition at room temperature. One report suggests 3% degradation in 36 days.[4]

The manufacturer indicates that the reconstituted injection decomposes by zero order kinetics.[2] Thus, at ambient temperature, this report anticipated losses of 6% in three hours, whilst at 4°C losses of 4% in 24 hours are to be expected (the pH of the reconstituted injection is 5.6–6.0).

Studies[5,6] indicate that carmustine is most stable in aqueous buffered solutions between pH 3.5 and 5.0. In more acid conditions, there is a small increase in degradation rate whilst at pH above 4.8, degradation rates increase rapidly. For example at pH 5.0 (buffer) $t_{95\%}$ = 5 hours (24°C) or 60 hours (4°C), but at pH 7.3 (buffer) $t_{95\%}$ = 40 minutes (22°C) or 9 hours (4°C). Degradation may also be accelerated by buffering agents, especially phosphates.[1] The pH will rise during degradation in unbuffered medium, causing an acceleration in degradation rate with time. It has been suggested that because of the importance of pH, diluted solutions will be more stable in 5% glucose than in 0.9% sodium chloride.[6]

Effect of light: Fredriksson et al.[6] have shown that carmustine is relatively light sensitive. Under artificial laboratory conditions using a light cabinet, the reaction rates at various light intensities were reported. Samples were placed in covered Petri dishes, not accurately reflecting degradation rates in practice. The authors reported a value for $t_{90\%}$ of 2.9 hours at an intensity of 1000 lux (a relatively high light intensity). The light-induced degradation rate is reduced in a bulk solution packed in a glass or plastic infusion container. Degradation may also occur during passage of the infusion through the administration set. Unfortunately the data from this report cannot be used to predict the outcome of light-exposure in practice, but they do indicate the need to protect the drug from light-exposure during storage after reconstitution and dilution into infusions. Information summarized from the manufacturer suggests, in contrast, that the drug is stable for 8 hours at 25°C exposed to fluorescent light.[2]

Effect of freezing: One report suggests that the drug is stable in infusions when in the frozen state,[6] but further studies are necessary to confirm this observation since evidence is somewhat conflicting.[7]

Container compatibility: Benvenuto et al.[8] indicated that infusions of carmustine in 5% glucose may be less stable in PVC than in glass containers. Some sorption to plastic containers (PVC Viaflex) was indicated. Losses of the order of 10% after 0.5 to 1 hour and 35% after 4 hours were evident (drug concentration = 1.25 mg/ml in 5% glucose at pH 4.4). However, these tests were carried out in 50 ml bags; in 500 ml bags, the surface area to volume ratio is lower so absorption rates may be reduced.

More recent studies[5] suggest that carmustine interacts with PVC, EVA and polyurethane administration sets, whilst no sorption to polyethylene was apparent. Tests under simulated infusion conditions from glass bottles suggest that if 500 ml of drug (0.20 mg/ml) is infused over one hour, about 4.6% (4.6 mg) of the dose is lost by sorption, but over two hours 6.5% (6.5 mg) will be lost.

However, all of these tests were conducted at a drug concentration of about 0.2 mg/ml. No studies on the effect of drug concentration were reported. It is likely that the losses may be substantially reduced (as a proportion of the total dose) at higher drug concentrations.

The evidence, therefore, indicates that carmustine binds to some plastics, especially PVC, but the full clinical implications regarding dose delivery from an infusion are yet to be fully quantified. In practice, it may be relatively unimportant.

Compatibility with other drugs: No further information available.

Stability in clinical practice

After reconstitution in the vial the injection can be stored for up to two days in the refrigerator. After dilution in 0.9% sodium chloride or 5% glucose in glass or polyethylene containers, the resulting infusion may be stored for up to two days in the refrigerator.[2] If diluted in an infusion in a PVC container, it should not be stored, but used as soon as possible.

Carmustine is unstable after addition to any infusion containing sodium bicarbonate (due to alkaline pH).

4 Clinical Use

Type of cytotoxic: Nitrosourea, alkylating agent.

Main indications: Brain tumours. In combination therapy for multiple myeloma, Hodgkin's disease and other lymphomas.

Dosage: 200 mg/m^2 every six weeks as a single agent, but adjusted if necessary according to haematological response. Lower doses are used in combination with other chemotherapeutic agents.

5 Preparation of Injection

Dilution: To each vial add 3 ml diluent (absolute ethanol), dissolve contents and then dilute with 27 ml water for injections. Resulting solution contains 3.3 mg in 1 ml of 10% ethanol. Dissolution may be faster if vial and diluent are allowed to equilibrate at room temperature.

Bolus administration: Not recommended but if essential, inject very slowly via the bolus site of a fast-running drip infusion.

Intravenous infusion: Dilute in 5% glucose (up to 500 ml), preferably in a glass or polyethylene (eg Polyfusor) container and administer over one to two hours as a slow infusion. Protect the contents from light by covering the infusion with a light-protecting overwrap if infused over two hours, or exposed to sunlight. Do not store in a PVC container but use immediately after preparation. Non-PVC containing sets (eg Sureset, Avon Medical) are recommended.

Extravasation: Vesicant; damaging (*see* Chapter 9).

6 Destruction of Drug or Contaminated Articles

Incineration: 1000°C.[2]

Chemical: 8.4% sodium bicarbonate solution/24 to 48 hours.

Contact with skin: Wash with copious amounts of water. In some cases of local irritancy apply sodium bicarbonate solution.

References

1. Montgomery, J.A. *et al.* (1967). The modes of decomposition of 1,3-bis (2-chloro-ethyl)-1-nitrosourea and related compounds. *J. Med. Chem.* **10**, 668–674.
2. *ABPI Data Sheet Compendium 1991–92.* (1991). Datapharm Publications Ltd, London.
3. Trissel, L.A. (1992). *Handbook on injectable drugs*, 7th edn. American Society of Hospital Pharmacists, Bethesda, Maryland, USA.
4. Kleinman, L.M. *et al.* (1976). Investigational drug information. *Drug Intell. Clin. Pharm.* **10**, 48–49.
5. Lasker, P.A. and Ayres, J.W. (1977). Degradation of carmustine in aqueous media. *J. Pharm. Sci.* **66**, 1073–1076.
6. Fredriksson, K. *et al.* (1986). Stability of carmustine—kinetics and compatibility during administration. *Acta Pharm. Suec.* **23**, 115–124.

7. Bosanquet, A.G. (1985). Stability of solutions of antineoplastic agents during preparation and storage for *in vitro* assays. General considerations and nitrosoureas and alkylating agents. *Cancer Chemother. Pharmacol.* **14**, 83–95.
8. Benvenuto, J.A. *et al.* (1981). Stability and compatibility of antitumour agents in glass and plastic containers. *Am. J. Hosp. Pharm.* **38**, 1914–1918.

Prepared by M.C. Allwood

CISPLATIN

1 General Details

Approved names: Cisplatin, cis DDP.

Proprietary names: Cisplatin.

Manufacturers or suppliers: David Bull Laboratories Ltd (DBL), Farmitalia Carlo Erba Ltd, Lederle Laboratories Ltd. Lederle supplies cisplatin as both solution and powder.

The powder is either freeze-dried or lyophilized (see Table 1). The solution is clear, practically colourless and is supplied in amber glass vials. The pH of both is usually between 3.5 and 5.5.

Presentation and formulation details: Some preparations contain mannitol to aid diuresis and renal clearance of cisplatin. Sodium chloride is added to improve chemical stability (*see* Stability Profile for further information).

Storage and shelf-life of unopened container: Both the powder and the solution preparations should be stored at controlled room temperature (15 to 30°C) and protected from direct bright sunlight. Protection from normal room fluorescent light is also recommended.[9] Unopened vials of the drug are stable for 2 to 3 years (depending on the manufacturer).

2 Chemistry

Type: Platinum-containing complex.

Molecular structure: The platinum atom is surrounded in a plane by two chloride atoms and 2 ammonia molecules, in the cis position, platinum diammino dichloride.

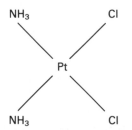

Molecular weight: 300.1.

Solubility: 1 mg/1 ml in water; 1 g in 42 ml of dimethyl formamide.

3 Stability Profile

Physical and chemical stabilty

Cisplatin is unstable in an aqueous vehicle unless chloride ions are present. For example, losses of 30 to 35% in four hours, or 70 to 80% in 24 hours at 25°C have been reported.[1] The minimum concentration of sodium chloride providing an acceptable level of stability is about 0.3% w/v[2].

Solutions of cisplatin in 0.9% sodium chloride are relatively stable for at least 24 hours at ambient temperatures. It should be noted that an equilibrium will be established between cisplatin and chloride ions in solution (see below). In 0.9% sodium chloride, approximately 97% cisplatin will be present at

Table 1: *Forms of cisplatin available*

Manufacturer	Form	Amount of Cisplatin	Strength of Solution	Strength of Solution after Reconstitution	Mannitol per ml of Solution	NaCl per ml of Solution
DBL	Solution	10 mg	1 mg/ml		10 mg	9 mg
	Solution	25 mg	1 mg/ml		10 mg	9 mg
	Solution	50 mg	1 mg/ml		10 mg	9 mg
Farmitalia	Freeze-dried powder	10 mg		1 mg/ml	30 mg	4.5 mg
	Powder	50 mg		1 mg/ml	30 mg	4.5 mg
Lederle	Solution	10 mg	1 mg/ml		10 mg	12 mg
	Solution	25 mg	1 mg/ml		10 mg	12 mg
	Solution	50 mg	1 mg/ml		10 mg	12 mg
	Lyophilized powder	10 mg		1 mg/ml	10 mg	9 mg
	Lyophilized powder	50 mg		1 mg/ml	10 mg	9 mg

equilibrium.[1,3] This level of degradation does not seriously compromise therapeutic efficacy or toxicity profiles. Other studies have indicated that dilutions of cisplatin injection in 0.9% sodium chloride are chemically stable (< 5% degradation) for four days at 4°C, two days at 25°C or 30 days at −15°C.[4] The pH does not appear to be an important factor in cisplatin injection stability after dilution in recommended infusion fluids. Cisplatin is also stable in 0.9% sodium chloride in the presence of magnesium sulphate and potassium chloride for up to 24 hours.[9]

Degradation pathways: Cisplatin undergoes nucleophilic displacement of the chloride ligand by water in aqueous media[3,5] (*see* Figure 1). It is believed that the major route of decomposition involves the displacement of one chloride ion. The loss of the second chloride ion may not contribute substantially to the overall decomposition rate. The reaction is reversible. When enough liberated chloride ions accumulate in the medium, the reaction reaches an equilibrium. The equilibrium drug concentration depends on the concentration of chloride ions present. (Cisplatin can re-form in decomposed drug solutions with the addition of sufficient amounts of chloride.)

The reactions can be described by first order kinetics, dependent principally on chloride ion concentration. Only the first reaction is of practical significance.[1,3]

Effect of light: Cisplatin is relatively sensitive to daylight, but reports confirm that the drug is not adversely affected by normal room lighting after dilution in 0.9% sodium chloride[1,9] (*see* Table 2). The solutions at the concentration of 150 mg cisplatin per 1000 ml 0.9% sodium chloride injection remained clear, colourless and free from particulate matter during the testing period.

Effect of temperature: Temperature appears to have little influence on the stability of cisplatin after dilution. However, because of limited solubility of cisplatin, especially in chloride-containing solutions, the cooling of diluted solutions can lead to precipitation. Studies have also shown that precipitates of cisplatin may be redissolved without further degradation by placing in a water bath heated to 70°C for four hours.[9] Concentrations of 1 mg/ml remain in solution at ambient temperature, while refrigeration can lead to precipitation within one hour.[4,6] Solutions stored in a refrigerator should contain NMT 0.6 mg/ml if stored for 24 hours or NMT 0.5 mg/ml if stored for 24 to 72 hours.[7] Further studies have shown that solutions containing 0.05 to 0.2 mg/ml remain potent for four days at 4°C.[4]

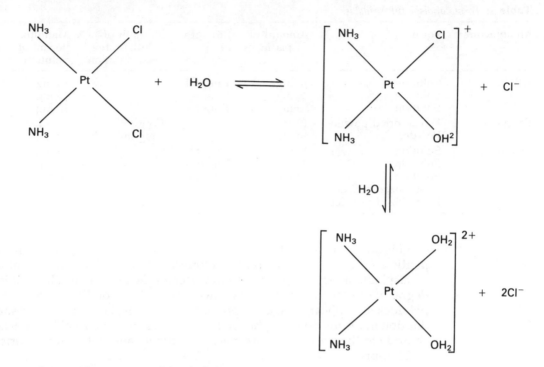

Figure 1: *Degradation pathways proposed for cisplatin*

Table 2: *Stability of cisplatin injection in 0.9% sodium chloride*

Time	Storage Condition 20°C			
	Viaflex Container/bag		Glass Bottle	
	Exposed to Light: % Cisplatin	Protected from Light: % Cisplatin	Exposed to Light: % Cisplatin	Protected from Light: % Cisplatin
0 day	100.0 pH 4.60	100.0 pH 4.90	100.0 pH 4.90	100.0 pH 4.95
4 days	89.2 + 0.2* pH 5.90	100.0 + 0.1 pH 4.87	83.8 + 0.2 pH 6.76	99.5 + 0.1 pH 5.35
7 days	85.9 + 0.2	100.5 + 0.3 pH: not recorded	79.0 + 0.1	100.2 + 0.1
14 days	77.2 + 0.2 pH 6.85	99.8 + 0.1 pH 4.70	70.1 + 0.2 pH 7.23	99.5 + 0.3 pH 4.86

* The figures represent the mean + standard deviation.

Container compatibility: Cisplatin diluted in 0.9% sodium chloride is stable in glass or PVC containers.[2,4] Cisplatin reacts with aluminium and care should be taken to avoid contact of injections with metal items containing aluminium. Stainless steel is compatible.[8]

Compatibility with other drugs: Cisplatin injection is compatible with mannitol and magnesium sulphate injection.[4] However, it has been suggested that mannitol–cisplatin complexes may form if diluted mixtures are stored for several days.[5]

Mannitol should therefore be added immediately before administration if 'diuresis' doses are required. Cisplatin has been reported to be physically compatible with fluorouracil,[10,11] etoposide[10,12] and cytarabine.[10]

Stability in clinical practice

Reconstituted or diluted cisplatin injections are stable, if diluted in 0.9% sodium chloride, for 20 hours at 25°C but will precipitate on refrigeration.[7] In practice, the appropriate dose should be diluted in 2 l 0.9% sodium chloride infusion, giving concentrations in the range 0.1 to 0.2 mg/ml. At such concentrations precipitation will not occur on refrigeration. Such dilute infusions are stable for four days at 4°C in PVC containers.[4]

The stability of cisplatin solutions (1 and 1.6 mg/ml) in plastic infusion bags was studied for up to 14 days at 25, 37 and 60°C. No evidence of any decomposition product was seen. Some precipitation was seen in the 1.6 mg/ml solution at temperatures below 37°C.[13]

Cisplatin 1 mg/ml in 0.9% sodium chloride in the medication cassette (CADD-1 pump, Deltec, Pharmacia) stored at 25°C has been reported to be stable for seven days, although 10% loss was recorded after 14 days.[14]

4 Clinical Use

Type of cytotoxic: platinum-containing complex. The exact mechanism of action has not been determined conclusively but the drug has biochemical properties similar to those of alkylating agents.

Main indications: Cisplatin is used for many indications and in varying doses, commonly 20–100 mg/m².

5 Preparation of Injection

Reconstitution: Cisplatin powder should be dissolved in water for injection to give a 1 mg/ml solution. The manufacturer recommends cisplatin solution to be added to 2 l of 0.9% sodium chloride solution or 4%/0.18% glucose/sodium chloride solution. At The Royal Marsden Hospital, doses of up to 100 mg/m² cisplatin are added to as little as 250 ml of 0.9% sodium chloride solution. Larger doses are added to 500 ml to 1000 ml. The resulting infusion bag should be protected from light and stored at room temperature.

Bolus administration: Must not be used.

Intravenous infusion: The manufacturers recommend that cisplatin solution be infused over six to eight hours, although at The Royal Marsden Hospital a dose of less than 100 mg in 250 ml 0.9% sodium chloride is infused over 30 minutes. Larger doses are often given over one to two hours or longer if renal function is particularly poor. Pre- and post-hydration are essential to induce diuresis during and after the cisplatin infusion. This is to ensure adequate renal clearance of cisplatin and varies according to the dose.

Below are The Royal Marsden Hospital procedures for pre- and post-hydration, for doses of cisplatin between 20–100 mg/m².

▼ Pre-hydrate with 1 l 0.9% sodium chloride + 20 mmol KCl over 12 hours, followed by 200 ml mannitol 20% over 30 minutes.

▼ Post-hydration regimen: 2 l 0.9% sodium chloride + 20 mmol KCl + 1 g magnesium sulphate over 12 hours.

Extravasation: Irritant (*see* Chapter 9).

6 Destruction of Drug or Contaminated Articles

Incineration: 800°C.

Chemical: Dilute in large volume of water, allow to stand for 48 hours.

Contact with skin: Wash with copious amounts of water. Apply a cream if transient stinging is experienced. (NB: Some individuals are sensitive to platinum and a skin reaction may occur.)

References

1. Hincal, A.A. *et al.* (1979). Cisplatin stability in aqueous parenteral vehicles. *J. Parenteral Drug. Assoc.* **33**, 107–116.
2. Cheung, Y.H. *et al.* (1987). Stability of cisplatin, iproplatin, carboplatin and tetraplatin in commonly used intravenous solutions. *Am. J. Hosp. Pharm.* **44**, 124–130.
3. Le Rey, R.H. (1970). Some quantitative data on cis-dichlorodiammineplatinum (II) species in solution. *Cancer Treat. Rep.* **63**, 231–233.
4. La Follette, J.M. *et al.* (1985). Stability of cisplatin admixtures in polyvinyl chloride bags. *Am. J. Hosp. Pharm.* **42**, 2652.
5. Trissel, L.A. (1992). *Handbook on injectable drugs*, 7th edn. American Society of Hospital Pharmacists, Bethesda, Maryland, USA.
6. Green, R.F. *et al.* (1979). Stability of cisplatin in aqueous solution. *Am. J. Hosp. Pharm.* **36**, 38–43.
7. *ABPI Data Sheet Compendium 1991–92.* (1991). Datapharm Publications Ltd, London, pp. 453–454 (Farmitalia Carlo Erba Ltd), pp. 726–727 (Lederle Laboratories).
8. Bohart, R.D. and Ogawa, G. (1979). An observation on the stability of cis-dichlorodiammineplatinum (II): A caution regarding its administration. *Cancer Treat. Rep.* **63**, 2117–2118.
9. DBL Ltd. Personal communications. Unpublished data.
10. Salamone, F.R. and Muller, R.J. (1990). Intravenous admixture compatibility of cancer chemotherapeutic agents. *Hosp. Pharm.* **25**, 567–570.
11. Stewart, C.F. and Fleming, R.A. (1990). Compatibility of cisplatin and fluorouracil on 0.9% sodium chloride injection. *Am. J. Hosp. Pharm.* **47**, 1373–1377.
12. Stewart, C.F. and Hampton, E.M. (1989). Stability of cisplatin and etoposide in intravenous admixtures. *Am. J. Hosp. Pharm.* **46**, 1400–1404.
13. Hrubisko, M. *et al.* (1992). Suitability of cisplatin solutions for 14-day continuous infusion by ambulatory pump. *Cancer Chemother. Pharmacol.* **29**, 252–255.
14. Pharmacia Deltec Inc. (1991). Personal communication. *Am. J. Hosp. Pharm.* **46**, 1400–1404.

Prepared by T. Root and D. Kan

CYCLOPHOSPHAMIDE

1 General Details

Approved names: Cyclophosphamide, cyclophospham.

Proprietary names: Endoxana, Cyclophosphamide.

Manufacturers or suppliers: ASTA Medica Ltd, Farmitalia Carlo Erba Ltd.

Presentation and formulation details: Sterile, white powder in vials containing: 107 mg, 214 mg, 535 mg or 1069 mg of cyclophosphamide BP, equivalent to 100 mg, 200 mg, 500 mg or 1000 mg respectively, of anhydrous cyclophosphamide. Sodium chloride is also present to render the solution isotonic after reconstitution with the recommended amount of water for injections.[1,2]

Storage and shelf-life of unopened container: Five years, below 25°C, protected from light.[1,2]

2 Chemistry

Type: A cytotoxic which is converted in the body to an active alkylating agent with properties similar to those of mustine.[3]

Cyclophosphamide (Farmitalia Carlo Erba Ltd)

Molecular structure: Contains 2-[bis (2 chloroethyl) amino]-perhydro-1,3,2 oxazaphosphorine-2-oxide monohydrate.

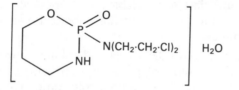

Formula: $C_7H_{15}Cl_2N_2O_2P.H_2O$

Molecular weight: 279.1.

Melting point: 49.5 to 53°C.[3]

Endoxana (ASTA Medica Ltd)

Molecular structure: Contains the anhydrous salt 2-[bis (2 chloroethyl) amino]-tetrahydro-2H-1,3,2 oxazaphosphorine-2-oxide.

Formula: $C_7H_{15}N_2O_2PCl_2$

Molecular weight: 261.08.

Melting point: 41 to 45°C.[4]

Solubility: Cyclophosphamide is soluble 1 in 25 parts of water and 0.9% sodium chloride and 1 in 1 of alcohol.[3,5]

3 Stability Profile

Physical and chemical stability

The manufacturer recommends that the reconstituted solution (20 mg/ml) is used within 8 hours when stored at room temperature (25°C).[1] A review of the literature reveals that cyclophosphamide may be chemically stable for longer periods if stored at 4°C.

The loss of cyclophosphamide monohydrate from aqueous solution results from hydrolysis, loss of a chloride ion, or both.[6–9] Degradation follows first order kinetics and is accompanied by a slight downward shift in pH which does not appear to affect the kinetics of drug loss.[10] During degradation the solution remains colourless.[10] Increase in temperature accelerates the rate of breakdown, as can the presence of benzyl alcohol.[10]

Effect of pH: Hirata *et al.*[6] showed that the rate constant for drug loss at 75°C was independent of pH (pH 2 to 10). Outside these limits acidic and basic catalysis was observed. In solutions between pH 2 and pH 14 cyclophosphamide degrades via a bicyclic compound, and a number of secondary intermediates, to give N-(2-hydroxyethyl)-N'-(3-hydroxypropyl) ethylenediamine.[7,11,12] The mechanism for hydrolysis of cyclophosphamide proposed by Chakrabarti and Friedman[11] is shown in Figure 1.

Under more acidic conditions (pH ≤ 1) cyclophosphamide degrades via a different mechanism to yield bis (2-chloroethyl) amine and 3-aminopropan-1-ol.[6,12]

Effect of light: There are no published data which have systematically compared photodegradation of cyclophosphamide with degradation in identical solutions stored in the dark. Two studies have examined degradation in solutions of cyclophosphamide which were not protected from light. Gallelli[13] observed that cyclophosphamide, 4 mg/ml in 0.9% sodium chloride, stored in glass vials, exhibited 3.5% decomposition over a period of 24 hours at room temperature. Benvenuto *et al.*[14] observed that solutions of cyclophosphamide, 6.6 mg/ml in 5% glucose in both PVC and glass, were stable for 24 hours at room temperature. From these data it is difficult to draw conclusions about the effect of light on the stability of cyclophosphamide.

Effect of temperature: If heated above 32°C cyclophosphamide may decompose to a damp-looking gel which should not be used.[1] The effect of briefly heating cyclophosphamide has been studied. Heating a solution containing 21 mg/ml of cyclophosphamide to 50 or 60°C for 15 minutes resulted in a negligible loss of potency.[15] However, heating to 70 or 80°C for 15 minutes resulted in approximately 10 and 23% decomposition respectively.[15] For this reason, the use of heat to speed up dissolution of cyclophosphamide is not recommended since decomposition may result.[15]

Brooke *et al.*[10] observed a 2% loss in potency in a solution of cyclophosphamide, 20 mg/ml, in glass vials, after four days storage at room temperature (24 to 27°C) and an 8% loss after 17 weeks at 4°C. The rate constants for drug loss recorded in that study were not significantly different for solutions reconstituted with water for injections, 5% glucose or glucose/saline admixtures.

Kirk *et al.*[16] studied the stability of cyclophosphamide in glass ampoules, polypropylene syringes and PVC infusion containers. In PVC infusion bags (Viaflex, Baxter), polypropylene syringes (Becton Dickinson, Plastipak), and glass ampoules, cyclophosphamide showed no appreciable degradation after four weeks at 4°C. After 19 weeks at 4°C, 5.7% and 8% degradation was observed in solutions stored in syringes and minibags respectively.

The effect of freezing cyclophosphamide was also investigated by Kirk *et al.*[16] Results showed that, in syringes, PVC minibags or glass ampoules, no appreciable degradation occurred after four weeks storage at −20°C. After 19 weeks, 4% and 8% degradation was observed in syringes and infusion bags respectively.

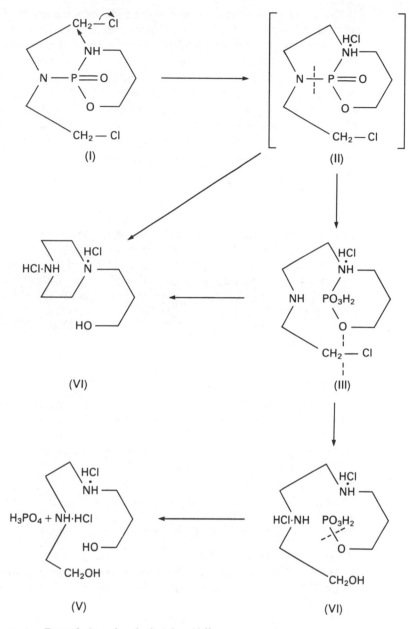

Figure 1: *Degradation of cyclophosphamide*[11]

However, two problems were encountered with freezing cyclophosphamide. First, at higher concentrations (20 mg/ml) precipitation occurred during thawing. Although dissolution occurred after vigorous shaking, the possibility arises of injecting particles into the patient. Secondly, during freezing, the integrity of polypropylene syringes was compromised by a marked contraction of the plungers, allowing seepage of fluid past the plunger and on to the inner surface of the barrel. Although this probably represents a negligible drug loss, the potential risk of microbial contamination is unacceptable. Therefore, freezing of cyclophosphamide in plastic syringes is not recommended.

The effect of thawing cyclophosphamide in a microwave has also been investigated.[16] Results indicated that during microwave thawing uneven distribution of energy may occur and lead to overheating and consequent degradation. For this reason, thawing solutions in a microwave is not recommended.

Container compatibility: Cyclophosphamide is compatible with glass, PVC and polypropylene.[16] It is not adsorbed on to either PVC or polypropylene. Adsorption onto glass has not been documented. In clinical practice, when cyclophosphamide is used at concentrations of approximately 20 mg/ml, adsorptive losses during storage are likely to be negligible.[16]

Compatibility with other drugs: The manufacturers recommend that no other drugs are mixed with cyclophosphamide.

Stability in clinical practice

Cyclophosphamide is compatible with, and may be infused in 5% glucose, 0.9% sodium chloride or mixtures of glucose and saline.[17] It is compatible with glass, PVC and polypropylene containers and appears to be chemically stable for at least 28 days at 4°C. Solutions of cyclophosphamide should not be frozen.[16] Cyclophosphamide (2 to 20 mg/ml) appears to be chemically stable for 15 days in 0.9% sodium chloride at 4°C in the Baxter Infusor. At a concentration of 20 mg/ml in water for injections it is also stable in the CADD pump for 14 days at 4°C and 24 hours at 35°C.[18]

4 Clinical Use

Main indications: As a single agent, and in combination chemotherapy, cyclophosphamide has been used successfully to induce and maintain regressions in a wide range of neoplastic diseases, including leukaemias, lymphomas, soft tissue and osteogenic sarcomas, paediatric malignancies and adult solid tumours, in particular breast and lung carcinoma.[2]

Dosage and administration: The dose, route and frequency of administration should be determined by the tumour type and stage, the general condition of the patient and whether other chemotherapy or radiation is to be administered concurrently. The following sample regimens may serve as guides:

▼ Low dose: 80 to 240 mg/m² (2 to 6 mg/kg) as a single dose intravenously each week or in divided doses orally.
▼ Medium dose: 400 to 600 mg/m² (10 to 15 mg/kg) as a single dose intravenously each week.
▼ High dose: 800 to 1600 mg/m² (20 to 40 mg/kg) as a single dose intravenously at 10 to 20-day intervals.
▼ Higher doses should be used only at the discretion of a physician experienced in cytotoxic chemotherapy.

It is recommended that the dose of cyclophosphamide is reduced when given in combination with other antineoplastic agents or radiotherapy, and in patients with bone marrow depression. Cyclophosphamide should also been used with caution in patients with renal and/or hepatic failure.[1,2]

Cyclophosphamide is metabolized to a compound (acrolein) which is toxic to the bladder. During treatment, a large urine output (a minimum of 100 ml/hr) should be maintained to avoid haemorrhagic cystitis.[1] In addition, intravenous or oral mesna may be given concurrently.[1]

5 Preparation of Injection

Reconstitution: The contents of a vial are reconstituted with water for injections (5 ml per 100 mg of anhydrous cyclophosphamide). After addition of the diluent and vigorous shaking, the contents of the vial will dissolve to produce a solution of 20 mg/ml. Formation of a solution may be delayed because of the slow dissolution rate of cyclophosphamide in aqueous media. The pH of an aqueous solution is between 4.0 and 6.0.[1] Water for injections preserved with benzyl alcohol should not be used for preparation.[10,19]

Bolus administration: Cyclophosphamide is usually given directly into a vein, over two or three minutes, or directly into the tubing of a fast running intravenous infusion. Cyclophosphamide injection may also be given intraperitoneally or intrapleurally, but these routes offer no therapeutic advantage over the intravenous route.[1] Cyclophosphamide has also been given intra-arterially and by local perfusion.

Intravenous infusion: High doses of cyclophosphamide may be added to an infusion of 5% glucose, 0.9% sodium chloride or glucose/saline and infused over one to two hours. Both prolonged, intermittent and continuous infusion of cyclophosphamide have been studied.[20–24] In a phase I study of a 72-hour continuous infusion, patients received 300 mg/m^2/day to 750 mg/m^2/day.[22] Another study employed a five-day continuous infusion at a rate of 400 mg/m^2/day.[20] Protracted infusion of cyclophosphamide has been reported by Lokich *et al.*[24] at doses of 50 to 100 mg/m^2/day for periods of 28 days or more.

Extravasation: Non-irritant (*see* Chapter 9).

6 Destruction of Drug or Contaminated Articles

Incineration: 900°C.[4,25]

Chemical: 0.2 M potassium hydroxide in methanol solution/one hour or 5% sodium hypochlorite solution/24 hours.[4,25]

Contact with skin: Wash well with water, or soap and water. If the eyes are contaminated, immediate irrigation with 0.9% sodium chloride should be carried out.[1,2]

References

1. *ABPI Data Sheet Compendium 1991–92.* (1991). Datapharm Publications Ltd, London, 363–364.
2. *ABPI Data Sheet Compendium 1991–92.* (1991). Datapharm Publications Ltd, London, 454–455.
3. Anon. (1989). *The Extra Pharmacopoeia*, 29th edn. Reynolds, J.E.F. (ed.), Pharmaceutical Press, London, pp. 610–614.
4. ASTA Medica Ltd. Personal communication.
5. Dorr, R.T. and Fritz, W.L. (1980). *Cancer Chemotherapy Handbook*. Elsevier, Amsterdam, p. 342.
6. Hirata, M. *et al.* (1967). Studies on cyclophosphamide: Part 1. Chemical determination and degradation kinetics in aqueous media. *Shionogi Kenkyusho Nempo* **17**, 107–113.
7. Friedman, O.M. (1967). Recent biologic and chemical studies of cyclophosphamide (NSC 26271). *Cancer Chemother. Rep.* **51**, 327–333.
8. Arnold, H. and Klose, H. (1961). Die hydrolyse hexacyclisher N-lostphosphamidester in gepufferten system. *Arzneimittel-Forsch.* **11**, 159–163.

9. Friedman, O.M. (1965). Studies on the hydrolysis of cyclophosphamide: I. Identification of N-(2-hydroxyethyl)-N'-(3-hydroxypropyl) ethylenediamine as the main product. *J. Am. Chem. Soc.* **87**, 4978–4979.

10. Brooke, D. *et al.* (1973). Chemical stability of cyclophosphamide in parenteral solutions. *Am. J. Hosp. Pharm.* **30**, 134–137.

11. Chakrabarti, J.K. and Friedman, O.M. (1973). Studies on the hydrolysis of cyclophosphamide: II. Isolation and characterization of intermediate hydrolytic products. *J. Heterocyclic Chem.* **10**, 55–58.

12. Zon, G. *et al.* (1977). High resolution nuclear magnetic resonance investigations of the chemical stability of cyclophosphamide and related phosphoramidic compounds. *J. Am. Chem. Soc.* **99**, 5785–5795.

13. Gallelli, J.F. (1967). Stability studies of drugs used in intravenous solutions: Part 1. *Am. J. Hosp. Pharm.* **24**, 425–433.

14. Benvenuto, J.A. *et al.* (1981). Stability and compatibility of antitumour agents in glass and plastic containers. *Am. J. Hosp. Pharm.* **38**, 1914–1918.

15. Brooke, D. *et al.* (1975). Effect of briefly heating cyclophosphamide solutions. *Am. J. Hosp. Pharm.* **32**, 44–45.

16. Kirk, B. *et al.* (1984). Chemical stability of cyclophosphamide injection. The effect of low temperature storage and microwave thawing. *Br. J. Parent. Ther.* 90–97.

17. Trissel, L.A. (1992). *Handbook on injectable drugs*, 7th edn., American Society of Hospital Pharmacists, Bethesda, Maryland, USA.

18. Baxter Healthcare Ltd. Personal communication.

19. D'Arcy, P.F. (1983). Handling anticancer drugs. *Drug Intell. Clin. Pharm.* **17**, 532–538.

20. Tchekmedyian, N.S. *et al.* (1986). Phase I clinical and pharmacokinetic study of cyclophosphamide administered by 5-day continuous intravenous infusion. *Cancer Chemother. Rep.* **18**, 33–38.

21. Solidoro, A. *et al.* (1981). Intermittent continuous IV infusion of high dose cyclophosphamide for remission induction in acute lymphocytic leukaemia. *Cancer Treat. Rep.* **65**, 213–218.

22. Bedikian, A.Y. and Bodey, G.P. (1983). Phase I study of cyclophosphamide (NSC 26271) by 72-hour continuous intravenous infusion. *Am. J. Clin. Oncol.* **6**, 365–368.

23. Smith, D.B. *et al.* (1986). A Phase II study of cyclophosphamide as a 24-hour infusion in advanced non-small cell lung cancer. *Eur. J. Cancer Clin. Oncol.* **22**, 435–437.

24. Lokich, J.J. and Botha, A. (1984). Phase I study of continuous infusion cyclophosphamide for protracted duration: A preliminary report. *Cancer Drug Deliv.* **1**, 329–332.

25. Farmitalia Carlo Erba Ltd. Personal communication.

Prepared by M.J. Wood

CYTARABINE

1 General Details

Approved names: Cytarabine, arabinosylcytosine, ara-C, cytosinearabinoside.

Proprietary names: Alexan, Alexan 100, Cytosar, Cytarabine.

Manufacturers or suppliers: Pfizer Ltd, Upjohn Ltd, David Bull Laboratories Ltd (DBL).

Presentation and formulation details:

▼ Alexan: 2 ml and 5 ml ampoules of an isotonic solution of cytarabine 20 mg/ml. Inactive excipients include sodium chloride, sodium lactate and sodium hydroxide.

▼ Alexan 100: 1 ml and 10 ml ampoules of a hypertonic solution of cytarabine 100 mg/ml. Inactive excipients include sodium lactate and sodium hydroxide.

All solutions of Alexan and Alexan 100 are preservative free.[1]

▼ Cytosar: An off-white freeze-dried cake of 100 mg or 500 mg cytarabine in a vial. Cytosar is supplied as a single vial with diluent (water for injections) or as ten vials without diluent.[2]

▼ Cytarabine: Vials containing 100 mg, 500 mg and 1000 mg with preserved diluent supplied.[3]

Storage and shelf-life of unopened container: Alexan solution in unopened ampoules is stable for three years from the date of manufacture when stored below 15°C.[1,4] Vials of Cytosar and Cytarabine (DBL) are stable for three and two years respectively from the date of manufacture when stored at room temperature.[3,5]

2 Chemistry

Type: A pyrimidine nucleoside analogue that kills cells undergoing DNA synthesis. Its actions are specific for the S phase of the cell cycle.[6]

Molecular structure: 4-amino-1-β-D arabinofuranosylpyrimidin-2-(1H)-one.

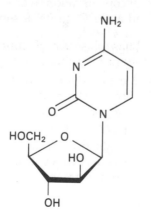

Molecular weight: 243.2.

Formula: $C_9H_{13}N_3O_5$

Solubility: Cytarabine is soluble 1 in 10 parts of water and is very slightly soluble in alcohol.[6]

3 Stability Profile

Physical and chemical stability

The manufacturer states that ampoules of Alexan should be discarded within 24 hours of opening. Alexan and Alexan 100 are stable for at least 24 hours following dilution with 0.9% sodium chloride or 5% glucose infusion.[1] After reconstitution, the manufacturers recommend that Cytosar should be discarded immediately and not stored.[2] A review of the literature reveals that cytarabine may be chemically stable for longer periods.

Effect of pH: In aqueous buffered solution, cytarabine is broken down by hydrolytic deamination to uracil arabinoside.[7]

Cytarabine is most stable in the neutral pH region and has been calculated to retain 90% potency for six and a half months in 0.06 M phosphate buffer, pH 6.9, at 25°C. The rate of degradation of cytarabine in alkaline solution is approximately 10 times as great as in acidic solution.[8]

In aqueous buffered solutions, cytarabine (I) has been shown to undergo hydrolytic deamination to form the inactive nucleoside arabinosyluracil (II). In the acid to neutral region, pH 0 to 7.8, I undergoes deamination to yield II via an intermediate, which is formed in maximum yield at pH 2 to 3, and is not formed in detectable yields at pH 5.5 to 7.8. The observed rate constant for the loss of I in the absence of buffer catalysis was found to pass through a maximum value at approximately pH 2.8. The proposed mechanism for the acid-catalysed degradation of cytarabine in aqueous solution, from Notari *et al.*[8] is shown in Figure 1.

The loss of I in alkaline solution is not accompanied by a corresponding increase in the concentration of II. Instead the degradation of I in alkaline solution is characterized by a complete loss of UV absorption spectra. This suggests that the pyrimidine ring is hydrolysed. Figure 2 illustrates the probable reaction pathways for loss of I in alkaline solution proposed by Notari *et al.*[8] based on the work of Fox *et al.*[9]

Effect of light: At a concentration of 5 mg/ml in Elliots B and lactated Ringer's solution, cytarabine exhibited no change in concentration over seven days, under fluorescent light, at room temperature and at 30°C. In 0.9% sodium chloride no decomposition occurred after 24 hours, but a 3% loss at room temperature, and a 6% loss at 30°C, was observed over seven days.[10] Benvenuto *et al.*[11] studied the stability of cytarabine (2 mg/ml) in glass and PVC bags (Viaflex, Baxter) in 5% glucose stored at room temperature and exposed to normal daylight. Results showed that cytarabine was stable for 24 hours. These data indicate that photodegradation of cytarabine does not appear to be significant.

Effect of temperature: At a concentration of 800 mg/l, one group suggests that cytarabine, in 0.9% sodium chloride and 5% glucose, showed no significant loss of activity over a period of 13 days,[4] whereas at a concentration of 500 mg/l, in the same solvents, another group indicates that cytarabine is stable for up to 48 hours.[5]

Gannon and Sesin[12] studied the stability of cytarabine in glass and polypropylene syringes at 25°C and 5°C. Results showed that cytarabine (20 mg/ml) was more stable at 5°C in glass than plastic. The maximum decrease in potency over the seven-day period of study in any of the containers was 2.9%. However,

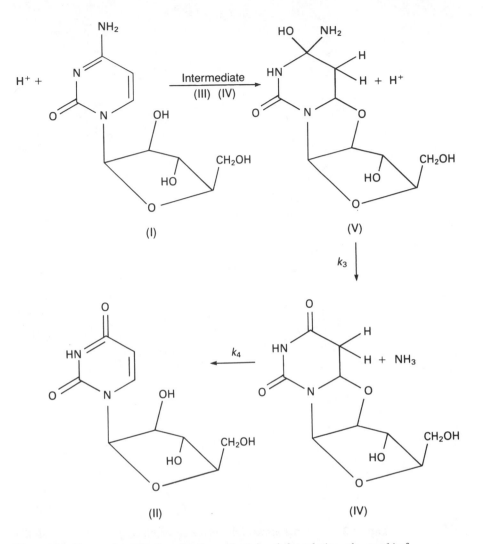

Figure 1: *Proposed mechanism for the acid-catalysed degradation of cytarabine[8]*

in that study, cytarabine concentration was measured using ultraviolet spectrophotometric assay. High-performance liquid chromatographic (HPLC) assay is a more accurate, specific and reliable method of quantitation of drug concentration. Those authors indicated that further study was warranted using HPLC assay to confirm the overall stability of cytarabine.

Munson *et al.*[13] studied the stability of cytarabine in 5% glucose and glucose/saline in glass and PVC containers, with added sodium bicarbonate, at 22 and 8°C. Stability in water for injections in plastic syringes (Pharmaseal) was also studied at 22, 8 and −10°C. Results showed that in plastic syringes, cytarabine, 20 mg/ml and 50 mg/ml, was chemically stable for one week at all temperatures studied. Addition of sodium bicarbonate, 50 mEq/l, to solutions had no effect on the chemical stability of cytarabine for at least one week at either 22 or 8°C.[13] In a recently published study, Weir and Ireland[14] observed that cytarabine (100 mg in 5 ml, 500 mg in 10 ml and 1 g in 20 ml) in polypropylene syringes was chemically stable for at least 30 days at 4 and 21°C.

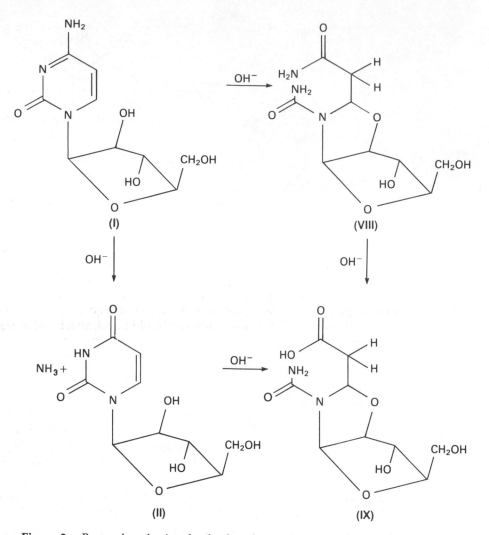

Figure 2: *Proposed mechanism for the degradation of cytarabine in alkaline solution*[8]

In another study, cytarabine, 40 mg/ml and 80 mg/ml, reconstituted with water for injections, was shown to be stable in 5 ml (Becton-Dickinson Plastipak) syringes for at least 15 days when stored at 4 and 25°C and for seven days at 37°C, however storage at −20°C resulted in precipitation.[5] Kirk *et al.*[15] noted that freezing cyclophosphamide in polypropylene syringes resulted in contraction of the plunger and seepage of the drug past the barrel. Although this probably represents a negligible drug loss the potential risk of microbial contamination is unacceptable. For this reason freezing of cytarabine in polypropylene syringes is not recommended.

Rochard *et al.* investigated the stability of cytarabine (25 and 1.25 mg/ml) in 0.9% sodium chloride and 5% glucose solution in an 80 ml EVA reservoir (RES80 A, Celsa Laboratories, Chasseneuil, France). Results indicated that it was stable at both concentrations in both solvents for 28 days at 4 and 22°C and for seven days at 35°C.[16]

Container compatibility: Cytarabine is compatible with glass, PVC and polypropylene.[12,13] Adsorption of cytarabine on to glass has not been documented.

Adsorption on to PVC is negligible at concentrations ≥ 0.5 mg/ml.[5] In clinical practice, when cytarabine is used at concentrations between 0.5 mg/ml and 20 mg/ml, adsorptive losses during storage and delivery are likely to be negligible.

Compatibility with other drugs: Cytarabine appears to be physically compatible with methotrexate, sodium 5-fluorouracil and heparin sodium and many other drugs.[17] The manufacturers recommend, however, that no other drugs are mixed with cytarabine.

Stability in clinical practice

Cytarabine appears to be chemically stable for at least one week, and possibly one month, when reconstituted with water for injections, the enclosed diluent, 5% glucose or 0.9% sodium chloride when stored at 4°C.[5,13] Cytarabine (20 mg/ml) is stable in 0.9% sodium chloride in the CADD Pump for 14 days at 4°C.[18] Cytarabine (25 and 1.25 mg/ml) is also stable in 0.9% sodium chloride and 5% glucose solution in EVA reservoirs (RES80 A, Celsa Laboratories, Chasseneuil, France) for 28 days at 4 and 22°C and for seven days at 35°C.[16] It is important to note that bacterially contaminated intrathecal injections could pose very grave risks and consequently such solutions should be administered as soon as possible after reconstitution.[19]

4 Clinical Use

Main indications: Induction of clinical remission and/or maintenance therapy in patients with acute myeloid leukaemia, acute non-lymphoblastic leukaemias, acute lymphoblastic leukaemias, blast crises of chronic myeloid leukaemia and diffuse histiocytic lymphomas (non-Hodgkin's lymphomas of high malignancy).[6]

Dosage for Alexan: For remission induction the dose is 100 to 200 mg/m²/day or 3 to 6 mg/kg/day. For remission maintenance the following doses are recommended:

▼ Leukaemias: 75 to 100 mg/m²/day or 1.5–3 mg/kg/day for five consecutive days once a month or for one day each week.
▼ CNS leukaemias: 10 to 30 mg/m² three times weekly, intrathecally.

Dosage for Alexan 100: Evidence suggests that the maximum tolerated dose is 3 g/m² every 12 hours for six days. High dose Alexan is reserved for the treatment of resistant or refractory cases of leukaemia.[1]

Dosage for Cytosar: For continuous treatment a dose of 2 mg/kg/day for 10 days, as a starting dose is given by bolus injection. If no antileukaemic effect and no toxicity is observed the dose may be increased to 4 mg/kg/day until a therapeutic response or toxicity occurs. Alternatively, 0.5 to 1.0 mg/kg/day may be given as an infusion of up to 24 hours' duration. After 10 days the dose may be increased to 2 mg/kg/day subject to toxicity. Treatment is continued until remission or toxicity occurs.[2]

For intermittent treatment an intravenous dosage of 3 to 5 mg/kg/day is administered on each of five consecutive days. After a two to nine day rest period a further course is given. Treatment is continued until a response or toxicity occurs.[2] Remissions which have been induced by cytarabine may be maintained by intravenous or subcutaneous injection of 1 mg/kg once or twice weekly.

5 Preparation of Injection

Reconstitution: The contents of the vial (Cytosar) may be reconstituted with water for injections, 0.9% sodium chloride or 5% glucose. When reconstituted with the accompanying diluent (water for injections) gentle shaking of the contents will produce a solution containing 20 mg/ml (100 mg vial) or 50 mg/ml (500 mg vial) of cytarabine.[2]

Bolus administration: Alexan is administered by intravenous, intrathecal, intramuscular and subcutaneous injection. For intrathecal injection it is recommended that 5 to 8 ml of cerebrospinal fluid (CSF) is drawn up, mixed with the injection solution in the syringe and slowly re-injected. Intramuscular and subcutaneous injections are usually used only in maintenance therapy.[1]

Subcutaneous injection of Alexan 100 is not recommended at present due to a lack of clinical data. Intrathecal or intramuscular use of Alexan 100 is contra-indicated due to slight hypertonicity of the formulation.[1] Cytarabine (Cytosar) may be administered by intravenous infusion or injection or by subcutaneous injection.[2]

Intravenous infusion: In high dose schedules Alexan 100 should be administered by continuous intravenous infusion in either 0.9% sodium chloride or 5% glucose solution. To reduce toxicity the duration of the infusion should not be less than one hour.[1] Continuous infusions of cytarabine have ranged from eight to 12 hours to 120 to 168 hours.[1,20] Kreis *et al.*[21] investigated a low dose infusion given over 21 days. Slevin *et al.*[22] compared intravenous and subcutaneous infusions. Results in that study showed that subcutaneous infusion was well tolerated without any local discomfort or excoriation. Continuous infusions (compared to bolus doses) show more pronounced gastrointestinal side-effects.[1]

Extravasation: Mildly irritant (*see* Chapter 9).

6 Destruction of Drugs or Contaminated Articles

Incineration: 1000°C.[1,3,5]

Chemical: Hydrochloric acid pH 2 for 24 hours.[1,3,5]

Contact with skin: Wash with water, or soap and water. If the eyes are contaminated immediate irrigation with sodium chloride 0.9% should be carried out.[1,3,5]

References

1. *ABPI Data Sheet Compendium 1991–92.* (1991). Datapharm Publications Ltd, London, pp. 1128–1130.
2. *ABPI Data Sheet Compendium 1991–92.* (1991). Datapharm Publications Ltd, London, pp. 1626–1627.
3. David Bull Laboratories. Personal communication. Unpublished data.
4. Pfizer Ltd. Personal communication. Unpublished data.
5. Upjohn Ltd. Personal communication. Unpublished data.
6. Anon. (1989). *The extra pharmacopoeia*, 29th edn. Reynolds, J.E.F. (ed.), The Pharmaceutical Press, London, pp. 619–621.
7. Notari, R.E. (1967). A mechanism for the hydrolytic deamination of cytosine arabinoside in aqueous buffer. *J. Pharm. Sci.* **56**, 804–809.
8. Notari, R.E. *et al.* (1972). Arabinosylcytosine stability in aqueous solutions: pH profile and shelf-life predictions. *J. Pharm. Sci.* **61**, 1189–1196.

9. Fox, J.J. *et al.* (1966). Nucleosides XXXVI. Transformation of arabinopyrimidine nucleosides (1). *Tetrahedron Lett.* **40**, 4927–4934.

10. Cradock, J.C. *et al.* (1978) Evaluation of some pharmaceutical aspects of intrathecal methotrexate sodium, cytarabine and hydrocortisone sodium succinate. *Am. J. Hosp. Pharm.* **35**, 402–406.

11. Benvenuto, J.A. *et al.* (1981). Stability and compatibility of antitumor agents in glass and plastic containers. *Am. J. Hosp. Pharm.* **38**, 1914–1918.

12. Gannon, P.M. and Sesin, G.P. (1983). Stability of cytarabine following repackaging in plastic syringes and glass containers. *Am. J. Intravenous Ther. Clin. Nutrition* **10**, 11–16.

13. Munson, J.W. *et al.* (1982). Cytosine arabinoside stability in intravenous admixtures with sodium bicarbonate and in plastic syringes. *Drug Intell. Clin. Pharm.* **16**, 765–767.

14. Weir, P.J. and Ireland, D.S. (1990). Chemical stability of cytarabine and vinblastine injection. *Br. J. Pharm. Pract.* **12**, 53–56.

15. Kirk, B. *et al.* (1984). Chemical stability of cyclophosphamide injection: The effect of low temperature storage and microwave thawing. *Br. J. Parent. Ther.* 90–97.

16. Rochard, E.B. *et al.* (1992). Stability of fluorouracil, cytarabine, or doxorubicin hydrochloride in ethylene vinylacetate portable infusion-pump reservoirs. *Am. J. Hosp. Pharm.* **49**, 619–623.

17. Trissel, L.A. (1992). *Handbook on injectable drugs*, 7th edn. American Society of Hospital Pharmacists, Bethesda, Maryland, USA.

18. Baxter Healthcare Ltd. Personal communication.

19. Sarubbi, F.A. *et al.* (1978). Nosocomial meningitis and bacteraemia due to contaminated Amphotericin B. *J. Am. Med. Assoc.* **35**, 402–406.

20. Spriggs, D.R. *et al.* (1985). Continuous infusion of high dose cytarabine a phase I and pharmacological study. *Cancer Res.* **45**, 3932–3936.

21. Kreis, W. *et al.* (1985). Pharmacokinetics of low dose 1-β-D arabinofuranosylcytosine given by continuous IV infusion over 21 days. *Cancer Res.* **45**, 6498–6501.

22. Slevin, M.L. *et al.* (1983). Subcutaneous infusion of cytosine arabinoside – A practical alternative to intravenous infusion. *Cancer Chemother. Pharmacol.* **10**, 112–114.

Prepared by M.J. Wood

DACARBAZINE

1 General Details

Approved name: Dacarbazine.

Proprietary name: DTIC-Dome.

Manufacturer or supplier: Bayer (UK) Ltd.

Presentation and formulation details: A colourless or ivory-coloured powder in amber glass vials containing 100 mg or 200 mg dacarbazine as the citrate salt. The 100 mg vial contains 100 mg citric acid and 50 mg mannitol. The 200 mg vial contains 100 mg citric acid and 37.5 mg mannitol. The vials do not contain any preservatives.

Storage and shelf-life of unopened container: Three years stored at 2 to 8°C and protected from light.

2 Chemistry

Type: Triazene, alkylating agent.

Molecular structure: 5-(3,3-dimethyl-1-1-triazeno) imidazole-4-carboxamide.

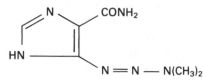

Molecular weight: 182.2.

Solubility: 1 mg/ml in water and 60 mg/ml in 10% citric acid.

3 Stability Profile

Physical and chemical stability

Dacarbazine is relatively stable after reconstitution and further dilution, the reconstituted drug being stable for at least 72 hours if stored at 2 to 8°C.[1] After further dilution in 0.9% sodium chloride or 5% glucose, there is less than 1% degradation after 24 hours storage at 4°C, if protected from light.[1,2]

Dacarbazine is very sensitive to daylight.[3-6] Exposure to sunlight causes rapid degradation.[4] However, exposure to artificial (fluorescent) light or diffuse daylight is far less detrimental. Kirk,[4] in a detailed study, has shown that approximately 4 to 6% losses were recorded during administration under conditions of 'normal' room lighting (diffuse daylight and fluorescent light), whilst solutions exposed to strong daylight showed losses of the order of 12% in 90 minutes. Photodegradation is indicated by a colour change from yellow to pink.

Degradation pathways: The mechanisms described by Kirk[4] have been elucidated by Horton and Stevens.[7] The degradation route of dacarbazine (DTIC) in solutions of different pH either exposed to daylight or maintained in the dark are shown in Figure 1; the principal degradation products are 5-diazoimidazole-4-carboxamide (DIAZO-IC: II), 2-azahypoxanthine (III), a metastable intermediate carbene moiety (IV) and 4-carbamoylimidazolium-5-olate (V).

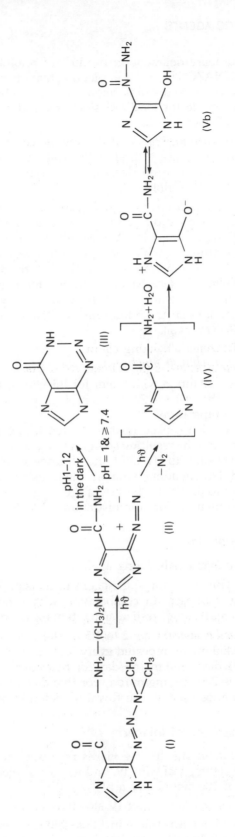

Figure 1: *The degradation route of dacarbazine (DTIC) in solutions of different pH either exposed to daylight or maintained in the dark*

The primary degradation product of photolysis is 5-diazoimidazole-4-carbox-amide (DIAZO-IC). Further degradation then occurs to conjugated polymers, which give rise to the pink colouration. It has been suggested that these polymers are responsible for localized side-effects at the site of injection.[3] This has not been confirmed.

Container compatibility: Dacarbazine is compatible with PVC containers and administration sets[4,5,8] and with Amberset (Avon Medical Ltd).[4] There is no further information on dacarbazine's compatibility with other delivery systems such as plastic syringes.[5]

Compatibility with other drugs: Dacarbazine forms an immediate precipitate with hydrocortisone sodium succinate, but not with hydrocortisone sodium phosphate nor with lignocaine 1 to 2%.[9] Dacarbazine is physically compatible with heparin in 5% dextrose.[9] A white precipitate has been observed when tubing containing dacarbazine (25 mg/ml) was flushed with heparin (100 units/ml).[10] Physical compatibility of dacarbazine with the following drugs has been documented: bleomycin, carmustine, cyclophosphamide, cytarabine, dactinomycin, doxorubicin, methotrexate and 5-fluorouracil.[11] No details of concentrations or conditions are, however, available.[11]

Stability in clinical practice

After reconstitution with water for injections, the resulting 10 mg/ml solution is stable in the vial for 72 hours at 4°C, protected from light, or eight hours at normal temperature.[1,2,5]

This solution can be further diluted in 5% glucose or 0.9% sodium chloride infusions and the resulting solution is stable for 24 hours at 2 to 8°C. Dacarbazine is very sensitive to UV light and all unnecessary exposure to daylight should be avoided. During administration, the infusion container should be protected from exposure to daylight. The use of a UV light-protecting administration set should be recommended for administration in daylight conditions.[4]

4 Clinical Use

Type of cytotoxic: Alkylating agent.

Main indications: As a single agent in metastatic malignant melanoma, sarcoma, Hodgkin's disease. In combination with other drugs for carcinoma of colon, ovary, breast, lung, testicular teratoma and some solid tumours in children.

Dosage and administration: 2 to 4.5 mg/kg/day for 10 days repeated every 28 days. 650 to 1450 mg/m² repeated every four to six weeks. 750 to 1200 mg/m² repeated every 21 days. 250 mg/m²/day for five days repeated every 21 days. Paediatric dosage is 200–250 mg/m²/day for five days, repeated every 28 days. (These are the regimens used at The Royal Marsden Hospital.)

5 Preparation of Injection

Reconstitution: The 100 mg vial is reconstituted with 9.9 ml water for injections and the 200 mg vial with 19.7 ml water for injections, both giving a final concentration of 100 mg/ml and a pH of 3.0 to 4.0.

Bolus administration: Inject IV slowly over one to two minutes.

Intravenous infusion: Dilute in 125 to 250 ml 0.9% sodium chloride or 5% glucose. Infuse over 15 to 30 minutes.

Extravasation: Moderately damaging. No specific antidote.

6 Destruction of Drug or Contaminated Articles

Incineration: 500°C.

Chemical: 10% sulphuric acid for 24 hours.

Contact with skin: Wash with water.

References

1. *ABPI Data Sheet Compendium 1991–92.* (1991). Datapharm Publications Ltd, London, p. 132.
2. Trissell, L.S. (1992). *Handbook on injectable drugs,* 7th edn. American Society of Hospital Pharmacists, Bethesda, Maryland, USA.
3. Baird, S.M. and Willoughby, M.L.N. (1978). Photodegradation of dacarbazine. *The Lancet* **ii**, 681.
4. Kirk, B. (1987). The evaluation of a light-protecting giving set. *Intensive Ther. & Clin. Monitor.* **8**, 78–86.
5. Bayer (UK) Ltd. Personal communication. Unpublished data.
6. Institute of Cancer Research, London. (1988). Personal communication. Unpublished data.
7. Horton, J.K. and Stevens, M.F.G. (1981). A new light on the photodecomposition of the antitumour drug DTIC. *J. Pharm. Pharmacol.* **33**, 808–811.
8. Benvenuto, J.A. *et al.* (1981). Stability and compatibility of antitumor agents in glass and plastic containers. *Am. J. Hosp. Pharm.* **38**, 1914–1918.
9. Dorr, R.T. (1979). Incompatibilities with parenteral anticancer drugs. *Am. J. Intravenous Ther.* **6**, 42–52.
10. Nelson, R.W. *et al.* (1987). Visual incompatibility of dacarbazine and heparin. *Am. J. Hosp. Pharm.* **44**, 2028.
11. Salamone, F.R. and Muller, R.J. (1990). Intravenous admixture compatibility of cancer chemotherapeutic agents. *Hosp. Pharm.* **25**, 567–570.

Prepared by T. Root and D. Kan

DACTINOMYCIN

1 General Details

Approved names: Dactinomycin, actinomycin D.

Proprietary name: Cosmegen Lyovac.

Manufacturer or supplier: Merck, Sharpe & Dohme Ltd.

Presentation and formulation details: Yellow lyophilized powder in vial, containing 500 µg dactinomycin. Each vial contains 20 mg mannitol.

Storage and shelf-life of unopened container: Five years when stored in cool, dry place protected from light.

2 Chemistry

Type: Antibiotic.

Molecular structure: Actinomycin(thr-val-pro-sar-meval).

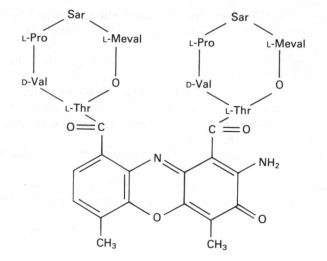

Molecular weight: 1255.5.

Solubility: Soluble in water.

3 Stability Profile

Physical and chemical stability

Degradation in aqueous solution is pH dependent. The pH of reconstituted drug is 5.5 to 7.0 and it is most stable between pH 5 and 7. One report indicates approximately 2 to 3% degradation in six days at 25°C at these pH values (30 µg/ml).[1] At pH 9.0, 80% loss was noted under the same conditions.[1]

Degradation pathways: Alkaline conditions – ring opening of the acridine-like centre.[2]

Physical: Degradation is reduced at lower temperatures. In aqueous solution, degradation at 2 to 6°C is negligible over a six day period.[1]

Container compatibility: Syringes – no information available. Dactinomycin is reported to be compatible with glass and PVC containers for infusions.[3]

No information is available on the compatibility of administration sets, but it should be noted that dactinomycin is compatible with PVC.[2]

There is evidence of dactinomycin binding to certain types of in-line filters.[4] For example, when 500 μg was diluted in 500 ml infusion fluid a total of 67 μg (approximately 13%) was subsequently bound to the in-line cellulose acetate membrane filter. Binding to polycarbonate filters has also been reported.[4] When dactinomycin, 500 μg/ml,[5] was injected through a 0.2 μm nylon filter (Utipor, Pall) 87% of the drug was delivered.[6]

Compatibility with other drugs and excipients: No further information available. Incompatible with benzyl alcohol and other preservatives; avoid preserved diluents for reconstitution.

Stability in clinical practice

The drug is relatively stable after reconstitution in water for injections and may be stored at 2 to 6°C for seven days. The drug is also reasonably stable after further dilution in 0.9% sodium chloride or 5% glucose showing less than 10% degradation after 24 hours at ambient temperature.[3] It should be protected from daylight during storage. The reconstituted drug is also stable when frozen.[7]

4 Clinical Use

Type of cytotoxic: Cytotoxic antibiotic.

Main indications: Wilms' tumour; rhabdomyosarcoma; carcinoma of testis or uterus.

Dosage: Adults, up to 500 μg/day, for up to five days; children, 15 μg/kg, for up to five days.

5 Preparation of Injection

Reconstitution: Add 1.1 ml water for injections and shake to dissolve. The injection may be stored for up to seven days at 2 to 6°C.

Bolus administration: Inject into the tubing of a fast-running infusion of 5% glucose or 0.9% sodium chloride.

Intravenous infusion: Add to up to 500 ml 0.9% sodium chloride or 5% glucose. The infusion may be stored for 24 hours at 2 to 6°C.

Stability in plastic syringes: No information available.

Extravasation: Very damaging (*see* Chapter 9).

6 Destruction of Drug or Contaminated Articles

Incineration: 1000°C.

Chemical: 5% trisodium phosphate, or 20% sodium hydroxide/24 hours.

Contact with skin: Wash in water or sodium phosphate solution.

References

1. Crevar, G.E. and Slotnick, I.J. (1964). A note on the stability of actinomycin D. *J. Pharm. Pharmacol.* **16**, 429.
2. Johnson, A.W. (1960). The chemistry of antinomycin D and related compounds. *Ann. New York Acad. Sci.* **89**, 336–341.

3. Benvenuto, J.A. *et al.* (1981). Stability and compatibility of antitumor agents in glass and plastic containers. *Am. J. Hosp. Pharm.* **38**, 1914–1918.
4. Rusmin, S. *et al.* (1977). Effect of inline filtration on the potency of drugs administered intravenously. *Am. J. Hosp. Pharm.* **34**, 1071–1074.
5. *ABPI Data Sheet Compendium 1991–92.* (1991). Datapharm Publications Ltd, London, pp. 905–907.
6. Ennis, C.E. *et al.* (1983). *In vitro* study of inline filtration of medication commonly administered to paediatric patients. *J. Parenter. Enteral. Nutr.* **7**, 156–158.
7. Bosanquet, A.G. (1986). Stability of solutions of antineoplastic agents during preparation and storage for *in vitro* assays II. Assay methods, adriamycin and other antitumour antibiotics. *Cancer Chemother. Pharmacol.* **17**, 1–10.

Prepared by M.C. Allwood

DAUNORUBICIN

1 General Details

Approved name: Daunorubicin.

Proprietary name: Cerubidin.

Manufacturer and supplier: Rhône-Poulenc Rorer UK Ltd.

Presentation and formulation details: Sterile, pyrogen-free, orange-red, freeze-dried powder in vials of 20 mg of daunorubicin as the hydrochloride, with mannitol as a stabilizing agent.[1]

Storage and shelf-life of unopened container: Three years, stored at room temperature protected from sunlight.[1]

2 Chemistry

Type: A cytotoxic antibiotic consisting of an amino sugar daunosamine linked through a glycosidic bond to the C7 of a tetracyclic aglycone, daunorubicinone. It forms a stable complex with DNA and interferes with the synthesis of nucleic acids. The cytotoxic effects of daunorubicin are most marked on cells in the S phase.[2]

Molecular structure: (1S,3S)-3-acetyl-1,2,3,4,6,11-hexahydro-3,5,12-trihydroxy-10-methoxy-6,11-dioxonaphthacen-1-yl-3-amino-2,3,6-trideoxy-α-L-lyxopyranoside hydrochloride.

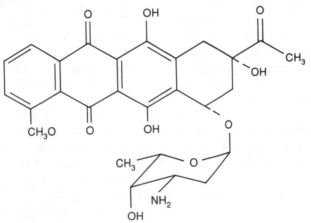

Molecular weight: 564.00.

Formula: $C_{27}H_{29}NO_{10}HCl$.

Solubility: Daunorubicin is soluble in water for injections, 5% glucose, 0.9% sodium chloride, partially soluble in methanol and ethanol and practically insoluble in chloroform, ether and other organic solvents.[2]

3 Stability Profile

Physical and chemical stability

The manufacturer states that the reconstituted solution is stable for up to 24 hours, at 2 to 8°C, when protected from strong daylight. The literature reveals that daunorubicin may be chemically stable for longer periods although few data have been published.[3–5]

The stability of daunorubicin depends on a number of factors. Degradation in aqueous solution is pH-dependent. Daunorubicin is also light sensitive and adsorbs onto glass and certain plastics.

Effect of pH: Daunorubicin becomes progressively more stable as the pH of the drug vehicle becomes more acidic (pH 7.4 to 4.5).[4] Maximum stability is observed at about pH 5.[6]

Decomposition in acidic solution has been studied by Beijnen *et al.*[7] Acidic hydrolysis of daunorubicin (pH below 3.5) (Figure 1) yields a red-coloured, water-insoluble aglycone, daunorubicinone and a water-soluble amino sugar, daunosamine. The rate of cleavage of the glycosidic bond in acidic media is strongly dependent on structural modifications in the amino sugar moiety and unaffected by structural modifications in the aglycone portion of the molecule.[8] As doxorubicin and daunorubicin both possess daunosamine as the amino sugar moiety, the rate of degradation of these two analogues is similar in acidic solution.[7]

At pH values above 3.5 two major degradation products are formed, both of which are aglycones, 7,8-dehydro-9,10-desacetyldaunorubicinone and 7,8-9,10-bisanhydrodaunorubicinone.[6,8] The proposed mechanism for this degradation is shown in Figure 2.

On addition to strongly alkaline solution, a colour change from red to a deep blue-purple is observed and rapid degradation of daunorubicin occurs. Analysis of the decomposition of daunorubicin at pH 8.0 showed the formation of seven possible degradation products; the three major ones were, 7,8-9,10-bisanhydro-daunorubicinone (I), 7 deoxydaunorubicinone (II) and 7,8,-dehydro-9,10-des-acetyldaunorubicinone (III). The structures of these products are shown in Figure 3. Low yields of the remaining four compounds prevented full characterization and structure elucidation.[9]

The rate of degradation of the anthracyclines in alkaline media is affected by structural differences in the aglycone portion of the molecule and unaffected by structural differences in the amino sugar moiety.[8] Daunorubicin has been observed to be more stable than doxorubicin in alkaline solution.[8] As the only difference between doxorubicin and daunorubicin is a C14 proton in dauno-rubicin versus a hydroxyl group in doxorubicin this structural difference must hold the key to the differences in stability of these two drugs.[8]

Effect of light: Data on the kinetics of degradation of doxorubicin in fluorescent light have been published[10] but, until recently, there were no data available for daunorubicin. Results from a study in which the rates of photodegradation of doxorubicin, daunorubicin and epirubicin were compared indicated that the rate of photodegradation of all three analogues was similar.[11] This suggests that the rate of photodegradation of daunorubicin may be significant at concentrations below 100 µg/ml if solutions are exposed to light for sufficient time.[11] However, at higher concentrations, such as those used for cancer chemotherapy (at least 500 µg/ml), no special precautions are necessary to protect freshly prepared solutions of daunorubicin from light.[11]

Effect of temperature: Studies designed to investigate the effect of temperature on the rate of degradation of daunorubicin in buffers at pH 8.0 and pH 1.5 between 40 and 60°C showed that the Arrhenius equation was obeyed.[6] Results from stability studies at room temperature (normally 25°C), in the refrigerator (about 4°C) or in the freezer (about −20°C) are presented below.

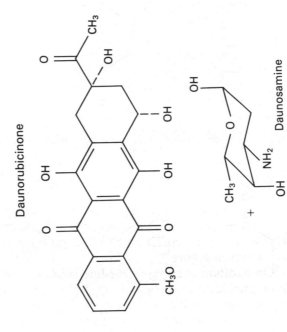

Daunorubicinone

Daunosamine

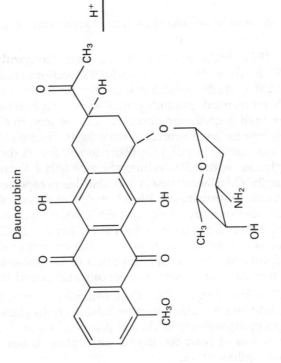

Daunorubicin

Figure 1: *Degradation pathway of daunorubicin in acidic solution*

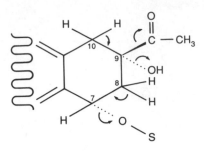

Figure 2: *Degradation scheme of daunorubicin (pH above 4) (S refers to the daunosamine sugar moiety)* [6]

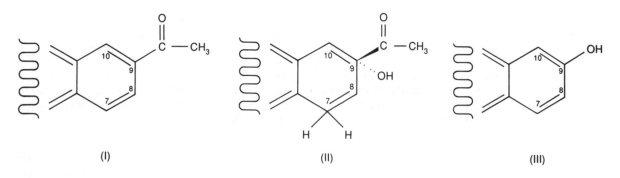

Figure 3: *Structures of the major degradation products of daunorubicin at pH 8.0* [9]

Poochikian *et al.*[4] observed that daunorubicin (20 µg/ml) was stable for 72 hours in 5% glucose and 0.9% sodium chloride in glass containers at 21°C. In that study, solutions were not protected from light and, at the low concentrations used, photodegradation may represent a considerable proportion of the overall degradation observed. Conversely, in a well-controlled study, where the solutions were protected from light, Beijnen *et al.*[5] reported that daunorubicin was stable, in polypropylene tubes, for 28 days in 5% glucose (pH 4.7), 3.3% glucose with 0.3% sodium chloride (pH 4.4) and 0.9% sodium chloride (pH 7.0) at 25°C.[5] Daunorubicin has also been reported to be stable for seven days at room temperature.[3] Wood *et al.*[12] observed that daunorubicin was stable in 5% glucose (pH 4.36) and 0.9% sodium chloride (pH 5.20 and 6.47) in PVC minibags for at least 43 days at 25, 4 and −20°C. Repeated freezing and thawing of solutions stored at −20°C did not cause degradation. In the same study, daunorubicin was also reported to be stable for at least 43 days when reconstituted with water for injections and stored in polypropylene syringes at 4°C.

Container compatibility: Daunorubicin is compatible with polypropylene, PVC and glass.[12,13] Daunorubicin adsorbs onto glass but not onto siliconized glass or polypropylene.[14] In clinical practice, when daunorubicin is used at concentrations of at least 500 µg/ml, adsorptive losses during storage and delivery are negligible.[12,13]

Compatibility with other drugs: Daunorubicin is physically incompatible with dexamethasone, sodium phosphate and heparin sodium.[1] The manufacturer recommends that no other drugs are mixed with daunorubicin.

Stability in clinical practice

Daunorubicin is compatible with polypropylene, PVC and glass.[12,13] Dauno-rubicin appears to be chemically stable for at least 28 days in PVC minibags (100 µg/ml) in 5% glucose and 0.9% sodium chloride stored at 4 and −20°C and for at least 28 days in polypropylene syringes (2 mg/ml) at 4°C.[12]

4 Clinical Use

Main indications: Daunorubicin and cytarabine (with or without thioguanine) are particularly effective in inducing remission in acute myeloblastic leukaemia. A combined treatment regimen of daunorubicin, prednisolone and vincristine has been used in acute lymphoblastic leukaemia. Daunorubicin also has some effect in disseminated neuroblastoma, rhabdomyosarcoma and carcinoma of the rectum and/or colon.[1] Daunorubicin should not be used in patients recently exposed to, or with existing, chicken pox or herpes zoster.[1]

Dosage and administration: The dosage of each individual injection may vary from 0.5 to 3 mg/kg. Doses of 0.5 to 1.0 mg/kg may be repeated at intervals of one or more days; doses of 2 mg/kg should be spaced four or more days apart; high doses of 2.5 or 3 mg/kg should only be given at seven to 14 day intervals. In acute myeloblastic leukaemia, each dose should be about 2 mg/kg, repeated at four to seven day intervals, according to the response. In acute lymphoblastic leukaemia doses of 1 mg/kg may be repeated, according to tolerance and effect, at one- to four-day intervals.

For dosages calculated in terms of body surface area the manufacturer recommends a dose of 50 mg/m^2 (for adults) on alternate days, for a course of up to three injections. The number of injections required varies between patients and must be determined in each case by response and tolerance. A dosage reduction of up to 50% is recommended in the elderly. The dosage for children over one year is the same as for adults, and for children below one year, 75% of the adult dose is recommended.[1]

Dosage should be reduced in patients with impaired hepatic or renal function. A 25% reduction is recommended in patients with serum bilirubin concentrations between 20 and 50 µmol/l and a 50% reduction in patients with serum bilirubin levels above 50 µmol/l or creatinine levels above 265 µmol/l.

When administered with other cytotoxic agents with overlapping toxicity, dosage should be suitably reduced. A cumulative dose of 550 mg/m^2 should not be exceeded, as above this level the risk of irreversible congestive cardiac failure increases greatly.[1] The cumulative dose should be limited to 400 mg/m^2 when there has been previous radiation to the mediastinum.

5 Preparation of Injection

Reconstitution: The contents of the 20 mg vial are reconstituted with 4 ml of water for injections. After addition of the diluent and gentle shaking, the contents of the vial will dissolve to produce a solution of 5 mg/ml.[1]

Bolus administration: Administration is only by the intravenous route. The manufacturer recommends that the calculated dose is further diluted with 0.9% sodium chloride to give a final concentration of 1 mg/ml. This solution should be injected, over a 20 minute period, into the side arm of a freely-running intravenous infusion of 0.9% sodium chloride. This technique minimizes the risk of thrombosis or perivenous extravasation, which can lead to severe cellulitis or vesication.[1]

Intravenous infusion: Although daunorubicin has been used as a continuous infusion in a phase I trial in previously treated patients with leukaemia, no phase II evaluation was conducted because of somewhat limited antileukaemic activity in patients who had previously received other anthracycline therapy.[15] In a study where fractionated daunorubicin was given to 16 patients with acute myeloid leukaemia a good response rate was obtained, coupled with a low incidence of side-effects. In addition, no significant cardiotoxicity was observed despite total doses of up to 1363 mg/m² of daunorubicin.[16]

Extravasation: Potent vesicant (*see* Chapter 9).

6 Destruction of Drug or Contaminated Articles

Incineration: 700°C.[17]

Chemical: 10% sodium hypochlorite (1% available chlorine)/24 hours.[1]

Contact with skin: Wash well with water, soap and water, or sodium bicarbonate solution. If the eyes are contaminated, immediate irrigation with 0.9% sodium chloride should be carried out.[1]

References

1. Daunorubicin: Package insert. (1992). May and Baker Pharmaceuticals, Rhône-Poulenc UK Ltd.
2. Anon. (1989). *The Extra Pharmacopoeia*. 29th edn. Reynolds J.E.F. (ed.), Pharmaceutical Press, London, p. 622.
3. Trissel, L.A. (1992). *Handbook on injectable drugs*, 7th edn. American Society of Hospital Pharmacists, Bethesda, Maryland, USA.
4. Poochikian, G.K. *et al.* (1981). Stability of anthracycline antitumor agents in four infusion fluids. *Am. J. Hosp. Pharm.* **38**, 483–486.
5. Beijnen, J.H. *et al.* (1985). Stability of anthracycline antitumor agents in infusion fluids. *J. Parent. Sci. Technol.* **39**, 220–222.
6. Beijnen, J.H. *et al.* (1986). Aspects of the degradation kinetics of daunorubicin in aqueous solution. *Int. J. Pharm.* **31**, 75–82.
7. Beijnen, J.H. *et al.* (1985). Aspects of the chemical stability of daunorubicin and seven other anthracyclines in acidic solution. *Pharm. Weekbl. (Sci.)* **7**, 109–116.
8. Beijnen, J.H. *et al.* (1986). Aspects of the degradation kinetics of doxorubicin in aqueous solution. *Int. J. Pharm.* **32**, 123–131.
9. Beijnen, J.H. *et al.* (1987). Structure elucidation and characterization of daunorubicin degradation products. *Int. J. Pharm.* **34**, 247–257.
10. Tavoloni, N. *et al.* (1980). Photolytic degradation of adriamycin. *J. Pharm. Pharmacol.* **32**, 860–862.
11. Wood, M.J. *et al.* (1990). Photodegradation of doxorubicin, daunorubicin and epirubicin measured by high-performance liquid chromatography. *J. Clin. Pharm. Ther.* **15**, 291–300.
12. Wood, M.J. *et al.* (1990). Stability of doxorubicin, daunorubicin and epirubicin in plastic syringes and minibags. *J. Clin. Pharm. Ther.* **15**, 279–289.
13. Wood, M.J. (1989). M. Phil. Thesis. University of Aston, Birmingham, UK.
14. Bosanquet, A.G. (1986). Stability of solutions of antineoplastic agents during preparation and storage for *in vitro* assays: II. Assay methods, adriamycin and the other antitumour antibiotics. *Cancer Chemother. Pharmacol.* **17**, 1–10.

15. Legha, S.S. *et al.* (1987). Anthracyclines. In Lokich, J.J. (ed.): *Cancer chemotherapy by infusion*. MTP Press Ltd, Lancaster.
16. Donohue, S.M. and Boughton, B.J. (1989). Fractionated anthracycline therapy in acute myeloblastic leukaemia in adults. *Cancer Chemother. Pharmacol.* **23**, 401–402.
17. May and Baker Pharmaceuticals; Rhône Poulenc Ltd. Personal communication.

Prepared by M.J. Wood

DOXORUBICIN

1 General Details

Approved name: Doxorubicin.

Proprietary names: Doxorubicin Rapid Dissolution, Doxorubicin Solution for Injection.

Manufacturer and supplier: Farmitalia Carlo Erba Ltd.

Presentation and formulation details:

▼ Doxorubicin Rapid Dissolution: Sterile, pyrogen-free, orange-red, freeze-dried powder in vials containing 10 mg and 50 mg of doxorubicin hydrochloride with lactose and hydroxybenzoate. The inclusion of hydroxybenzoate 0.02% (which is a sub-preservative concentration) is to prevent gel formation, which used to occur occasionally on reconstitution of Adriamycin. Adriamycin has been replaced by Doxorubicin Rapid Dissolution.[1]

▼ Doxorubicin Solution for Injection: Sterile, red, mobile solution in vials of 10 mg and 50 mg, each containing doxorubicin hydrochloride as a 2 mg/ml solution in 0.9% sodium chloride injection.[2] The solution is adjusted to pH 3 with 0.5 M hydrochloric acid.[2]

Storage and shelf-life of unopened container:

▼ Doxorubicin Rapid Dissolution: Three years, at room temperature protected from light.[3]

▼ Doxorubicin Solution for Injection: Stored in the refrigerator (2 to 8°C). Eighteen months at 2 to 8°C. Once removed from the refrigerator the shelf-life is one month.[3]

2 Chemistry

Type: A cytotoxic antibiotic consisting of an amino sugar, daunosamine, linked through a glycosidic bond to the C7 of a tetracyclic aglycone, doxorubicinone. Doxorubicin may act by forming a stable complex with DNA and interfering with the synthesis of nucleic acids. It is most active against cells in the S phase.[4]

Molecular weight: 580.0.

Formula: $C_{27}H_{29}NO_{11}HCl$.

Solubility: Doxorubicin is soluble in water for injections, 5% glucose and 0.9% sodium chloride, partially soluble in methanol and ethanol and practically insoluble in chloroform, ether and other organic solvents.[4]

3 Stability Profile

Physical and chemical stability

The manufacturer states that reconstituted solutions of Doxorubicin Rapid Dissolution are chemically stable for up to 48 hours at room temperature in normal artificial light.[1] Doxorubicin Solution for Injection, which has a pH of 3, is stable for 18 months at 2 to 8°C and for one month at room temperature.[3] A review of the literature reveals that doxorubicin appears to be chemically stable for longer periods[5-12] but data are limited and contradictory and require critical assessment.

Molecular structure: (1S,3S)-3-Glycoloyl-1,2,3,4,6,11-hexahydro-3,5,12-trihy-droxy-10-methoxy-6,11-dioxonaphthacen-1-yl 3-amino-2,3,6-trideoxy-α-L-lyxo-pyranoside hydrochloride.

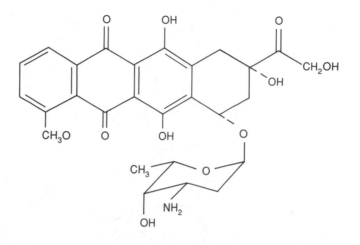

The stability of doxorubicin depends on a number of factors, the most important of which are temperature, pH and the type of solvent used for reconstitution.[13,14] Doxorubicin is also light sensitive and adsorbs onto glass and certain plastics.

Effect of pH: Doxorubicin becomes more stable as the pH of the drug infusion fluid admixture becomes more acidic (pH 7.4 to 4.5).[6] Maximum stability is observed at about pH 4.[15]

Decomposition in acidic solution has been studied by several authors.[16,17] Acidic hydrolysis of doxorubicin (pH below 4), which is shown in Figure 1, yields a red-coloured, water-insoluble aglycone, doxorubicinone and a water-soluble amino sugar, daunosamine. Degradation follows first order kinetics.[17] The first order rate constant is directly proportional to the hydrogen ion concentration (0.01 M to 0.5 M).[16]

The rate of cleavage of the glycosidic bond in acidic media is strongly dependent on structural modifications in the amino sugar moiety and is unaffected by structural modifications in the aglycone portion of the molecule. As doxorubicin and daunorubicin both possess daunosamine as the sugar moiety, the rate of degradation of these two analogues is similar in acidic solution.[15]

At pH values above 4, the degradation pattern of doxorubicin has not been elucidated completely. On addition to strongly alkaline solution, a colour change from red to deep blue-purple is observed and rapid degradation of doxorubicin occurs. Abdeen *et al.*[18] observed that a solution of doxorubicin in 2 M sodium hydroxide was initially blue and slowly turned yellow as degradation occurred. Acidification and extraction of this mixture afforded at least five components which were not identified. Analysis of degradation mixtures at pH 8.0 by Beijnen *et al.*[15] showed one major degradation product, 7,8-dehydro-9,10-des-acetyldaunorubicinone and minor quantities of other fluorescing compounds. The proposed scheme for this conversion is shown in Figure 2.

At pH values less than or equal to 9.5, degradation has been shown to be accelerated by acetate, phosphate and carbonate buffers. At pH values above 10, buffer catalysis has not been observed.[15]

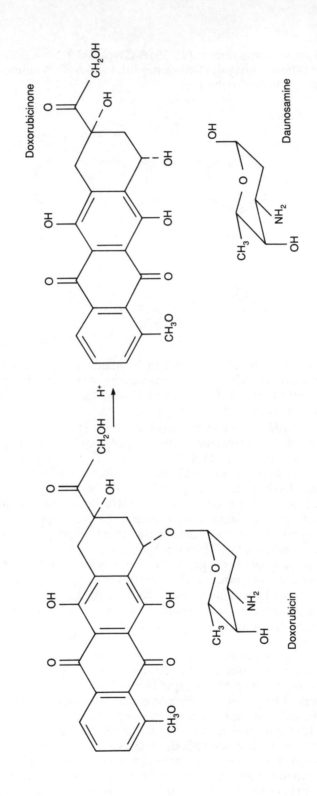

Figure 1: *Degradation pathway of doxorubicin in acidic solution*

In alkaline solution, the rate of degradation of the anthracyclines is affected by structural modifications in the aglycone portion of the molecule but not by structural modifications in the amino sugar moiety. As doxorubicin and epirubicin possess identical aglycones the rate of degradation of these two analogues is similar in alkaline solution. Conversely, the rate of degradation of daunorubicin, which possesses a different aglycone, is substantially different.[15]

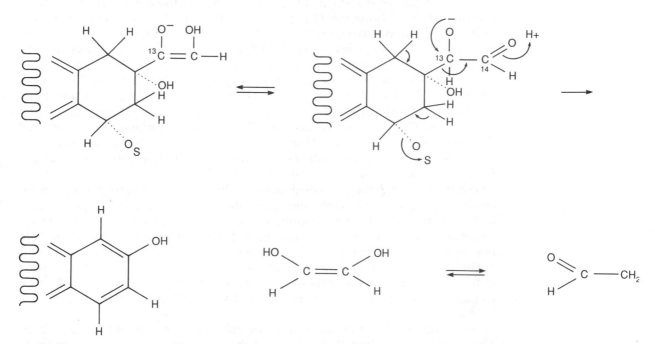

Figure 2: *Proposed degradation scheme for the conversion of doxorubicin to 7,8-dehydro-9,10-desacetyldaunorubicinone[15] (S refers to the daunosamine moiety)*

Effect of light: The large differences in stability which have been reported by different groups for virtually identical experiments[6,19] may be partially explained by poor control of photodegradation. Photodegradation of doxorubicin may be substantial at concentrations below 100 μg/ml, if solutions are exposed to light for sufficient time.[19,20] However, at higher concentrations, such as those used for cancer chemotherapy (at least 500 μg/ml), no special precautions are necessary to protect freshly prepared solutions of doxorubicin from light.[19,20]

Effect of temperature: Studies designed to investigate the effect of temperature on the rate of degradation of doxorubicin in buffers show that the Arrhenius relationship was obeyed for solutions between pH 4 and pH 10 between 30 and 70°C.[15] Results from stability studies at room temperature (normally 25°C), in the refrigerator (about 4°C) or in the freezer (about −20°C) are presented below.

In a well-controlled study Beijnen *et al.*[9] reported that doxorubicin was stable in 5% glucose (pH 4.7) and 3.3% glucose with 0.3% sodium chloride (pH 4.4), in polypropylene tubes, for 28 days at 25°C in the dark. However, in 0.9% sodium chloride (pH 7.0) significant degradation occurred after six days at the same temperature.

Wood *et al.*[21] reported that doxorubicin was stable in 0.9% sodium chloride (pH 6.47) in PVC minibags stored in the dark for 20 days at 25°C. In 5% glucose (pH 4.36) and 0.9% sodium chloride (pH 5.20 and pH 6.47) doxorubicin was stable in PVC minibags for at least 43 days at 4°C. In the same study, doxorubicin was also observed to be stable when reconstituted with water for injections and stored in polypropylene syringes at 4°C.[21]

Stiles and Allen[22] investigated the stability of both the commercially available preparations of doxorubicin (2 mg/ml) in portable pump reservoirs (Pharmacia Deltec Medication Cassette 602100A). Results showed that both formulations were stable for up to 14 days at 3 and 23°C and for an additional 28 days at 30°C.

Rochard *et al.*[23] investigated the stability of doxorubicin (500 µg/ml and 1.25 mg/ml) in 0.9% sodium chloride and 5% glucose solution in an 80 ml EVA reservoir (RES80 A, Celsa Laboratories, Chasseneuil, France). Results showed that both concentrations of doxorubicin were stable in both solvents for 14 days at 4 and 22°C and for seven days at 35°C. Finally, Hoffman *et al.*[5] observed that solutions of doxorubicin (2 mg/ml) in water for injections, were stable for six months at 4°C. Those authors indicated that filtration through a 0.22 µm filter would ensure sterility without loss of drug.

Several authors have published data on the effects of freezing doxorubicin. Hoffman *et al.*[5] observed that aqueous solutions of doxorubicin (2 mg/ml) could be frozen and stored for one month at −20°C without significant degradation but indicated that doxorubicin reconstituted with 0.9% sodium chloride should not be frozen. Conversely, doxorubicin has been reported to be stable in 0.9% sodium chloride, for 30 days[8] and two weeks,[12] respectively, at −20°C. Wood *et al.*[21] reported that doxorubicin was stable in 5% glucose (pH 4.36), 0.9% sodium chloride (pH 5.20 and pH 6.47) in PVC minibags for at least 43 days at −20°C.

The effects of thawing doxorubicin by microwave radiation have also been investigated.[8,12] Karlsen *et al.*[8] observed that the concentration of doxorubicin in PVC minibags declined significantly after four re-thawings in a microwave. Keusters *et al.*[12] compared the effects of freezing and thawing doxorubicin at room temperature with thawing in the microwave. Results showed that doxorubicin was stable for two weeks at −20°C when thawed by either method. After re-freezing and subsequent re-thawing a small, but significant, decrease in concentration was observed in solutions thawed by both methods. Alternatively, Hoffman *et al.*[5] observed that aqueous solutions of doxorubicin could be frozen and thawed at room temperature, seven times, without significant loss of potency. Wood *et al.*[21] also observed that repeated freezing and thawing of solutions of doxorubicin in PVC minibags at room temperature did not lead to significant degradation.

Uneven distribution of energy can occur during microwave thawing which may overheat solutions and lead to degradation.[24] For this reason, thawing in a microwave is not recommended. If frozen, doxorubicin should be thawed at room temperature.

Container compatibility: Doxorubicin is compatible with polypropylene, PVC and glass.[21,25] It has been reported to be more stable in plastic (PVC) than glass.[7] Doxorubicin adsorbs onto glass and polyethylene but not onto siliconized glass or polypropylene.[10,25] Solutions which contain concentrations of 2 mg/ml do not adsorb to membrane filters but with more dilute solutions, especially when associated with small volumes, greater than 95% of doxorubicin adsorbs to cellulose ester membranes and about 40% binds to polytetrafluoroethylene

(PTFE) membranes.[26,27] In clinical practice, when doxorubicin is used at concentrations of at least 500 μg/ml, adsorption during storage and delivery is negligible.[21,25]

Compatibility with other drugs: Doxorubicin is physically incompatible with heparin, dexamethasone sodium phosphate, hydrocortisone sodium succinate and diazepam. The manufacturers recommend that no other drugs are mixed with doxorubicin. Combinations of doxorubicin and fluorouracil or aminophylline result in a colour change from red to blue-purple which indicates the onset of rapid degradation of doxorubicin.[28]

A combination of doxorubicin and vincristine in 0.9% sodium chloride, and in a mixture of 2.5% glucose with 0.45% sodium chloride, appears to be stable for at least seven days.[29] A mixture of doxorubicin and vinblastine in 0.9% sodium chloride appears to be relatively stable for at least five days.[30]

Stability in clinical practice

Doxorubicin is compatible with polypropylene, polyethylene, PVC and glass.[21,25] Doxorubicin appears to be chemically stable in PVC minibags (100 μg/ml) for at least 28 days in 5% glucose or 0.9% sodium chloride when stored at 4°C and −20°C, and in polypropylene syringes (2 mg/ml) for at least 28 days at 4°C.[21] Both the commercially available preparations of doxorubicin are stable in portable pump reservoirs (Pharmacia Deltec Medication Cassette 602100A) for up to 14 days at 3 and 23°C and for an additional 28 days at 30°C.[22] Doxorubicin (500 μg/ml and 1.25 mg/ml) is stable in 0.9% sodium chloride or 5% glucose solution in EVA reservoirs (RES80 A, Celsa Laboratories, Chasseneuil, France) for 14 days at 4 and 22°C and for seven days at 35°C.[23] Doxorubicin (200 μg/ml to 5 mg/ml) is stable in 0.9% sodium chloride for at least 15 days in the Baxter Infusor at 4°C. At a concentration of 2 mg/ml it is also stable in the CADD pump for 14 days at 4°C.[31]

4 Clinical Use

Main indications: Successfully used to produce regression in acute leukaemia, lymphomas, soft tissue and osteogenic sarcomas, paediatric malignancies and adult solid tumours, in particular breast and lung carcinomas. Doxorubicin is frequently used in combination regimens with other cytotoxics.[1]

Dosage: Dosage is usually calculated on the basis of body surface area. For single agent therapy, 60 to 75 mg/m^2 is given every three weeks. When administered in combination with other agents which possess overlapping toxicity, dosage may need to be reduced to 30 to 40 mg/m^2 every three weeks. If the dosage is to be calculated on the basis of body weight 1.2 to 2.4 mg/kg is given as a single dose every three weeks. The total dose for the cycle may be divided over three successive days (20 to 25 mg/m^2 on each day). Administration of doxorubicin on a weekly regimen (20 mg/m^2) has been shown to be as effective as the three-weekly regimen. Dosage may need to be reduced in patients who have had prior treatment with other cytotoxics, in children and the elderly. If hepatic function is impaired, doxorubicin dosage should be reduced by 50% if serum bilirubin concentrations are between 1.2 and 3 mg/100 ml and by 75% if serum bilirubin concentrations are greater than 3 mg/100 ml. A cumulative dose of 450 mg to 550 mg/m^2 should only be exceeded with extreme caution, as above this level the risk of irreversible congestive cardiac failure increases greatly.[1,2]

5 Preparation of Injection

Reconstitution: With Doxorubicin Rapid Dissolution, the contents of the 10 mg vial are reconstituted with 5 ml of water for injections or 0.9% sodium chloride, and the 50 mg vial with 25 ml of the same solvent. After addition of the diluent and gentle shaking without inversion the contents of the vial will dissolve within 30 seconds to produce a solution of 2 mg/ml.[1]

Bolus administration: Administration is most frequently by the intravenous route. The manufacturer recommends that the reconstituted solution is given over two to three minutes, via the tubing of a freely-running intravenous infusion of 0.9% sodium chloride, 5% glucose or sodium chloride with glucose. This technique minimizes the risk of thrombosis or perivenous extravasation, which can lead to severe cellulitis or vesication. Doxorubicin may also be administered by the intra-arterial or intravesical route.[1,2]

Intravenous infusion: Although the optimum schedule of continuous infusion of doxorubicin has not been established, most current investigations can be grouped into two broad categories. Most experience has been acquired using a schedule of short-term infusions given over one to four days with cycles repeated every three to four weeks. The most thoroughly investigated short-term infusion has been the 96-hour cycle which generally takes five days to complete. In more recent studies, patients have received infusions for several months or longer.

Based on the marked decrease in the cardiac toxicity seen with short-term infusions of doxorubicin, a number of investigators have recently initiated studies with low dose doxorubicin given as a continuous infusion on a more protracted basis.[32-35] With a daily dose of 1 to 2 mg/m² the maximum total daily dose has varied between 3 and 5 mg/m² for periods of several weeks to several months in responding patients. Some investigators have used higher daily doses for two-week cycles of therapy, followed by two weeks without chemotherapy to allow for recovery from side-effects.[36]

Extravasation: Potent vesicant (*see* Chapter 9).

6 Destruction of Drug or Contaminated Articles

Incineration: 700°C.[3]

Chemical: 10% sodium hypochlorite (1% available chlorine)/24 hours.[1]

Contact with skin: Wash well with water, soap and water, or sodium bicarbonate solution. If the eyes are contaminated, immediate irrigation with saline should be carried out.[1]

References

1. *ABPI Data Sheet Compendium 1991–92.* (1991). Datapharm Publications Ltd, London, pp. 455–456.
2. *ABPI Data Sheet Compendium 1991–92.* (1991). Datapharm Publications Ltd, London, pp. 457–458.
3. Farmitalia Carlo Erba Ltd. Personal communication.
4. Anon. (1989). *The Extra Pharmacopoeia*, 29th edn. Reynolds, J.E.F. (ed.), Pharmaceutical Press, London, pp. 623–626.
5. Hoffman, D.M. *et al.* (1979). Stability of refrigerated and frozen solutions of doxorubicin hydrochloride. *Am. J. Hosp. Pharm.* **36**, 1536–1538.

6. Poochikian, G.K. *et al.* (1981). Stability of anthracycline antitumor agents in four infusion fluids. *Am. J. Hosp. Pharm.* **38**, 483–486.
7. Benvenuto, J.A. *et al.* (1981). Stability and compatibility of antitumor agents in glass and plastic containers. *Am. J. Hosp. Pharm.* **38**, 1914–1918.
8. Karlsen, J. *et al.* (1983). Stability of cytotoxic intravenous solutions subjected to freeze-thaw treatment. *Nor. Pharm. Acta* **45**, 61–67.
9. Beijnen, J.H. *et al.* (1985). Stability of anthracycline antitumor agents in infusion fluids. *J. Parenter. Sci. Technol.* **39**, 220–222.
10. Bosanquet, A.G. (1986). Stability of solutions of antineoplastic agents during preparation and storage for *in vitro* assays: II. Assay methods, adriamycin and the other antitimour antibiotics. *Cancer Chemother. Pharmacol.* **17**, 1–10.
11. Bouma, J. *et al.* (1986). Anthracycline antitumour agents: A review of physicochemical, analytical and stability properties. *Pharm. Weekbl. (Sci.)* **8**, 109–135.
12. Keusters, L. *et al.* (1986). Stability of solutions of doxorubicin and epirubicin in plastic minibags for intravesical use after storage at −20°C and thawing by microwave radiation. *Pharm. Weekbl. (Sci.)* **8**, 194–197.
13. Gupta, P.K. *et al.* (1988). Investigation of the stability of doxorubicin hydrochloride using factorial design. *Drug Dev. Indust. Pharm.* **14**, 1657–1671.
14. Janssen, M.J.H. *et al.* (1985). Doxorubicin decomposition on storage: Effect of pH, type of buffer and liposome encapsulation. *Int. J. Pharm.* **23**, 1–11.
15. Beijnen, J.H. *et al.* (1986). Aspects of the degradation kinetics of doxorubicin in aqueous solution. *Int. J. Pharm.* **32**, 123–131.
16. Wasserman, K. and Bundgaard, H. (1983). Kinetics of the acid catalysed hydrolysis of doxorubicin. *Int. J. Pharm.* **14**, 73–78.
17. Beijnen, J.H. *et al.* (1985). Aspects of the stability of doxorubicin and seven other anthracyclines in acidic solution. *Pharm. Weekbl. (Sci.)* **7**, 109–116.
18. Abdeen, Z. *et al.* (1985). Degradation of adriamycin in aqueous sodium hydroxide: Formation of a ring-A oxabicyclononenone. *J. Chem. Res. (S)*, 254–255.
19. Tavoloni, N. *et al.* (1980). Photolytic degradation of adriamycin. *J. Pharm. Pharmacol.* **32**, 860–862.
20. Wood, M.J. *et al.* (1990). Photodegradation of doxorubicin, daunorubicin and epirubicin measured by high-performance liquid chromatography. *J. Clin. Pharm. Ther.* **15**, 291–300.
21. Wood, M.J. *et al.* (1990). Stability of doxorubicin, daunorubicin and epirubicin in plastic syringes and minibags. *J. Clin. Pharm. Ther.* **15**, 279–289.
22. Stiles, M.L. and Allen, L.V. (1991). Stability of doxorubicin hydrochloride in portable pump reservoirs. *Am. J. Hosp. Pharm.* **48**, 1976–1977.
23. Rochard, E.B. *et al.* (1992). Stability of fluorouracil, cytarabine, or doxorubicin hydrochloride in ethylene vinylacetate portable infusion-pump reservoirs. *Am. J. Hosp. Pharm.* **49**, 619–623.
24. Williamson, M. and Luce, J.K. (1987). Microwave thawing of doxorubicin hydrochloride admixtures not recommended. *Am. J. Hosp. Pharm.* **44**, 505, 510.
25. Wood, M.J. (1989). M. Phil. Thesis, University of Aston, Birmingham, UK.
26. Pavlik, E.J. *et al.* (1982). Sensitivity of anticancer agents *in vitro*, standardising the cytotoxic response and characterising the sensitivities of a reference cell line. *Gynecol. Oncol.* **14**, 243–261.

27. Pavlik, E.J. *et al.* (1984). Stability of doxorubicin in relation to chemosensitivity determinations: Loss of lethality and retention of antiproliferative activity. *Cancer Invest.* **2**, 449–458.
28. Trissel, L.A. (1992). *Handbook on injectable drugs*, 7th edn. American Society of Hospital Pharmacists, Bethesda, Maryland, USA.
29. Beijnen, J.H. *et al.*. (1986). Stability of intravenous admixtures of doxorubicin and vincristine. *Am. J. Hosp. Pharm.* **43**, 3022–3027.
30. Gaj, E. and Sesin, P. (1984). Compatibility of doxorubicin hydrochloride and vinblastine sulphate. The stability of a solution stored in Cormed reservoir bags or Monoject plastic syringes. *Am. J. Intraven. Ther. Clin. Nutr.* **11**, 8–20.
31. Baxter Healthcare Ltd. Personal communication.
32. Garnick, M.B. *et al.* (1983). Clinical evaluation of long term continuous infusion doxorubicin. *Cancer Treat. Rep.* **67**, 133–142.
33. Bowen, J. *et al.* (1981). Phase I study of adriamycin by 5-day continuous intravenous infusion. *Proc. Am. Assoc. Cancer Res.* **22**, 354 (C-84).
34. Lokich, J.J. *et al.* (1983) Constant infusion schedule for adriamycin: A phase I–II clinical trial of a 30-day schedule by ambulatory pump delivery system. *J. Clin. Oncol.* **1**, 24–28.
35. Vogelsang, W.J. *et al.* (1984). Continuous doxorubicin infusion using an implanted lithium battery-powered drug administration device system (DADS, Medtronic, Inc.). *Proc. Am. Soc. Clin. Oncol.* **3**, 263 (C-1030).
36. Legha, S.S. *et al.* (1987). Anthracyclines. In Lokich, J.J. (ed.): *Cancer chemotherapy by infusion*. MTP Press Ltd, Lancaster.

Prepared by M.J. Wood

EPIRUBICIN

1 General Details

Approved name: Epirubicin.

Proprietary name: Pharmorubicin Rapid Dissolution, Pharmorubicin Solution for Injection.

Manufacturer and supplier: Farmitalia Carlo Erba Ltd.

Presentation and formulation details:

▼ Pharmorubicin Rapid Dissolution: Sterile, pyrogen-free, red, freeze-dried powder in vials containing 10 mg, 20 mg and 50 mg of epirubicin hydrochloride with lactose and hydroxybenzoate. The inclusion of hydroxybenzoate 0.04% (which is a sub-preservative concentration) is to prevent gel formation which used to occur occasionally on reconstitution of Pharmorubicin. Pharmorubicin has been replaced by Pharmorubicin Rapid Dissolution.[1]

▼ Pharmorubicin Solution for Injection: Sterile, red, mobile solution in vials containing 10 mg, 20 mg and 50 mg of epirubicin hydrochloride as a 2 mg/ml solution in 0.9% sodium chloride.[2]

Storage and shelf-life of unopened container:

▼ Pharmorubicin Rapid Dissolution: Three years when protected from sunlight at room temperature.[3]

▼ Pharmorubicin Solution for Injection: Stored between 2 and 8°C[2] the shelf-life is 18 months. Once removed from the refrigerator the shelf-life is 48 hours.[3]

2 Chemistry

Type: A cytotoxic antibiotic consisting of an amino sugar, acosamine, linked through a glycosidic bond to the C7 of a tetracyclic aglycone, doxorubicinone.

Molecular structure: (8S,10S)-10-(3-Amino-2,3,6-trideoxy-α-L-arabino-hexopyranosyloxy)-8-glycoloyl-7,8,9,10-tetrahydro-6,8,11-trihydroxy-1-methoxynaphthacene-5,12-dione hydrochloride.

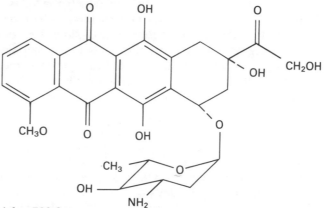

Molecular weight: 580.0.

Formula: $C_{27}H_{29}NO_{11}HCl$.

Solubility: Epirubicin is soluble in water for injections, 5% glucose and 0.9% sodium chloride, partially soluble in methanol and ethanol and practically insoluble in chloroform, ether and other organic solvents.[4]

3 Stability Profile

Physical and chemical stability

The manufacturer states that reconstituted solutions of Epirubicin Rapid Dissolution are chemically stable for up to 48 hours at 2 to 8°C, or 24 hours at room temperature.[1] Epirubicin Solution for Injection is stable for 18 months at 2 to 8°C and for 48 hours at room temperature.[3] The literature indicates that epirubicin may be chemically stable for longer periods, although few data have been published.[5,6]

The stability of epirubicin depends on a number of factors. Degradation in aqueous solution is pH dependent. Epirubicin is also light sensitive and adsorbs to glass and certain plastics.

Effect of pH: Acidic hydrolysis of epirubicin (pH below 4) which is shown in Figure 1, yields a red-coloured, water-insoluble aglycone, doxorubicinone, and a water-soluble amino sugar, acosamine. The rate of cleavage of the glycosidic bond in acidic media is strongly affected by structural differences in the amino sugar moiety and unaffected by structural differences in the aglycone portion of the molecule. As doxorubicin and epirubicin possess different amino sugar residues the rate of degradation of these two analogues in acidic solution is different.[7]

At pH values above 4, the degradation pathway of epirubicin has not been elucidated. However, on addition to strongly alkaline solution a colour change from red to deep blue-purple is observed and rapid degradation occurs. Data on the degradation of epirubicin in alkaline solution have recently been published indicating that at pH 8.0 the main degradation product is 7,8,-dehydro-9,10-des-acetyldaunorubicinone.[7] The structure of this compound is shown in Figure 2.

In alkaline solution, the rate of degradation of the anthracyclines is affected by structural differences in the aglycone portion of the molecule and unaffected by structural differences in the amino sugar moiety. As epirubicin and doxorubicin possess the same aglycone their rates of degradation in alkaline solution are similar.[7]

Effect of light: Data on the kinetics of degradation of doxorubicin in fluorescent light have been published[8] but until recently there were no available data for epirubicin. Results from a study in which the rates of photodegradation of doxorubicin, daunorubicin and epirubicin were compared indicated that the rate of photodegradation of epirubicin was similar to doxorubicin. This suggests that photodegradation of epirubicin may be significant at concentrations below 100 µg/ml if solutions are exposed to light for sufficient time.[9] However, at higher concentrations, such as those used for cancer chemotherapy (at least 500 µg/ml), no special precautions are necessary to protect freshly prepared solutions of epirubicin from light.[9]

Effect of temperature: In a well-controlled study Beijnen *et al.*[7] reported that epirubicin was stable, in polypropylene tubes, in 5% glucose (pH 4.7) and 3.3% glucose with 0.3% sodium chloride (pH 4.4) for 28 days at 25°C, when stored in the dark. However, in 0.9% sodium chloride (pH 7.0) significant degradation occurred after eight days at the same temperature.[7]

Wood *et al.*[10] reported that epirubicin was stable for at least 43 days in PVC minibags in 5% glucose (pH 4.36) and 0.9% sodium chloride (pH 5.20) at 25 and 4°C. When dissolved in 0.9% sodium chloride (pH 6.47) epirubicin was stable for 24 days at 25°C and at least 43 days at 4°C. In the same study epirubicin was reported to be stable for at least 43 days, when reconstituted with water for injections and stored in polypropylene syringes at 4°C.

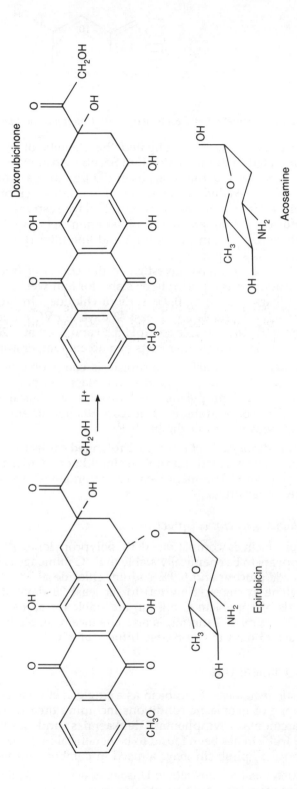

Figure 1: *Degradation pathway of epirubicin in acidic solution*

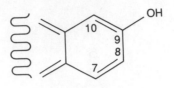

Figure 2: *Structure of 7,8,-dehydro-9,10-desacetyldaunorubicinone*[7]

De Vroe *et al.*[11] investigated the stability of epirubicin during storage and simulated continuous infusion. Sorption to administration sets was also studied. Results showed that epirubicin (50 µg/ml) was stable in PVC, glass and high density polyethylene (HDPE) in 0.9% sodium chloride (pH 5.5) and 5% glucose (pH 4.26) for periods of 24 and 25 days respectively at 4°C. No sorption onto infusion containers or administration sets was observed during simulated infusion. Infusion through an end-line filter (Pall ELD-96 LL) resulted in negligible loss of potency.

Two studies have investigated the effects of freezing epirubicin. In the first, epirubicin was reported to be stable for four weeks when frozen at −20°C in PVC minibags containing 0.9% sodium chloride.[6] In the second, epirubicin was observed to be stable for at least 43 days in PVC minibags in 5% glucose (pH 4.36) and 0.9% sodium chloride (pH 5.20 and 6.47) at −20°C.[10] Repeated freezing and re-thawing of these minibags at ambient temperature did not cause degradation.

Container compatibility: Epirubicin is compatible with polypropylene, PVC and glass.[10–12] Epirubicin adsorbs onto glass and polyethylene but not to siliconized glass or polypropylene.[10,12] However, in clinical practice, when epirubicin is used at concentrations of at least 500 µg/ml, adsorptive losses during storage and delivery are negligible.[10–12]

Compatibility with other drugs: Prolonged contact with any solution of alkaline pH should be avoided. Epirubicin should not be mixed with heparin as a precipitate may form.[1,2] The manufacturers recommend that epirubicin is not mixed with any other drugs.

Stability in clinical practice

Epirubicin is compatible with polypropylene, PVC and glass.[10–12] Epirubicin appears to be chemically stable in PVC minibags (100 µg/ml) for at least 28 days in 5% glucose and 0.9% sodium chloride at 4°C and −20°C, and in polypropylene syringes (2 mg/ml) for at least 28 days at 4°C.[10] After reconstitution, vials of epirubicin (2 mg/ml) are stable for at least 14 days at 4°C.[12] Epirubicin (200 µg/ml to 1 mg/ml) is also chemically stable in 0.9% sodium chloride for at least 15 days in the Baxter Infusor at 4°C.[13]

4 Clinical Use

Main indications: Epirubicin as a single agent has produced regression in a wide range of neoplastic conditions including breast, ovarian, gastric and colorectal carcinomas, lymphomas, leukaemias and multiple myeloma. Intravesical epirubicin has been found to be beneficial in the treatment of superficial bladder cancer. Epirubicin may be used in combination with other cytotoxic agents.[1,2]

Dosage and administration: Dosage is usually calculated on the basis of body surface area. For single agent intravenous therapy, the dose range most commonly used is 75 to 90 mg/m^2 every three weeks. The total dose for the cycle may be divided over two successive days. When epirubicin is used in combination therapy with other cytotoxics the dosage should be reduced. Dosage should also be reduced in hepatic impairment.[1] In moderate hepatic impairment (bilirubin 1.2 to 3 mg/100 ml) dosage should be reduced by 50%, and in severe impairment (bilirubin above 3 mg/100 ml) dosage should be reduced by 75%.

Epirubicin can be administered intravenously on a weekly regimen, particularly for the palliative treatment of poor-risk patients for whom the toxicity of a conventional three-weekly regimen would be unacceptable. For these patients, the most commonly used dose is 20 mg per week.[1]

Epirubicin can be used intravesically to treat papillary transitional cell carcinoma of the bladder and carcinoma-in-situ. However, it should not be used to treat invasive bladder tumours which have penetrated the bladder wall, where systemic therapy or surgery is more appropriate. Epirubicin has also been used successfully intravesically as a prophylactic agent after transurethral resection of superficial tumours in order to prevent recurrences.

Many regimens of intravesical therapy have been used. However, the following may serve as a guide: For therapy, weekly instillations of 50 mg in 50 ml of 0.9% sodium chloride or water for injections are given for eight weeks. If local toxicity occurs (chemical cystitis) a dose reduction to 30 mg in 50 ml is advised. For carcinoma-in-situ the dose may be increased to 80 mg in 50 ml (depending on patient tolerance). For prophylaxis, weekly administration of 50 mg in 50 ml for four weeks is followed by monthly instillations for 11 months at the same dosage.

The solution should be retained intravesically for one hour. During the instillation, the patient should be rotated occasionally and should be instructed to void at the end of the instillation time.[1]

A cumulative dose of 900 to 1000 mg/m^2 should only be exceeded with extreme caution, as above this level the risk of irreversible congestive cardiac failure increases greatly. A lower cumulative dose of epirubicin is recommended for patients with prior or concomitant mediastinal radiation, or therapy with related anthracycline compounds such as doxorubicin, daunorubicin or anthracene derivatives.[1,2]

5 Preparation of Injection

Reconstitution: The contents of the 10 mg vial are reconstituted with 5 ml of water for injections, the 20 mg vial with 10 ml, and the 50 mg vial with 25 ml of the same solvent. After addition of the diluent and gentle shaking, the contents, without inversion of the vial, will dissolve to produce a solution of 2 mg/ml.[1]

Bolus administration: The reconstituted solution is given, over three to five minutes, via the tubing of a freely-running intravenous infusion of 0.9% sodium chloride. This technique minimizes the risk of thrombosis or perivenous extravasation, which can lead to severe cellulitis or vesication.[1,2] Administration of epirubicin by intravesical, intra-arterial, intrapleural and intraperitoneal routes has been investigated in clinical trials.[14–16]

Intravenous infusion: Continuous infusion schedules of epirubicin have been investigated. At New York University, epirubicin has been given as a six-hour infusion.[17] At the MD Anderson Center, a 48-hour infusion of doxorubicin (60 to 70 mg/m^2) has been compared with a 48-hour infusion of epirubicin (90 to 105 mg/m^2).[18]

Extravasation: Potent vesicant (*see* Chapter 9).

6 Destruction of Drug or Contaminated Articles

Incineration: 700°C.[3]

Chemical: 10% sodium hypochlorite (1% available chlorine)/24 hours.[1,2]

Contact with skin: Wash well with water, soap and water, or sodium bicarbonate solution. If the eyes are contaminated, immediate irrigation with 0.9% sodium chloride solution should be carried out.[1,2]

References

1. *ABPI Data Sheet Compendium 1991–92.* (1991). Datapharm Publications Ltd, London, pp. 463–465.
2. *ABPI Data Sheet Compendium 1991–92.* (1991). Datapharm Publications Ltd, London, pp. 465–466.
3. Farmitalia Carlo Erba Ltd. Personal communication.
4. Anon. (1989). *The Extra Pharmacopoeia.* 29th edn. Reynolds, J.E.F. (ed.), Pharmaceutical Press, London, p. 626.
5. Beijnen, J.H. *et al.* (1985). Stability of anthracycline antitumor agents in infusion fluids. *J. Parenter. Sci. Technol.* **39**, 220–222.
6. Keusters, L. *et al.* (1986). Stability of solutions of doxorubicin and epirubicin in plastic minibags for intravesical use after storage at −20°C and thawing by microwave radiation. *Pharm. Weekbl. (Sci.)* **8**, 194–197.
7. Beijnen, J.H. *et al.* (1986) Aspects of the degradation kinetics of doxorubicin in aqueous solution. *Int. J. Pharm.* **32**, 123–131.
8. Tavoloni, N. *et al.* (1980). Photolytic degradation of adriamycin. *J. Pharm. Pharmacol.* **32**, 860–862.
9. Wood, M.J. *et al.* (1990). Photodegradation of doxorubicin, daunorubicin and epirubicin measured by high-performance liquid chromatography. *J. Clin. Pharm. Ther.* **15**, 291–300.
10. Wood, M.J. *et al.* (1990). Stability of doxorubicin, daunorubicin and epirubicin in plastic syringes and minibags. *J. Clin. Pharm. Ther.* **15**, 279–289.
11. De Vroe, C. *et al.* (1990). A study on the stability of three antineoplastic drugs and on their sorption by IV delivery systems and end-line filters. *Int. J. Pharm.* **65**, 49–56.
12. Wood, M.J. (1989). M. Phil. Thesis, University of Aston, Birmingham, UK.
13. Baxter Healthcare Ltd. Personal communication.
14. Ferrazzi, E. *et al.* (1982). Preliminary phase II experience with 4'epidoxorubicin. In Muggia, F.M., Young, C.W., Carter, S.K. (eds): *Anthracycline antibiotics in cancer therapy*, Martinus Nijhoff, The Hague, p. 562.
15. Strocchi, E. *et al.* (1983). 4'epidoxorubicin in locoregional therapy: Pharmacokinetic study after intrahepatic arterial and intraperitoneal administration. *Proc. 4th NCI-EORTC Symposium*, Brussels, Abst. 108.
16. Friedman, M.A. and Ignoffo, R.J. (1984). Intra-arterial use of adriamycin. In Ogawa, M., Muggia, F.M., Rozencweig, M. (eds): *Adriamycin: Its expanding role in cancer treatment*, Excerpta Medica, Tokyo, p. 387.
17. Muggia, F.M. and Green, M.D. (1984). Special modes of administration: In Bonnadonna, G. (ed.): *Advances in anthracycline chemotherapy: Epirubicin.* Masson, Milano, pp. 149–152.
18. Bodey, G.P. *et al.* (1983). Clinical trials with 4'epidoxorubicin. *Proc. 13th International Congress of Chemotherapy, Vienna*, part 215/23, Masson, Canada.

Prepared by M.J. Wood

ETOPOSIDE

1 General Details

Approved name: Etoposide.

Proprietary name: Vepesid.

Manufacturer or supplier: Bristol-Myers Squibb Pharmaceuticals Ltd.

Presentation and formulation details: Glass vials containing 100 mg etoposide in 5 ml solution, 20 mg/ml. Each vial also contains: polyethylene glycol 300, ethyl alcohol, polysorbate 80, benzyl alcohol and citric acid.

Storage and shelf-life of unopened container: Five years from the date of manufacture when stored at room temperature and protected from light.

2 Chemistry

Type: Semi-synthetic podophyllotoxin derivative.

Molecular structure: 4-o-Demethyl-1-1 o-(4,6-o-Ethylidene-β-D-glucopyranosyl)-epi-podophyllotoxin.

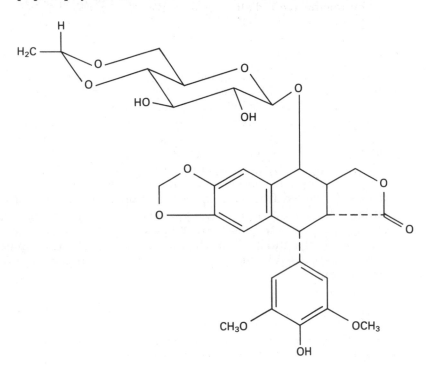

Molecular weight: 588.6.

Solubility: Highly insoluble in water, soluble in organic solvents.[1] In dilutions with 0.9% sodium chloride, the concentration of etoposide should not exceed 0.25 mg/ml.[2] In other reports, however, it is suggested that concentrations up to 0.4 mg/ml are acceptable in clinical practice.[3,4] Occasional precipitation of drug has been reported in infusions where etoposide concentration exceeded 0.4 mg/ml.[4]

3 Stability Profile

Physical and chemical stability

Etoposide degrades by hydrolytic cleavage of the glucopyranosyl moiety, or by epimerization to the cis-lactone.

Effect of pH: Maximum stability is found at 5.0.[5] The aglycone may hydrolyse in acid, while based-catalysed epimerization occurs in alkali.[5]

Effect of light: Etoposide should be protected from light during storage[1] and from strong daylight during administration.

Container compatibility: Glass or PVC containers are recommended,[2] and polypropylene syringes are also acceptable.[6,7] Etoposide is incompatible with cellulose acetate membrane filters but compatible with nylon or fluripore type membranes.[8] Undiluted etoposide injection has been implicated in the formation of hairline cracks in infusion devices constructed of plastics produced from the monomers acrylonitrile, butadiene and styrene.[9] The effect on these plastics (known collectively as ABS plastic) has been attributed to the action of polyethylene glycol (PEG) 300, a solubilizing agent in the injectable formulation. Caution should be exercised in the use of any plastic infusion device with undiluted etoposide injection.

Compatibility with other drugs: The manufacturer does not recommend mixing etoposide with any other drug.[1]

Stability in clinical practice

Etoposide infusions (0.4 mg/ml) in 5% glucose and in 0.9% sodium chloride are chemically stable for at least four days at room temperature.[10,11] As with an earlier report,[3] the stability of etoposide was not influenced by the type of container material (glass or PVC) or by normal room fluorescent lighting. One report, however, has suggested that the drug may be daylight-sensitive and is unstable beyond six hours in unprotected solutions.[12]

Etoposide infusions (0.2 mg/ml) in PVC containers of 0.9% sodium chloride or 5% glucose exhibited no loss of etoposide over 72 hours storage at 5 or 25°C.[6] It was concluded from this study that etoposide was not adsorbed on to the surface of the container. Polypropylene syringes containing etoposide infusion (1 mg/ml in water for injections) prepared for continuous infusion were chemically stable at 4 and 20°C for 28 days.[7] However, etoposide precipitated during administration and the clinical use of concentrated infusions cannot be recommended.

4 Clinical Use

Type of cytotoxic agent: Mitotic inhibitor which arrests the cell cycle in the G2 phase.

Main indications: Small cell carcinoma of the lung. Resistant non-seminomatous testicular carcinoma.

Dosage by injection: 60 to 120 mg/m² by IV infusion daily, for five consecutive days repeated every three to four weeks. Alternatively, 100 mg/m²/day on days 1, 2, 3, 5, every three to four weeks.

Oral: Twice the IV dose should be given on five consecutive days every three to four weeks, myelosuppression permitting.

5 Preparation of the Injection

Dilution: The injection should be diluted in 5% glucose or 0.9% sodium chloride solution to give a maximum concentration of 0.25 mg/ml etoposide in the infusion.

Bolus administration: Not recommended.

Intravenous infusion: The dose should be given by infusion over not less than 30 minutes.

Extravasation: Irritant (*see* Chapter 9).

6 Destruction of Drug or Contaminated Articles

Incineration: 1000°C.

Chemical: 10% sodium hypochlorite solution (1% available chlorine)/24 hours.

Contact with skin: Accidental exposure to etoposide may cause skin reactions. A soap and water wash should be employed.

References

1. Anon. (1982). *The Extra Pharmacopoeia*, 29th edn. Reynolds, J.E.F. (ed.), Pharmaceutical Press, London, pp. 208–209.
2. *ABPI Data Sheet Compendium 1991–92*. (1991). Datapharm Publications Ltd, London, pp. 269–270.
3. Phillips, N.C. and Lauper, R.D. (1983). Review of etoposide. *Clin. Pharm.* **2**, 112–119.
4. Arnold, A.M. (1979). Podophyllotoxin derivative VP 16–213. *Cancer Chemother. Pharmacol.* **3**, 71–80.
5. Lidenberg, W.J.M. *et al.* (1985). Analysis and degradation kinetics of etoposide (VP 16–213) in aqueous solution. *Pharmaceutish. Weekblad. Sci. Ed.* **1**, 291.
6. Sewell, G.J. (1988). Adsorption of etoposide (Vepesid) on to PVC of Viaflex infusion bags. Unpublished report, No. 67.
7. Adams, P.S. *et al.* (1987). Pharmaceutical aspects of home infusion therapy for cancer patients. *Pharm. J.* **238**, 46–478.
8. Forrest, S.C. (1984). Vepesid injection. *Pharm J.* **232**, 88.
9. Schwinghammer, T.L. and Reilly, M. (1988). Cracking of ABS plastic devices used to infuse undiluted etoposide injection (letter). *Am. J. Hosp. Pharm.* **45**, 1277.
10. Trissel, L.A. (1992) *Handbook on injectable drugs*, 7th edn. American Society of Hospital Pharmacists, Bethesda, Maryland.
11. Beijnen, J.H. *et al.* (1990). Chemical and physical stability of etoposide and tenoposide in commonly used infusion fluids. *J. Parenter. Sci. Technol.* **45**, 108–112.
12. Arnold, A.M. (1979). Podophyllotoxin derivative VP 16–213. *Cancer Chemother. Pharmacol.* **3**, 71–80.

Prepared by G.J. Sewell

FLUOROURACIL

1 General Details

Approved names: Fluorouracil, 5-fluorouracil.

Proprietary names: Fluoro-uracil.

Manufacturer or suppliers: Roche Products Ltd, David Bull Laboratories Ltd (DBL).

Presentation and formulation details: Colourless to slightly yellow solution in clear glass ampoules (Roche) or rubber-capped clear glass vials (DBL) containing 25 mg/ml fluorouracil; solution in water for injections with sodium hydroxide for pH adjustment.

Storage and shelf-life of unopened container: The shelf-life is two years when stored at room temperature and protected from light.

2 Chemistry

Type: Fluorinated pyrimidine.

Molecular structure: 5-Fluoro-2,4(1H,3H)pyrimidine-dione.

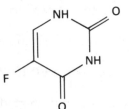

Molecular weight: 130.1.

Solubility: 12.5 mg/ml in water; 6 mg/ml in ethanol.

3 Stability Profile

Physical and chemical stability

Fluorouracil breakdown occurs by two routes: thermal and photochemical decomposition cause the opening of the pyrimidine ring between N3 and C4 and N1 and C5 to produce urea. Alkaline hydrolysis leads to the production of barbituric acid and uracil which further degrades to urea. The rate of alkaline hydrolysis increases rapidly above pH 9.0 so the injection is formulated within the pH range of 8.6 to 9.0. Although the drug is stable at acid pH, solubility is reduced.

The injection should be protected from strong daylight and temperatures above 25°C.

Container compatibility: Many studies has been made of container compatibility at various concentrations. At concentrations of 5 to 10 mg/ml, the drug has been shown to be stable for 16 weeks at 5°C in PVC containers. Similar and more concentrated solutions have been shown to be stable for up to 42 days at room temperature.[1,2,3] A small increase in concentration resulted from loss of moisture. Undiluted injections have been stored in a plastic syringe or glass vial without loss of potency.[4] Studies for the Exeter continuous chemotherapy infusion programme have shown the undiluted injection to be stable for 28 days at 5°C and 25°C in plastic syringes.[5]

Compatibility with other drugs: Compatible at an infusion 'Y' site with mannitol,[6] ondansetron,[7] potassium chloride, calcium gluconate, magnesium sulphate, heparin,[8] bleomycin,[9] prednisolone sodium phosphate, vincristine sulphate[10] and calcium leucovorin.[11] It is also compatible with methotrexate and cyclophosphamide.[12] Fluorouracil is incompatible in mixtures with acidic drugs or drugs that decompose in an alkaline environment (eg doxorubicin).[13] It is also incompatible with cytarabine,[10] diazepam,[13] cisplatin[14] and droperidol.[8] McRae and King[10] found that fluorouracil is incompatible with methotrexate, although this is contradicted by Lokich *et al.*[12]

Stability in clinical practice

The drug has been shown to be quite stable at pH values below 9.0 and when protected from strong daylight and temperatures above 25°C. In syringes and PVC containers, undiluted or diluted in 0.9% sodium chloride, the drug has been shown to be stable for at least 28 days. In 5% glucose, there is some conflicting evidence. Studies have indicated that the drug is stable for 16 weeks at 5°C[1] or five days at room temperature,[15] whereas other workers reported a loss of 10% in 43 hours.[16] If 5% glucose infusion has to be used, the shelf-life should be restricted to 36 hours.

Stability studies in ambulatory pump units and reservoirs have reported that fluorouracil injection (DBL), 25 mg/ml (undiluted), is stable for at least 14 days at 4 and 37°C in the Parker Micropump[17] and for at least seven days in four other ambulatory pumps.[18] Solutions of fluorouracil ranging from 5 to 42 mg/ml in 0.9% sodium chloride have been shown to be stable for at least 15 days in the Baxter Infusor when stored at 4°C.[19] The drug is also stable, after refrigerated storage for 15 days, during administration through a seven-day Infusor or Large Volume Intermate device (Baxter).[19]

4 Clinical Use

Type of cytotoxic: Antimetabolite.

Main indications: Palliative treatment of a variety of carcinomas both alone and in combination.

Dosage: Up to 15 mg/kg IV once weekly, maximum daily dose 1 g. Fluorouracil may be used as an induction once daily for five to seven days or in a three to four week cycle as part of combination therapy. Also, 5 to 7.5 mg/kg by continuous intra-arterial infusion over 24 hours has been used.

5 Preparation of Injection

Dilution: May be administered undiluted or diluted as an infusion.

Bolus administration: Administer injection slowly directly into the vein or via a fast-running drip.

Intravenous infusion: Diluted in 5% glucose or 0.9% sodium chloride and administered over four to 24 hours.

Extravasation: Non-irritant.

6 Destruction of Drug or Contaminated Articles

Incineration: 700°C.

Chemical: 10% sodium hypochlorite/24 hours.

Contact with skin: Wash thoroughly with soap and water.

References

1. Quebbeman, E.J. *et al.* (1984). Stability of fluorouracil in plastic containers used for continuous infusion at home. *Am. J. Hosp. Pharm.* **41**, 1153–1156.
2. Vincke, A.E. *et al.* (1989). Extended stability of 5-fluorouracil and methotrexate solutions in PVC containers. *Int. J. Pharm.* **54**, 181–189.
3. Allen, V.J. *et al.* (1988). Stability study of fluorouracil administered using a constant infusion pump. American Society of Hospital Pharmacists Meeting, **23**, 387.
4. Sesin, G.P. *et al.* (1982). Stability study of 5-fluorouracil following repackaging in plastic disposable syringes and multidose vials. *Am. J. Intraven. Ther. Clin. Nutrition*, **9**, 23–25, 29–30.
5. Sewell, G.J. (1988). Cancer chemotherapy by infusion: drug stability and compatibility considerations. *Proc. Int. Symposium on Oncological Pharmacy Practice*, Rotorua, New Zealand, 253–278.
6. Woloschuck, D.M.M. *et al.* (1991). Stability and compatibility of fluorouracil and mannitol during simulated Y-site administration. *Am. J. Hosp. Pharm.* **48**, 2158–2160.
7. Leak, R.F. and Woodford, J.D. (1989). Pharmaceutical development of ondansetron injection. *Eur. J. Cancer Clin. Oncol.* **25(Suppl.1)**, S76–S69.
8. Salamone, F.R. and Muller, R.J. (1990). Intravenous admixture compatibility of cancer chemotherapeutic agents. *Hosp. Pharm.* **25**, 567–570.
9. Dorr, R.T. *et al.* (1982). Bleomycin compatibility with selected intravenous medications. *J. Medicine*, **13**, 121–130.
10. McRae, M.P. and King, J.C. (1976). Compatibility of antineoplastic, antibiotic and corticosteroid drugs in intravenous admixtures. *Am. J. Hosp. Pharm.* **33**, 1010–1013.
11. Leonard, S.L. *et al.* (1988). Stability of 5-fluorouracil and leucovorin calcium combined in a single infusion for intravenous administration. American Society of Hospital Pharmacists Midyear Clinical Meeting **23**, 48.
12. Lokich, J. *et al.* (1989). Cyclophosphamide, methotrexate and 5-fluorouracil in a three-drug admixture. *Cancer* **63**, 822–824.
13. Dorr, R.T. (1979). Incompatibilities with parenteral and anticancer drugs. *Am. J. Intraven. Ther. Clin. Nutrition* **6**, 42,45,46,52.
14. Stewart, C.F. and Fleming, R.A. (1990). Compatibility of cisplatin and fluorouracil in 0.9% sodium chloride injection. *Am. J. Hosp. Pharm.* **47**, 1373–1377.
15. David Bull Laboratories. (1985). Personal communication.
16. Benvenuto, J.A. *et al.* (1981). Stability and compatibility of antitumor agents in glass and plastic containers. *Am. J. Hosp. Pharm.* **38**, 1914–1918.
17. Northcott, M. *et al.* (1991). The stability of carboplatin, diamorphine, 5-fluorouracil and mitozantrone infusions in an ambulatory pump under storage and prolonged 'in-use' conditions. *J. Clin. Pharm. Ther.* **16**, 123–129.
18. Stiles, M.L. *et al.* (1989). Stability of fluorouracil administered through four portable infusion pumps. *Am. J. Hosp. Pharm.* **46**, 2036–2040.
19. Baxter Healthcare. (1992). Personal communication.

Prepared by R.J. Needle

IDARUBICIN

1 General Details

Approved name: Idarubicin.

Proprietary name: Zavedos.

Manufacturer and supplier: Farmitalia Carlo Erba Ltd.

Presentation and formulation details: Sterile, pyrogen-free, orange-red, freeze-dried powder in vials containing 5 mg and 10 mg of idarubicin hydrochloride, with 50 mg and 100 mg of lactose respectively.[1] Capsules (5 mg and 10 mg) are also available on a named patient basis.[2]

Storage and shelf-life of unopened container: Three years at room temperature protected from sunlight.[2]

2 Chemistry

Type: A cytotoxic antibiotic consisting of an amino sugar daunosamine, linked through a glycosidic bond to the C7 of a tetracyclic aglycone, 4-demethoxy-daunorubicinone.

Molecular structure: (1S,3S)-3-acetyl-1,2,3,4,6,11-hexahydro-3,5,12-trihydroxy-6,11-dioxo-1-naphthacenyl-3-amino-2,3,6-trideoxy-α-L-lyso-hexopyranoside.

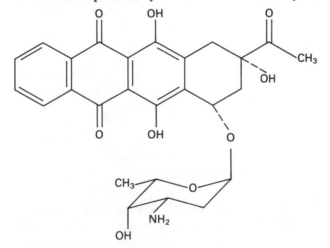

Molecular weight: 533.97.

Formula: $C_{26}H_{27}NO_9HCl$.

Solubility: Idarubicin is sparingly soluble in water for injections, 5% glucose and 0.9% sodium chloride, slightly soluble in ethanol and practically insoluble in non-polar organic solvents.[3]

3 Stability Profile

Physical and chemical stability

The manufacturer states that the reconstituted solution is chemically stable for at least 48 hours at 2 to 8°C and 24 hours at room temperature.[1] Very few data on the long-term stability of idarubicin are available.

The stability of the anthracyclines is dependent on a number of factors, including the pH of the medium. They are also light sensitive and adsorb onto glass and certain plastics.

Effect of pH: The rate of cleavage of the glycosidic bond in acidic media is strongly dependent on structural modifications in the amino sugar moiety and unaffected by structural modifications in the aglycone portion of the molecule.[4] As daunorubicin and idarubicin both possess daunosamine as the sugar moiety, the rate of degradation of these three analogues in acidic solution is expected to be similar. There are no published data available to confirm this hypothesis.

Acidic hydrolysis of idarubicin, which is shown in Figure 1, is expected to yield a red-coloured, water-insoluble aglycone, 4-demethoxydaunorubicinone, and a water-soluble amino sugar, daunosamine.

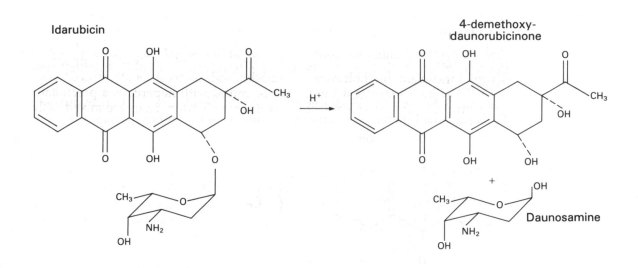

Figure 1: *Proposed degradation pathway for idarubicin in acidic solution*

In alkaline solution, the rate of degradation of the anthracyclines is affected by structural modifications in the aglycone portion of the molecule and unaffected by structural modifications in the amino sugar moiety.[4] As idarubicin possesses a unique aglycone, 4-demethoxydaunorubicinone, its stability in alkaline media cannot be predicted from existing data for the other anthracyclines. The manufacturers recommend that prolonged contact of idarubicin with any solution of alkaline pH should be avoided as it will result in degradation.[1]

Effect of light: Data on the photodegradation of doxorubicin have been published[5] but there are no data available for idarubicin. The rates of photodegradation of doxorubicin, daunorubicin and epirubicin have been reported to be similar and may be substantial at concentrations below 100 µg/ml if solutions are exposed to light for sufficient time.[6] At higher concentrations, such as those used for cancer chemotherapy (at least 500 µg/ml), no special precautions are necessary to protect freshly prepared solutions of doxorubicin, daunorubicin and epirubicin from light.[6] The manufacturers suggest that idarubicin is treated in a similar fashion to these other anthracyclines and that no precautions are necessary to protect freshly prepared solutions of idarubicin from light.[2]

Effect of temperature: A review of the literature reveals one well-controlled study, in which Beijnen *et al.*[7] reported that idarubicin was stable in polypropylene tubes, in 5% glucose (pH 4.7), 3.3% glucose with 0.3% sodium chloride (pH 4.4), lactated Ringer's solution (pH 6.8) and 0.9% sodium chloride (pH 7.0) for 28 days when stored in the dark at 25°C.

Container compatibility: Idarubicin is compatible with polypropylene, PVC and glass.[2] Doxorubicin, daunorubicin and epirubicin adsorb onto glass but not onto siliconized glass or polypropylene.[8,9] Therefore, idarubicin may behave in a similar manner. In clinical practice, when idarubicin is used at concentrations of at least 500 µg/ml, adsorptive losses during storage and delivery are expected to be negligible.

Compatibility with other drugs: Prolonged contact with any solution of alkaline pH should be avoided as it will result in degradation. Idarubicin has been observed to be physically incompatible with acyclovir, ceftazidime, clindamycin, dexamethasone, etoposide, frusemide, gentamicin, hydrocortisone, imipenem-cilastin, lorazepam, methotrexate, mezlocillin, sodium bicarbonate, vancomycin and vincristine.[10] Idarubicin should not be mixed with heparin as a precipitate may form.[1] The manufacturer recommends that no other drugs are mixed with idarubicin.[1]

Stability in clinical practice

Idarubicin (100 µg/ml) appears to be chemically stable for at least 28 days in 5% glucose, glucose/saline admixtures and 0.9% sodium chloride at 25°C.[7] After reconstitution, vials of idarubicin should be refrigerated and protected from light.[2]

4 Clinical Use

Main indications: Remission induction in untreated adults with acute non-lymphocytic leukaemia or for remission induction in relapsed or refractory patients. Idarubicin is also indicated in acute lymphocytic leukaemia as second line treatment in adults and children. It may be used in combination regimens with other cytotoxic agents.[1]

Dosage: Dosage is usually calculated on the basis of body surface area. The manufacturer gives the following recommendations for the intravenous preparation:

▼ Acute non-lymphocytic leukaemia: In adults, the dose schedule suggested is 12 mg/m² intravenously daily for three days in combination with cytarabine. Another dosage schedule in which idarubicin has been used as a single agent and in combination is 8 mg/m² intravenously daily for five days.

▼ Acute lymphocytic leukaemia: As a single agent the suggested dose is 12 mg/m² intravenously daily for three days in adults, and 10 mg/m² intravenously daily for three days in children.

Oral idarubicin has been used in various clinical trials in doses ranging from 20 mg/m² to 50 mg/m².[2,11]

All of the above dosage schedules should, however, take into account the haematological status of the patient and the dosages of other cytotoxic drugs when used in combination. Idarubicin therapy should not be started in patients with severe renal and liver impairment or patients with uncontrolled infections. In a number of phase III trials, treatment was not given if bilirubin levels exceeded 2 mg/100 ml. With other anthracyclines, a 50% dosage reduction is generally employed if bilirubin levels are in the range 1.2 to 2.0 mg/100 ml.[1]

On the basis of the recommended dosage schedules the total cumulative dose administered over two courses can be expected to reach 60 to 80 mg/m^2. Although a cumulative dosage limit cannot yet be defined, a specific cardiological evaluation in cancer patients showed no significant modifications of cardiac function in patients treated with idarubicin at a mean cumulative dosage of 93 mg/m^2.[1]

5 Preparation of Injection

Reconstitution: The contents of the 5 mg vial should be dissolved in 5 ml of water for injections and the 10 mg vial in 10 ml of the same solvent. After addition of the diluent and gentle shaking, the contents of the vial will dissolve to produce a solution of 1 mg/ml.[1]

Bolus administration: Administration is by the intravenous route only. The reconstituted solution should be given, over five to ten minutes, into the side arm of a freely-running intravenous infusion of 0.9% sodium chloride. This technique minimizes the risk of thrombosis or perivenous extravasation which can lead to severe cellulitis or necrosis.[1]

Intravenous infusion: The doses and duration of infusions of idarubicin that have been used in clinical trials range from 8 mg/m^2 to 16 mg/m^2 over four hours, 24 hours or 72 hours.[2,11–13]

Extravasation: Potent vesicant (*see* Chapter 9).

6 Destruction of Drug or Contaminated Articles

Incineration: 700°C.[2]

Chemical: 10% sodium hypochlorite (1% available chlorine) solution/24 hours.[1]

Contact with skin: Wash well with water, or soap and water. If the eyes are contaminated immediate irrigation with 0.9% sodium chloride should be carried out.[1]

References

1. *ABPI Data Sheet Compendium 1991–92.* (1991). Datapharm Publications Ltd, London, pp. 470–471.
2. Farmitalia Carlo Erba Ltd. Personal communication.
3. *Idarubicin: Summary of preclinical studies up to March 1980.* (1992). Cagnasso, M.G. (ed.), Farmitalia Carlo-Erba Ltd.
4. Beijnen, J.H. *et al.* (1986). Aspects of the degradation kinetics of doxorubicin in aqueous solution. *Int. J. Pharm.* **32**, 123–131.
5. Tavoloni, N. *et al.* (1980). Photolytic degradation of adriamycin. *J. Pharm. Pharmacol.* **32**, 860–862.

6. Wood, M.J. *et al.* (1990). Photodegradation of doxorubicin, daunorubicin and epirubicin measured by high-performance liquid chromatography. *J. Clin. Pharm. Ther.* **15**, 291–300.
7. Beijnen, J.H. *et al.* (1985). Stability of anthracycline antitumor agents in infusion fluids. *J. Parenter. Sci. Technol.* **39**, 220–222.
8. Bosanquet, A.G. (1986). Stability of solutions of antineoplastic agents during preparation and storage for *in vitro* assays: II. Assay methods, adriamycin and the other antitumour antibiotics. *Cancer Chemother. Pharmacol.* **17**, 1–10.
9. Wood, M.J. (1989). M.Phil. Thesis, University of Aston, Birmingham, UK.
10. Turowski, R.C. and Durthaler, J.M. (1991). Visual compatibility of idarubicin hydrochloride with selected drugs during simulated Y-site injection. *Am. J. Hosp. Pharm.* **48**, 2181–2184.
11. Speth, P.A.J. *et al.* (1986). Plasma and human leukaemic cell pharmacokinetics of oral and intravenous 4-demethoxydaunomycin. *Clin. Pharmacol. Ther.* **40**, 643–649.
12. Speth, P.A.J. *et al.* (1989). Idarubicin *vs* daunorubicin: Pre-clinical and clinical pharmacokinetic studies. *Semin. Oncol.* **16(Suppl.2)**, 2–9.
13. Vogler, W.R. *et al.* (1988). A phase III trial comparing daunorubicin or idarubicin combined with cytosine arabinoside in acute myelogenous leukaemia (AML). Abstract of two symposia, *XXII Congress of the International Society of Haematology*, Milan, Italy.

Prepared by M.J. Wood

IFOSFAMIDE

1 General Details

Approved names: Ifosfamide, iphosphamide, isophosphamide.

Proprietary name: Mitoxana.

Manufacturer or supplier: ASTA Medica Ltd.

Presentation and formulation details: White freeze-dried powder in glass vials containing 500 mg, 1 g or 2 g ifosfamide. Contains no excipients.

Storage and shelf-life of unopened container: Vials should be stored below 25°C, protected from light;[1] the intact vials are stable for at least five years at 22 to 25°C.[2]

2 Chemistry

Type: Nitrogen mustard.

Molecular structure: N,3-(2-chloroethyl)tetrahydro-2H-1,2,3 Oxaphosphorin-2-amine.

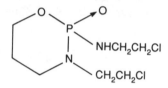

Molecular weight: 261.1.

Solubility: In water: 1 in 10; in methylene chloride up to 1 g/ml and in carbon disulphide 15 mg/ml. Readily soluble in ethanol.

3 Stability Profile

Physical and chemical stability

Ifosfamide is relatively stable after reconstitution.

Effect of pH: No information available.

Effect of light: Infusions should be protected from light during storage. Light protection during administration is not necessary.

Container compatibility: Compatible with glass, PVC and polypropylene containers.[3]

Compatibility with other drugs: Compatible with mesna (*see* Mesna monograph for details). No further information is available.

Reconstitution of ifosfamide with water for injections containing benzyl alcohol (0.9%) results in the formation of two separate liquid phases.[4] Ifosfamide should, therefore, be reconstituted with unpreserved water for injections.

Stability in clinical practice

Reconstituted solutions are chemically stable for seven days at room temperature and for six weeks under refrigeration.[2,3] Ifosfamide infusion 50 mg/ml in

10 ml polypropylene syringes showed no drug loss over seven days at 4 and 20°C.[5] Combinations of ifosamide (50 mg/ml) and mesna (40 mg/ml) in 10 ml syringes were stable for 28 days at 4 and 20°C.[5] Ifosamide (50 mg/ml) and combinations of ifosamide with mesna (each 50 mg/ml) showed no drug loss at 37°C over 24 hours.[6] In a further study,[7] ifosamide in aqueous solution (either alone or mixed with mesna) was found to be stable for nine days when stored in a dark environment at 27°C. Ifosamide, 20, 40 or 80 mg/ml in 0.9% sodium chloride, or 80 mg/ml in water for injections, was also reported to be stable for 8 days at 35°C stored in 100 ml PVC medication cassettes (Pharmacia device).[8]

Dilution of the reconstituted solution to ifosamide concentrations of 16 and 0.6 mg/ml in the following intravenous infusion solutions resulted in 1 to 5% decomposition over seven days at room temperature and no decomposition over six weeks under refrigeration:[2]

5% glucose in Ringer's injection, lactated
5% glucose in 0.9% sodium chloride
glucose in water
Ringer's injection, lactated
0.45% sodium chloride
0.9% sodium chloride
1/6 M sodium lactate

4 Clinical Use

Type of cytotoxic agent: Alkylating agent of the nitrogen-mustard type, activated by hepatic microsomal enzymes to produce anti-tumour metabolites.

Main indications: Tumours of the lung, ovary, cervix, breast and testis and soft-tissue sarcoma. Ifosamide also produces response in osteosarcoma, malignant lymphoma, carcinoma of the pancreas, head and neck tumours and acute leukaemias (except AML).

Dosage: Ifosamide should not be used without the concurrent administration of mesna (*see* Mesna monograph).

The usual dose for each course is 8 to 10 g/m^2, equally fractionated as single daily doses over five days or alternatively, 5 to 6 g/m^2 (maximum of 10 g) administered as a 24-hour infusion. Courses are normally repeated at intervals of two to four weeks for intermittent therapy or three to four weeks for 24-hour infusions. The white cell count should not be less than $4 \times 10^3/mm^3$ and the platelet count not less than $100 \times 10^3/mm^3$ before starting each course. Usually, four courses are given but up to seven (six by 24 hour infusion) have been administered.

5 Preparation of Injection

Reconstitution: The injection should be reconstituted to give a solution of approximately 8% (80 mg/ml) using:

▼ 6.5 ml water for injections with 500 mg ifosamide
▼ 12.5 ml water for injections with 1 g ifosamide
▼ 25 ml water for injections with 2 g ifosamide.

Bolus administration: Dilute to less than 4% and inject into the vein with the patient supine or inject directly into a fast-running infusion.

Intravenous infusion: Infuse in 5% glucose, glucose-saline or 0.9% sodium chloride infusion over 30 to 120 minutes, or infuse over 24 hours in 3 × 1 l glucose-saline or 0.9% sodium chloride. Increased doses of mesna are recommended in children and in patients with urothelial damage from previous therapies (*see* monograph on mesna).

Extravasation: Non-irritant.

6 Destruction of Drug or Contaminated Waste

Incineration: 1000°C.

Chemical: 2 N sodium hydroxide in dimethyl formamide/24 hours.

Contact with skin: Wash with water.

7 References

1. *ABPI Data Sheet Compendium 1991–92.* (1991). Datapharm Publications Ltd, London, pp. 365–366.
2. Trissell, L.A. *et al.* (1979). Investigational drug information: ifosfamide and semustine. *Drug Intell. Clin. Pharm.* **13**, 340–343.
3. Trissel, L.A. *et al.* (1985). *Investigational drugs pharmaceutical data.* NCI. Bethesda, Maryland, USA.
4. Behme, R.J. *et al.* (1988). Incompatibility of ifosfamide with benzyl-alcohol-preserved bacteriostatic water for injections. *Am. J. Hosp. Pharm.* **45**, 627–628.
5. Adams, P.S. *et al.* (1987). Pharmaceutical aspects of home infusion therapy for cancer patients. *Pharm, J.* **238**, 476–478.
6. Sewell, G.J. and Palmer, A. (1987). Internal report of Exeter Health Authority. *Cytotoxic drugs – stability under in-use conditions.*
7. Radford, J.A. *et al.* (1990). The stability of ifosfamide in aqueous solution and its suitability for continuous 7-day infusion by ambulatory pump. *Cancer Chemother. Pharmacol.* **26**, 144–146.
8. Munoz, M. *et al.* (1992). Stability of ifosfamide in 0.9% sodium chloride solution in water for injection in a portable IV pump cassette. *Am. J. Hosp. Pharm.* **49**, 1137–1139.

Prepared by G.J. Sewell

MELPHALAN

1 General Details

Approved names: Melphalan, phenylalanine mustard, L-sarcolysine.

Proprietary name: Alkeran.

Manufacturer or supplier: Wellcome Medical Division.

Presentation and formulation details: 100 mg sterile anhydrous melphalan BP in 20 ml vial with an ampoule of solvent containing 1.8 ml of 0.086 ml hydrochloric acid in 36% ethanol and an ampoule of sterile diluent containing 108 mg dipotassium phosphate, 6 ml propylene glycol and water for injections to 9 ml.

Storage and shelf-life of unopened container: The shelf-life is three years when stored between 15 and 25°C and protected from light.

2 Chemistry

Type: Alkylating agent related to nitrogen mustard.

Molecular structure: 4-[bis(2-chloroethyl)amino]-L-phenylalanine.

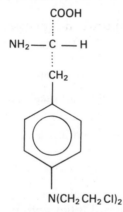

Molecular weight: 305.2 (base); 345.9 (hydrochloride).

Solubility: Practically insoluble in water, soluble in ethanol.

3 Stability Profile

Physical and chemical stability

The reconstituted drug is relatively unstable. The rate of degradation is influenced by temperature, aqueous vehicle and pH.[1] The degradation products are also less water-soluble than melphalan and a precipitate may form on standing, especially in the reconstituted vial.[2] The reconstituted injection retains 90% of its initial potency for approximately 19 hours.

Effect of pH: The drug is most stable at pH 3.0, stability is slightly reduced at pH 5 to 7 but substantially reduced at pH 9.0. Data from Tabibi and Cradock (1984)[2] have quantified this effect:

pH (buffer)	$t_{1/2}$
3.0	5.3 h
5.0	4.9 h
7.0	4.8 h
9.0	3.9 h

The addition of reconstituted injection to infusions will tend to acidify such solutions. The pH of infusions after adding melphalan injection (final concentration 40 μg/ml) are as follows:[1]

infusion fluid	pH
5% glucose	4.1
0.9% sodium chloride	4.2
Ringer's lactate	5.9

Effect of chloride ions: Studies have shown that chloride reduces the rate of hydrolysis of melphalan.[1,3,4,5] For example, $t_{90\%}$ of melphalan in 5% glucose is 1.5 hours and in 0.9% sodium chloride is 4.5 hours at 20°C. Hydrophobic interaction of melphalan with propylene glycol also contributes to greater stability.[5]

Studies[1] provide some evidence of the significance of storage temperature on rates of degradation. Increasing the temperature from 15 to 20°C raised the degradation rate by approximately 25% in various infusion fluids. Unfortunately no studies were conducted under refrigerated storage, but the manufacturer suggests the drug may precipitate on refrigeration.

Effect of light: No information available.

Degradation pathways: Melphalan is degraded to mono-hydroxy-melphalan (II), and then to di-hydroxy-melphalan (III).[2] The kinetics can be described as pseudo-first order (*see* Figure 1).[1,4]

Degradation products are said to be much less cytotoxic.[6]

Container compatibility: Melphalan is compatible with plastic containers, administration sets and plastic syringes.[6]

Compatibility with other drugs: No further information available.

Stability in clinical practice

Reconstituted vials must be used or further diluted within 30 minutes.[7] They can be further diluted on 0.9% sodium chloride and infused over two hours. The diluted drug should not be stored for longer than two hours at ambient temperature (refrigeration may cause precipitation). Melphalan is not absorbed by in-line filters.[8] It is also suggested that solutions of melphalan can be stored frozen in 0.9% sodium chloride for six months without undergoing significant degradation.[8]

No special precautions are required to protect the injection from normal lighting conditions; however, exposure to strong daylight should be avoided.

4 Clinical Use

Type of cytotoxic: Alkylating agent.

Main indications: Localized malignant melanomas; localized soft tissue sarcoma of the extremities.

Dosage: 1 mg/kg administered intravenously every four weeks, or by intra-arterial perfusion of 70 to 100 mg through the part of the body affected by the tumour.

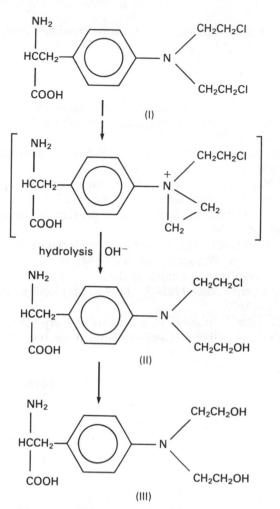

Figure 1: *Degradation of melphalan, 1st-step hydrolysis*

5 Preparation of Injection

Reconstitution: Add 1.8 ml acid-alcohol solvent to the vial containing 100 mg melphalan. Shake to dissolve (about two minutes), then add 9 ml diluent and shake.

Bolus administration: Inject within 30 minutes of preparation into the tubing of a fast-running infusion.

Infusion of local tissue by perfusion: Dilute in up to 500 ml of 0.9% sodium chloride to give a solution containing 0.4 mg/ml, and infuse slowly over two hours.[8] Consult relevant literature for details and alternative methods of tissue perfusion.

Extravasation: Not very irritant (*see* Chapter 9).

6 Destruction of Drug or Contaminated Articles

Incineration: 500°C.

Chemical: 5% sodium thiosulphate in sodium hydroxide solution/24 hours.
Contact with skin: Wash with water.

References

1. Flora, K.P. *et al.* (1979). Application of a simple HPLC method for the determination of melphalan in the presence of its hydrolysis products. *J. Chromatogr.* **177**, 91–97.
2. Tabibi, S.E. and Cradock, J.C. (1984). Stability of melphalan in infusion fluids. *Am. J. Hosp. Pharm.* **41**, 1380–1382.
3. Trissel, L.A. (1992). *Handbook on injectable drugs,* 7th edn. American Society of Hospital Pharmacists, Bethesda, Maryland, USA.
4. Chang, S.Y. *et al.* (1978). Hydrolysis and protein binding of melphalan. *J. Pharm. Sci.* **67**, 682–684.
5. Chang, S.Y. *et al.* (1979). The stability of melphalan in the presence of chloride ions. *J. Pharm. Pharmacol.* **31**, 853–854.
6. Calmic Medical Division. Unpublished data.
7. *ABPI Data Sheet Compendium 1991–92.* (1991). Datapharm Publications Ltd, London, pp. 1671–1672.
8. Bosanquet, A.G. (1985). Stability of solutions of melphalan during preparation and storage for *in vitro* chemosensitivity assays. *J. Pharm. Sci.* **74**, 348–351.

Prepared by M.C. Allwood

MESNA

1 General Details

Approved name: Mesna.

Proprietary name: Uromitexan.

Manufacturer or supplier: ASTA Medica Ltd.

Presentation and formulation details: Clear glass ampoules containing an aqueous solution of mesna, 400 mg in 4 ml and 1000 mg in 10 ml.[1]

Each ampoule also contains disodium edetate 0.25 mg/ml and sodium hydroxide as buffer.

Storage and shelf-life of unopened container: When stored below 30°C and protected from light, mensa has a shelf-life of five years.[1]

2 Chemistry

Type: Sulphydryl compound (not cytotoxic).

Molecular structure: sodium 2-mercapto-ethanesulphonate, HS-CH -CH -SO .Na.

Molecular weight: 164.2.

Solubility: Water soluble.

3 Stability Profile

Physical and chemical stability

Mesna degrades by oxidation to form dimesna. Mesna should be protected from light, but it is stable under normal lighting conditions during administration.[2]

Container compatibility: Compatible with glass, PVC and polypropylene.

Compatibility with other drugs: Compatible with ifosfamide in 0.9% sodium chloride, 5% glucose and Ringer's lactate infusions.[2]

Stability in clinical practice

Mesna is stable for up to 24 hours in a solution of 0.9% sodium chloride or in a solution of ifosfamide in 0.9% sodium chloride.[1] Mesna (3.3 g and 5 g/l) and ifosfamide (also at concentrations of 3.3 g and 5 g/l, respectively) were admixed in 5% glucose solution and Ringer's lactate injection. Mesna exhibited approximately 5% decomposition over 24 hours while ifosfamide showed no decomposition during this period.[2]

Admixtures of mesna (40 mg/ml) and ifosfamide (50 mg/ml) in water for injections (10 ml) were stable in polypropylene syringes at 4 and 20°C over 28 days, with less than 5% loss of each component present.[3] At 50 mg/ml the admixture was stable for 24 hours at 37°C,[4] thus enabling ambulatory continuous infusion of this regimen. The undiluted formulation of mesna was found to be stable when stored in polypropylene syringes at 5, 24 or 35°C for at least nine days.[5] (Mesna was also stable for at least one week when diluted 1:2 with various syrups for oral use and stored at 24°C.[5] Dilutions of mesna ranging from 1:2 to 1:100 in a variety of carbonated drinks, fruit juice and milk which were stored at 4°C exhibited no clinically significant change in drug concentration.[5])

4 Clinical Use

Type of cytotoxic: Non-cytotoxic, used in the prophylaxis of urothelial toxicity in patients treated with ifosfamide and cyclophosphamide.

Main indications: Cancer chemotherapy in combination with ifosfamide and cyclophosphamide.

Dosage: Where ifosfamide and cyclophosphamide are used as an intravenous bolus injection, mesna is given over 15 minutes at 20% w/w of the oxazaphosphorine and repeated after four and eight hours. The total dose = 60% w/w of oxazaphosphorine dose. This can be increased to 40% w/w given at 0, 3, 6 and 9 hours (total 160% w/w of oxazaphosphorine dose) in children and patients with damaged urothelium.

Where ifosfamide is used as a 24 hour infusion, mesna is used as a concurrent infusion. Initially, 20% (w/w) of the total ifosfamide dose is given as an intravenous bolus injection, then ifosfamide is infused over 24 hours, followed by a further 12 hour infusion of 60% w/w of the ifosfamide dose. This 12 hour infusion can be replaced with bolus injections at 28, 32, 36 hours, each of 20% of the ifosfamide dose, or by oral mesna.

Oral mesna can be used with intermittent oxazaphosphorine therapy or following 24 hour infusion.

The first dose of 40% w/w of mensa is given with the oxazaphosphorine or as the infusion is stopped and repeated at four and eight hours.

5 Preparation of Injection

Dilution: Use undiluted for bolus administration. Add to oxazaphosphorine infusion for 24 hour infusion regimens. For oral administration, mesna should be taken in a soft drink immediately after opening the ampoule.

Bolus administration: Mesna is given over 15 minutes as 20% of the oxazaphosphorine dose and is repeated after four and eight hours.

Intravenous infusion: Mesna is given as a concurrent infusion. Initially 20% of the oxazaphosphorine dose is given by intravenous bolus injection, followed by the oxazaphosphorine dose over 24 hours. A further infusion of 60% w/w of the oxazaphosphorine dose is then given.

Extravasation: Non-irritant.

6 Destruction of Drug or Contaminated Articles

Mesna is not cytotoxic.

References

1. *ABPI Data Sheet Compendium 1991–92.* (1991). Datapharm Publications Ltd, London, p. 369.
2. Trissel, L.A. *et al.* (1985). *Investigational drugs pharmaceutical data.* NCI, Bethesda, Maryland, USA.
3. Adams, P.S. *et al.* (1987). Pharmaceutical aspects of home infusion therapy for cancer patients. *Pharm. J.* **238**, 476–478.
4. Sewell, G.J. and Palmer, A. (1987). Internal report of Exeter Health Authority. *Cytotoxic drugs – stability under in-use conditions.*
5. Goren, M.P. *et al.* (1991). The stability of mesna in beverages and syrup for oral administration. *Cancer Chemother. Pharmacol.* **28**, 298–301.

Prepared by G.J. Sewell

METHOTREXATE

1 General Details

Approved name: Methotrexate.

Proprietary name: Methotrexate Injection, Methotrexate Powder for Injection.

Manufacturer or supplier: Lederle Laboratories Ltd, David Bull Laboratories Ltd (DBL).

Presentation and formulation details:

Methotrexate (Lederle): Solution for injection: A clear, yellow, aqueous, isotonic solution containing methotrexate sodium equivalent to 2.5 mg/ml (ampoule), 5 mg/2 ml, 25 mg/ml, 50 mg/2 ml, 100 mg/4 ml, 200 mg/8 ml, 500 mg/20 ml, 1 g/40 ml, 5 g/200 ml of methotrexate per vial, together with sodium chloride and sodium hydroxide to adjust the pH to approximately 8.5. Powder for injection: Vials containing yellow, lyophilized powder of methotrexate sodium, equivalent to 500 mg of methotrexate, which is reconstituted before use with 10 ml of water for injections. Sodium hydroxide and, if necessary, hydrochloric acid are used during the manufacturing process to adjust the pH to approximately 8.5. All formulations are preservative-free.

Methotrexate Injection (DBL): A clear, yellow solution of methotrexate in water for injections with sodium chloride to make the solution isotonic. The pH of the solution is 8.4. It is available in the following strengths and packs: 5 mg/2 ml, 50 mg/2 ml, 100 mg/4 ml, 500 mg/20 ml, 1 g/10 ml, 5 g/50 ml. All solutions are preservative-free.

Storage and shelf-life of unopened containers: Methotrexate preparations (Lederle) should be stored at controlled room temperature (15–30°C) and protected from direct sunlight. The 25 mg/ml solution has a shelf-life of three years from the date of manufacture. All other preparations have a shelf-life of two years from the date of manufacture.

Methotrexate Injection (DBL) should be stored below 25°C. It should be protected from light and freezing. All preparations have a shelf-life of two years from the date of manufacture.

2 Chemistry

Type: 4-amino-N-methyl analogue of folic acid.

Molecular structure:

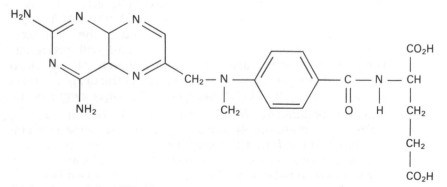

Molecular weight: 454.44.

Solubility: Practically insoluble in water. Very soluble in dilute solutions of alkaline hydroxides and carbonates.[1]

3 Stability Profile

Physical and chemical stability

Methotrexate is relatively stable in aqueous solution provided the recommended storage conditions are observed. The compound is susceptible both to hydrolytic and photolytic degradation. The rate of hydrolytic degradation increases with increase in pH, with minimum degradation occurring between pH 6.6–8.2.[2]

Degradation pathways: The major hydrolytic degradation compound is N-methyl-pteroylglutamic acid (methopterin). The major photolytic degradation compounds are p-aminobenzoylglutamic acid and 2-amino-4-hydroxypteridine-6-carboxylic acid.[3]

Effect of light: The drug is light sensitive and forms a yellow precipitate on prolonged exposure to direct sunlight. Polypropylene and styrene acrylonitrile syringes provide better light protection than glass ampoules when the drug is stored under controlled light conditions at 25°C.[4] In all cases, no precipitate was observed over a seven-day storage period. Samples stored in the dark showed no evidence of precipitation.[4]

McElnay *et al.*[5] studied the photodegradation of methotrexate 0.1% w/v in 0.9% w/v sodium chloride in three burette administration systems (a standard set, a 'light-protective' Amberset and a 'low adsorption' Sureset (Avon Medical)). Storage under normal lighting conditions (diffuse daylight/fluorescent tube room lighting) led to little change in drug concentration over the first 24 hours of storage although a decrease in concentration (maximum 12%) was noted in both the standard sets and Suresets by 48 hours. A much more rapid decrease in methotrexate concentration was demonstrated when the drug solution was exposed to sunlight. An 11% decline in methotrexate concentration occurred in the standard sets in seven hours (Suresets not investigated). The use of Ambersets or wrapping the standard sets in tinfoil prevented photodegradation over this period. Storage in the administration tubing of all three sets under normal lighting conditions resulted in greater than 10% degradation within 12 hours in the standard sets and Suresets and within 48 hours in the light-protected Suresets and Ambersets. All these results were obtained for a static system and it is difficult to extrapolate them to the dynamic situation of an intravenous administration.

Effect of pH: Methotrexate is a bicarboxylic acid with pK_a's in the range 4.8–5.5.[6] Hence, it is essentially ionized at physiological pH. At pH values between 2.6 and 6.6 the drug is converted to the bicarboxylic acid which is relatively insoluble in aqueous solution and will precipitate. Commercially available injection is stabilized to approximately pH 8.4, however, dilution in acidic solutions may result in precipitation of the drug. For this reason, dilutions in 5% glucose should be checked carefully for evidence of precipitation.

Container compatibility: At a pH value of 8.4, methotrexate injection is largely ionized and, therefore, is unlikely to exhibit sorption phenomena.

McElnay *et al.*[5] found the sorption of methotrexate, 0.1% w/v in 0.9% w/v sodium chloride, stored in 'low sorption' Suresets and standard or Ambersets (Avon Medical) to be negligible but were unable to explain the greater than 10% loss of drug when methotrexate was stored in light-protected polybutadiene and

PVC tubing for 48 hours at room temperature. No other studies have shown significant sorption to PVC containers. The sorption of methotrexate in 5% glucose to the latex reservoir of Baxter Infusors was also found to be negligible.[7]

Methotrexate 50 mg/100 ml, 0.9% w/v sodium chloride was not absorbed by a 0.2 μm endotoxin-retentive end-line filter (Pall Intravenous Set Saver, Pall Biomedical Ltd) when infused at a rate of 80 ml/hr.[8]

Although extraction into solution is possible, especially with plastic syringes, the extent and rate of leaching is likely to be low at room temperature.[9,10] It should be noted, however, that 2-mercaptobenzothiazole (a mercaptan present in the rubber plunger) is soluble in alkali and alkali carbonate solutions[11] and may leach into the alkaline methotrexate injection on prolonged storage in plastic syringes. Mercaptans may cause problems as analytical or toxicological contaminants.

Compatibility with other drugs: D'Arcy[12] found methotrexate to be chemically and physically incompatible with cytarabine, fluorouracil and prednisolone sodium phosphate. However, two other studies have shown the drug to be compatible and stable with cytarabine and fluorouracil under defined storage conditions. In the first study[13] the stability of cytarabine, methotrexate sodium and hydrocortisone sodium succinate admixtures was investigated. Two admixtures: (cytarabine 50 mg, methotrexate 12 mg (as the sodium salt) and hydrocortisone 25 mg (as the sodium succinate salt); and cytarabine 30 mg, methotrexate 12 mg (as the sodium salt) and hydrocortisone 15 mg (as the sodium succinate salt)) were prepared in one of four diluents (Elliott's B solution, 0.9% sodium chloride, 5% glucose and lactated Ringer's). The drugs were reconstituted according to manufacturers' instructions with the infusion fluid under test. After reconstitution the drug solutions were mixed in the desired proportions and diluted to 12 ml with the respective infusion fluid. Each admixture was filtered through a 0.45 μm membrane filter and placed in a 12 ml disposable syringe (type of plastic not identified) and kept at 25 ± 0.1°C in a water bath. Cytarabine and methotrexate were stable in the fluids studied for 24 hours at 25°C. Alteration in stability related to vehicles or drug concentration combinations was not evident and the stability of each of the drugs did not appear to be affected by the presence of the other two drugs. Hydrocortisone sodium succinate was found to be less stable in Elliott's B solution, with only 94.1% of the drug remaining in the first admixture, and 86% remaining in the second after 24 hours. Alkaline catalysis may explain the increased degradation of the drug in Elliott's B solution, which has a higher pH than the other vehicles. No precipitation was observed in either group of admixtures during 8 hours at 25°C, although storage for several days resulted in some precipitation. The nature of the precipitate was not identified.

At the concentrations studied, cytarabine, methotrexate and hydrocortisone sodium succinate may be mixed in 0.9% sodium chloride, 5% glucose or lactated Ringer's and stored in plastic disposable syringes for up to 24 hours at 25°C. Admixtures in Elliott's B solution should be used within 10 hours.

The second study[14] investigated the compatibility and stability of cyclophosphamide, methotrexate and 5-fluorouracil in a three-drug admixture. Cyclophosphamide (100 mg), methotrexate (1.5 mg), and 5-fluorouracil (500 mg) were reconstituted in a total volume of 60 ml of 0.9% sodium chloride. The solution was maintained at room temperature in PVC plastic reservoir bags (Lifecare 1500 System, Abbott). No significant loss of 5-fluorouracil or methotrexate was observed up to 14 days after reconstitution of the three-drug admixture. However, a 9.3% loss of cyclophosphamide was observed, accompanied by the appearance of a degradation product in the HPLC chromatogram after seven days. Control admixtures indicated that the cyclophosphamide and methotrexate were chemically incompatible and that there was a pH change in this admixture from 6.6 to 4.57. At this pH methotrexate stability is compromised.

Based on this information, it may be possible to administer cyclophosphamide, methotrexate and 5-fluorouracil as a three-drug admixture in an infusion pump, in the proportions reported, for up to seven days. However, solutions should be checked carefully for precipitation and such admixtures should not be used in implantable infusion pumps.

In addition, Trissel[15] lists a wide range of compatibility information. Although useful for reference purposes, much of the data relates to short-term physical compatibility of admixtures in the laboratory setting and is not applicable clinically.

Stability in clinical practice

Although the manufacturers do not recommend re-use of the methotrexate injection after opening, its relative stability in aqueous solution would suggest that, provided the injection is manipulated under aseptic conditions and is stored in the original container at 4–8°C in the absence of light once opened, chemical and physical stability will be preserved. In general, a shelf-life of one month at 4°C after opening would seem to be satisfactory.

Infusions: Information on the stability of the drug, when diluted in the recommended solutions for infusion, is variable. The manufacturers are limited by the terms of their product licences to recommend a maximum shelf-life of 24 hours at 25°C. However, a number of reports suggest that methotrexate is stable over a wide range of concentrations when stored in Viaflex (Baxter) containers for longer than 24 hours.[16–20] In particular, work carried out by Baxter Laboratories[17] indicated that, at a concentration of 1–10 mg/ml in 5% glucose and 1.25–12.5 mg/ml in 0.9% sodium chloride infusions, methotrexate is stable (< 10% degradation) for up to one month at 4°C and five days at 25°C when stored in both Baxter Infusors and Viaflex minibags. More recent data[18] indicate that solutions of methotrexate ranging from 1.25–12.5 mg/ml reconstituted with 0.9% sodium chloride are chemically stable for at least 15 days in the Baxter Infusor when stored at 4°C. However, due to lack of stability data at 33°C, the company advise that methotrexate is delivered using the half-day Infusor only.

Further studies[19] on the stability of methotrexate 1.25–12.5 mg/ml in 0.9% sodium chloride, stored in both glass and PVC containers (Viaflex, Baxter), have shown that the drug is physically and chemically stable for up to 15 weeks at 4°C followed by one week's storage at room temperature.

Although there is some evidence that methotrexate infusion solutions prepared in Viaflex (Baxter) minibags can be frozen to −20°C and stored for at least three months without significant reduction in methotrexate concentration or change in pH,[20] the use of microwave ovens to thaw solutions prior to use should not be undertaken without careful validation of the thawing process.

Syringe storage: Methotrexate injection, at a concentration of 50 mg/ml or less, stored in sealed Monoject (Sherwood Medical) or Plastipak (Becton-Dickinson) plastic disposable syringes in the absence of light at a temperature not exceeding 25°C, is stable (<10% degradation) for a period of up to eight months.[4] Storage in Sabre (Gillette) and Steriseal (NI Ltd) syringes should not exceed 70 days.[4]

Ambulatory infusion pumps: Methotrexate, over the concentration range 0.33–10.0 mg/ml in 0.9% w/v sodium chloride stored in an implantable infusion pump (Model 400, Shiley Infusaid Inc.) at 37°C, was found to be stable for up to 12 days.[21] The solutions were filtered through a 5 μm filter prior to addition to the pump.

Methotrexate (Lederle) at a concentration of 25 mg/ml in 0.9% sodium chloride stored in a Medication Cassette reservoir (Pharmacia Deltec) exhibited no evidence of degradation over seven days' storage at 25°C and 14 days' storage at 5°C.[22]

4 Clinical Use

Type of cytotoxic: Antimetabolite.

Main indications: Meningeal leukaemia, choriocarcinoma, non-Hodgkin's lymphomas, solid tumours, severe psoriasis.

Dosage and administration: Methotrexate injection may be given by the intramuscular, intravenous (bolus injection or infusion), intrathecal, intra-arterial or intraventricular routes. Subcutaneous administration of methotrexate has been evaluated.[23] Methotrexate administered by this route is well tolerated and well absorbed. Intratumour administration using implantable catheters and subcutaneous refillable pumps has also been investigated.[21]

Dosages vary considerably depending on the condition being treated and are based on the patient's body weight or surface area,[24] except in the case of intrathecal or intraventricular administration, when a maximum dose of 15 mg is recommended.

It must be noted that all preparations of methotrexate (Lederle) are suitable for intrathecal use, although it is recommended that only the low volume preparations are used to avoid possible confusion. Methotrexate Injection (DBL), 500 mg/20 ml, 1 g/10 ml and 5 g/50 ml, are not suitable for intrathecal use. The 1 g/10 ml and 5 g/50 ml solutions are hypertonic.

High doses may cause the precipitation of methotrexate and its metabolites in the renal tubules. Alkalinization of the urine to pH 6.5–7.0 by the oral or intravenous administration of sodium bicarbonate (eg 5 × 625 mg tablets every three hours) or acetazolamide (500 mg orally four times a day) is recommended as a preventive measure.[24]

Doses greater than 100 mg should be given by IV infusion over a period not exceeding 24 hours. Lower doses may be given by rapid IV bolus injection over two to three minutes or by infusion. The concentration of the final injection is not critical.

5 Preparation of Injection

Dilution: The drug may be diluted in 0.9% sodium chloride, 5% glucose, glucose/saline, compound sodium chloride, compound sodium lactate infusions or Elliott's B solution.

Extravasation: Irritant but does not cause tissue damage (*see* Chapter 9).

6 Destruction of Drug or Contaminated Articles

Incineration: 1000°C.[25]

Chemical: None recommended.

Contact with skin: Wash with water and soothe any transient stinging with a bland cream. Irrigate eyes with copious amounts of water or saline. If significant quantities are inhaled or injected, calcium folinate cover should be considered.

References

1. Anon. (1989). *The Extra Pharmacopoeia*, 29th edn. Reynolds, J.E.F. (ed.), The Pharmaceutical Press, London.
2. Hansen, J. *et al.* (1983). Kinetics of degradation of methotrexate in aqueous solution. *Int. J. Pharm.* **16**, 141–152.
3. Chatterji, D.C. and Gallelli, J.F. (1978). Thermal and photolytic decomposition of methotrexate in aqueous solution. *J. Pharm. Sci.* **67**, 526–531.
4. Wright, M.P. and Newton, J.M. (1988). Stability of methotrexate injection in prefilled plastic disposable syringes. *Int. J. Pharm.* **45**, 237–244.
5. McElnay, J.C. *et al.* (1988). Stability of methotrexate and vinblastine in burette administration sets. *Int. J. Pharm.* **47**, 239–247.
6. Bleyer, W.A. (1978). The clinical pharmacology of methotrexate. New applications of an old drug. *Cancer* **41**, 36–50.
7. Bertocchio, F. *et al.* (1986). Study of the viability of an infusion system. *J. Pharm. Clin.* **5**, 331–339.
8. Stevens, R.F. and Wilkins, K.M. (1989). Use of cytotoxic drugs with an endline filter: A study of four drugs commonly administered to paediatric patients. *J. Clin. Pharm. Ther.* **14**, 475–479.
9. Sherwood Medical Industries Ltd. (1984). Personal communication.
10. Gillette UK Ltd. (1984). Personal communication.
11. *The Merck Index*, 10th edn. (1983). Merck and Co. Inc., Rathway, New Jersey, USA.
12. D'Arcy, P.F. (1983). Reactions and interactions in handling anticancer drugs. *Drug Intell. Clin. Pharm.* **17**, 532–538.
13. Cheung, Y. *et al.* (1984). Stability of cytarabine, methotrexate sodium and hydrocortisone sodium succinate admixtures. *Am. J. Hosp. Pharm.* **41**, 1802–1806.
14. Lokich, J. *et al.* (1989). Cyclophosphamide, methotrexate, and 5-fluorouracil in a three-drug admixture. Phase I trial of 14-day continuous ambulatory infusion. *Cancer* **63**, 822–824.
15. Trissel, L.A. (1992). *Handbook on injectable drugs*, 7th edn. American Society of Hospital Pharmacists, Bethesda, Maryland, USA.
16. Roach, M. (1979). Methotrexate infusions. *Pharm. J.* **223**, 557.
17. Baxter Healthcare Ltd. (1985). Information chart.
18. Baxter Healthcare Ltd. (1992). Personal communication.
19. Vincke, B.J. *et al.* (1989). Extended stability of 5-fluorouracil and methotrexate solutions in PVC containers. *Int. J. Pharm.* **54**, 181–189.
20. Dyvik, O. *et al.* (1986). Methotrexate in infusion solutions: A stability test for the hospital pharmacy. *J. Clin. Hosp. Pharm.* **11**, 343–348.
21. Nierenberg, D. *et al.* (1991). Continuous intratumoral infusion of methotrexate for recurrent glioblastoma: A pilot study. *Neurosurgery* **28**, 752–761.

22. Landersjo, L. and Nyhammar, E. (1989). Stability and compatibility of methotrexate in medication cassettes. A study by Apoteksbolaget AB, Stockholm, Sweden.
23. Balis, F.M. *et al.* (1988). Pharmacokinetics of subcutaneous methotrexate. *J. Clin. Oncol.* **6**, 1882–1886.
24. *ABPI Data Sheet Compendium 1991–92.* (1991). Datapharm Publications Ltd, London, pp. 461–462, 737–738.
25. Bristol Myers Pharmaceuticals Ltd. (1985). Personal communication.

Prepared by M.P. Wright

MITOMYCIN

1 General Details

Approved names: Mitomycin C, Mitomycin X.

Proprietary name: Mitomycin C Kyowa.

Manufacturer or supplier: Martindale Pharmaceuticals Ltd.

Presentation and formulation details: Purple powder in vials containing 2 mg, 10 mg or 20 mg mitomycin C. The 2 mg vial contains 48 mg sodium chloride and the 10 mg vial contains 240 mg sodium chloride.

The diluent for the USP formulation is mannitol (Mutamycin, Bristol Laboratories Ltd).

Storage and shelf-life of unopened container: Four years at ambient temperature and protected from light.

2 Chemistry

Molecular Structure: 1 S-(1,8,8a,8b)-6-amino-8-(aminocarbonyl)oxy methyl-1,1, 2,8,8a,8b-hexahydro-methoxy-5-methyl-azirino 2′,3′,4,7, pyrrolo 1,2-indole-4, 7-dione.

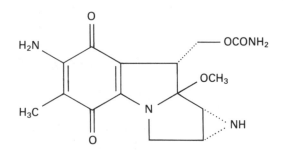

Molecular weight: 349.

Solubility: Sparingly soluble in water.

3 Stability Profile

Physical and chemical stability

Relatively unstable in aqueous solution, losing about 20% potency at room temperature in three days, according to the UK supplier. It should be noted that early studies[1] suggested that the reconstituted drug was stable for 72 hours at 2 to 6°C in water for injections. This information was not supported by adequate data. Stability is pH-dependent and is greatest between pH 7 and 8. Mitomycin is significantly less stable in acid conditions. One report has indicated a degradation rate constant of 5×10^{-6} s^{-1} at pH 4.9 and 20°C.[2]

Degradation pathways: See[2] for a recent summary.

In alkali the 7 amino group is replaced by an hydroxyl group while the remainder of the mitosane skeleton remains intact.

In acid the methoxy group is cleaved to form a 9-9a unsaturated bond. Also the 1,2 – fused aziridine ring is opened to give two isomeric compounds 1 and 2, with an hydroxyl group at position 1 and amino group at position 2:

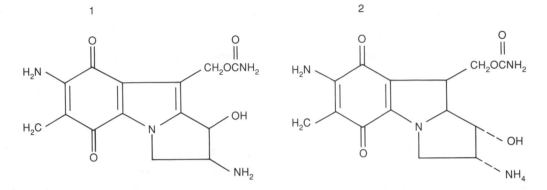

Degradation rate is related to temperature after reconstitution. The reconstituted drug is significantly more stable at 2 to 6°C compared to ambient conditions. However, solubility is reduced substantially in the refrigerator and solutions containing 0.5 mg/ml in water for injections may precipitate at 2 to 6°C. The reconstituted drug should be protected from daylight, although light-induced degradation would not normally be a significant factor during bolus administration.

Container compatibility: There is no information to indicate that stability or compatibility are affected by storage in plastic syringes.

Infusion containers: Studies suggest that stability is not greatly influenced by the nature of the container in which the drug is diluted (glass bottles, PVC containers, Viaflex), when the dilution vehicle is 0.9% sodium chloride infusion.[3]

Administration sets: No information available. However, the studies would suggest that mitomycin does not adsorb significantly to standard administration sets.[3]

Compatibility with other drugs: Mitomycin 10–50 µg/ml in 0.9% sodium chloride may be mixed with bleomycin 20–30 IU, if used immediately, but compatibility depends on concentration.[4] Some degradation of bleomycin was reported, mitomycin stability was not assessed. Trissel reported studies suggesting that mitomycin may be physically compatible with a number of other drugs.[1]

Stability in clinical practice

Current guidelines from the UK supplier recommend that reconstituted vials are stable for 12 hours if stored at room temperature. Refrigeration may cause precipitation and is not, therefore, recommended. The drug may be further diluted, preferably in 0.9% sodium chloride. In 5% glucose, the diluted infusion should be used immediately, whilst it may be stored for not more than 12 hours in 0.9% sodium chloride. Few studies have been reported on stability after dilution in infusion fluids. One report[3] indicates that degradation is more rapid in 5% glucose than in 0.9% sodium chloride. The studies suggest an initial rapid fall (about 10 to 15%) in content after dilution. However, these studies have not been repeated and remain controversial.

The stability of mitomycin was also studied in 0.9% sodium chloride and 5% glucose, with or without buffering, stored in PVC containers.[5] The drug, at a concentration of 50 µg/ml, was unstable in both (unbuffered) vehicles. There was about 75% degradation in 5% glucose after 12 hours storage at room temperature. In contrast, if vehicles were phosphate-buffered to pH 7.8, mitomycin appeared to be stable for more than 120 days at 5°C. These results, however, have been questioned.[6] In a further study, unbuffered solutions in 0.9% sodium chloride were reported to be stable when stored at −30°C for at least 28 days.[7] Sorption to PVC containers does not appear to occur.[8] Mitomycin 0.5 mg/ml in water for injections, stored at 2–6°C, may precipitate.[9]

4 Clinical Use

Type of cytotoxic: Anti-tumour antibiotic.

Main indications: Bladder, rectal and skin cancer.

Dosage: 4 to 10 mg (0.06–0.15 mg/kg) at one to six weekly intervals; up to 40 to 80 mg (2 mg/kg) cumulative doses have been given in some treatments.

5 Preparation of Injection

Reconstitution: solutions are formed rapidly.

```
 2 mg vial +  5 ml water for injections = 0.4 mg/ml
10 mg vial + 10 ml water for injections =   1 mg/ml
20 mg vial + 20 ml water for injections =   1 mg/ml
```

May be stored for up to 12 hours at room temperature (do not refrigerate).[9,10]

Bolus administration: Inject slowly into a vein or slow-running drip at a rate of approximately 1 ml/min or more rapidly into a fast-running drip of 0.9% sodium chloride or 5% glucose. The stability of reconstituted drug in plastic syringes is not known.

Intravenous infusion: Dilute with 0.9% sodium chloride (use within 12 hours) or 5% glucose (use immediately) and infuse over one hour.

Extravasation: Vesicant, very damaging (*see* Chapter 9).

6 Destruction of Drug or Contaminated Articles

Incineration: 1000°C.

Chemical: 2 to 5% of hydrochloric acid or sodium hydroxide/12 hours.

Contact with skin: Very irritant, neutralize with several washes of sodium bicarbonate solution (8.4%) followed by soap and water; avoid hand creams.

References

1. Trissel, L.A. (1992). *Handbook on injectable drugs*, 7th edn. American Society of Hospital Pharmacists, Bethesda, Maryland, USA.
2. Beijner, J.H. and Underberg, W.J.M. (1985). Degradation of mitomycin C in acidic conditions. *Int. J. Pharm.* **24**, 219–229.
3. Benuvento, J.A. *et al.* (1981). Stability and compatibility of antitumor agents in glass and plastic containers. *Am. J. Hosp. Pharm.* **38**, 1914–1918.

4. Dorr, R.T. *et al.* (1982). Bleomycin compatibility with selected intravenous medications. *J. Medicine* **13**, 121–130.
5. Quebberman, E.J. *et al.* (1985). Stability of mitomycin admixtures. *Am. J. Hosp. Pharm.* **42**, 1750–1754.
6. Keller, J.H. (1986). Stability of mitomycin admixtures. *Am. J. Hosp. Pharm.* **43**, 59–64.
7. Stole, L.M.L. *et al.* (1986). Stability after freezing and thawing of solutions of Mitomycin C in plastic minibags for intravesical use. *Pharm. Weekbl. (Sci.)* **8**, 286–288.
8. Quebberman, E.J. and Hoffman, N.E. (1986) Stability of mitomycin admixtures. *Am. J. Hosp. Pharm.* **43**, 64.
9. Martindale Pharmaceuticals Ltd. Personal communication.
10. *ABPI Data Sheet Compendium 1991–92.* (1991). Datapharm Publications Ltd, London, pp. 876–877.

Prepared by M.C. Allwood

MITOZANTRONE

1 General Details

Approved name: Mitozantrone.

Proprietary name: Novantrone.

Manufacturer or supplier: Lederle Laboratories Ltd.

Presentation and formulation details: Vials containing mitozantrone dihydro-chloride solution, equivalent to 2 mg/ml mitozantrone. Solutions of 20 mg in 10 ml, 25 mg in 12.5 ml and 30 mg in 15 ml are available.

Each vial also contains: sodium chloride 0.8% w/v, sodium metabisulphite 0.01% w/v and sodium acetate 0.005% w/v in water for injections.

Storage and shelf-life of unopened container: Store at controlled room temperature 15–25°C. Stable for two years from the date of manufacture.

2 Chemistry

Type: Anthracenedione.

Molecular structure: 1,4-Dihydroxy-5,8-bis-2-(2-hydroxyethyl) amino ethyl-amine-9,10-anthraquinone dihydrochloride.

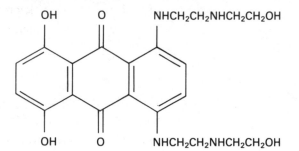

Molecular weight: 517.4.

Solubility: Water soluble.

3 Stability Profile

Physical and chemical stability

Mitozantrone degrades by oxidation of the phenylenediamine moiety to the corresponding quinoneimine, which then hydrolyses to the quinone.[1]

Effect of pH: Stability is optimal in acidic conditions.

Effect of light: Vials of mitozantrone may precipitate under refrigerated storage. Exposure of vials to sunlight for one month has little effect on the potency or appearance of the product.

Container compatibility: Mitozantrone adsorbs onto glass but not onto polypropylene or PVC.[2]

Compatibility with other drugs: Unstable in alkaline infusions. The injection should not be mixed with infusions containing heparin as precipitation may occur. Trissel[3] reported that hydrocortisone sodium phosphate or succinate may be compatible, but this may depend on the container.

Stability in clinical practice

Dilution to 5 mg/l in 0.9% sodium chloride or 5% glucose infusions produced solutions that were physically and chemically compatible, exhibiting no decomposition in 48 hours.[3] The Data Sheet[4] states that dilutions retain potency for 24 hours at room temperature. Polypropylene syringes containing mitozantrone diluted to 2 mg in 10 ml with water for injections (for use in continuous infusion schedules) were found to be stable for 14 days at 4 and 20°C[5] and for 24 hours at 37°C.[2] Mitozantrone infusions (0.2 mg/ml in water for injections) in PVC medication reservoirs (for use with an ambulatory infusion pump) were chemically and physically stable for 14 days at 4°C and under 'in-use' conditions at 37°C.[6] Mitozantrone infusions (0.1–0.5 mg/ml in 0.9% sodium chloride) in Single and Multiday Infusors (Baxter Healthcare) have been reported to be stable for two days at room temperature and for five days at 33°C.[7] Infusions containing 0.5 mg/ml mitozantrone in 0.9% sodium chloride have also been reported to be stable in the CADD Medication Cassette (Pharmacia Deltec) for ten days at 25°C or 14 days at 5°C.[8]

4 Clinical Use

Type of cytotoxic: Antibiotic anti-tumour agent.

Indications: Advanced breast cancer, non-Hodgkin's lymphoma, adult acute non-lymphocytic leukaemia in relapse and paediatric leukaemia, hepatoma.

Dosage: As a single agent, 14 mg/m^2 (12 mg/m^2 in patients with low bone marrow reserves).

5 Preparation of Injection

Dilute the required volume of mitozantrone solution to at least 50 ml in either 0.9% sodium chloride, 5% glucose or 0.18% sodium chloride and 4% glucose.

Bolus administration: Not recommended (mitozantrone must be diluted before administration).

Intravenous infusion: Mitozantrone infusion should be administered over not less than three minutes via the tubing of a freely-running IV infusion of the above fluids.

Extravasation: Mildly irritant (*see* Chapter 9).

6 Destruction of Drug or Contaminated Articles

Incineration: 800°C.

Chemical: 40% sodium hypochlorite solution (4% available chlorine)/24 hours.

Contact with skin: Wash with water.

References

1. Reynolds, D.L. *et al.* (1981). Clinical analysis for the antineoplastic agent 1,4-dihydroxy-5,8-bis-2(2-hydroxyethyl)aminoethyl)-amino. 9,10-anthracenedione dihydrochloride (NSC 301739) in plasma. *J. Chromatography* **222**, 225–240.
2. Sewell, G.J. *et al.* (1988). Pharmaceutical aspects of domiciliary continuous infusion chemotherapy. *Br. J. Cancer* **58**, 536.

3. Trissel, L.A. *et al.* (1985). *Investigational drugs, pharmaceutical data. Pharmaceutical aspects of home infusion therapy for cancer patients.* NCI, Bethesda, Maryland, USA.

4. *ABPI Data Sheet Compendium 1991–92.* (1991). Datapharm Publications Ltd, London, pp. 745–747.

5. Adams, P.S. *et al.* (1987). Pharmaceutical aspects of home infusion therapy for cancer patients. *Pharm. J.* **328**, 476–478.

6. Northcott, M. *et al.* (1991). The stability of carboplatin diamorphine, 5-fluorouracil and mitozantrone infusions in an ambulatory pump under storage and prolonged 'in-use' conditions. *J. Clin. Pharm. Ther.* **16**, 123–129.

7. Baxter Healthcare Ltd. (1992). Personal communication.

8. Pharmacia Deltec. (1991). Personal communication.

Prepared by G.J. Sewell

MUSTINE

1 General Details

Approved names: Chlormethine, mustine hydrochloride, mustagen, mechlorethamine hydrochloride, nitrogen mustard.

Proprietary name: Mustine Hydrochloride for Injection BP.

Manufacturer or supplier: Boots Company Plc.

Presentation and formulation details: White lyophilized powder in 20 ml vial, containing 10 mg mustine hydrochloride with no excipients.

Storage and shelf-life of unopened container: Two years when stored at 2 to 15°C.

2 Chemistry

Molecular structure: 2-chloro-N-(2-chloroethyl)-N-methylethanamine hydrochloride.

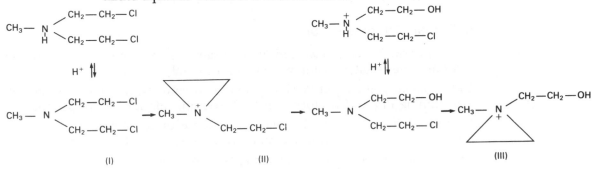

Molecular weight: 192.5 (hydrochloride).

Solubility: Very soluble in water.

3 Stability Profile

Physical and chemical stability

Degradation pathways: The degradation route of mustine hydrochloride (II) in dilute aqueous solution is shown below:

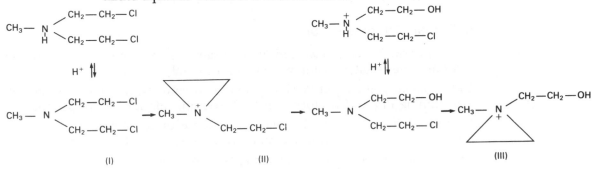

(I)　　　　　　　　(II)　　　　　　　　(III)

In aqueous solution mustine appears to lose alkylating activity relatively slowly. Alkylating activity arises from mustine together with compounds II and III in the degradation pathway. However, certain of these degradation products are either more carcinogenic than mustine or may be more neurotoxic.[1,2] Kirk[1] has recently reviewed the conflicting reports in the literature concerning the rate of degradation of mustine in aqueous solution. It is pointed out that almost all studies were carried out using a test for alkylating activity which was not fully stability-indicating. Certain of the products of degradation have alkylating activity *in vitro*. However, an analysis of previous studies indicates that degradation is very pH-dependent,[3] the compound degrading rapidly in neutral or alkaline conditions. An unbuffered solution of mustine has a pH of 3 to 5 and will be more stable. The recent study by Kirk[2] showed that solutions of mustine after reconstitution in 0.9% sodium chloride or water for injections (1 mg/ml) at room temperature, degrade by 8 to 10% in six hours, or by 3 to 6% at 4°C. Solutions diluted in 0.9% sodium chloride (18 to 36 µg/ml) exhibited 15% loss in six hours at room temperature, whilst in 5% glucose, about 11% loss was recorded.

Stability after reconstitution is decreased as the temperature is raised. Mustine is stable in the frozen state (−20°C) for four weeks, showing about 5% loss.[1,4]

Mustine does not appear to be unduly sensitive to light.

Container compatibility: Kirk[1] has shown recently that mustine does not appear to interact with styrene acrylonitrile syringes (Gillette) or PVC infusion containers.

Compatibility with other drugs: Incompatible with methohexital sodium.[5] No further information is available.

Stability in clinical practice

Reconstituted mustine injection (1 mg/ml) should be used within four hours at room temperature or six hours if stored in the refrigerator.[4] Mustine injection diluted in 500 ml of 0.9% sodium chloride should be administered within two hours, and dilutions in 500 ml of 5% glucose should be used within four hours.[1]

4 Clinical Use

Type of cytotoxic: Alkylating agent.

Main indications: Hodgkin's disease (with other agents).

Dosage: single dose of 0.4 mg/kg body-weight or a course of four daily doses of 0.1 mg/kg body-weight.

5 Preparation of Injection

Reconstitution: To each vial add 10 ml water for injections or 0.9% sodium chloride. The resulting solution contains 1 mg/ml.

Bolus administration: Inject IV slowly (over two minutes) into the bolus site of a fast-running drip of 5% glucose or 0.9% sodium chloride (60 drops/minute).

Intravenous infusion: Add the required volume of reconstituted injection to 500 ml of 0.9% sodium chloride and infuse slowly over 1 to 2 hours.

Extravasation: Vesicant, very damaging (*see* Chapter 9).

6 Destruction of Drug or Contaminated Articles

Incineration: 800°C.

Chemical:

Sodium hydroxide (SG1.5)	1 part) for
IMS	4 parts) 48
Water	3 parts) hours.
(Prepare 24 hours before use.)	

Contact with skin: Wash immediately with large amounts of water. Can be neutralized with sodium thiosulphate or sodium bicarbonate.

References

1. Kirk, B. (1986). Stability of reconstituted mustine injection BP during storage. *Br. J. Parent. Therap.* **7**, 86–92.
2. Kirk, B. (1987). A study of the stability of aqueous solutions of mustine hydrochloride using colorimetric and HPLC assay techniques. *Proc. of Guild.* **23**, 47–52.
3. Friedman, O.M. and Boger, E. (1961). Colorimetric estimation of nitrogen mustards in aqueous media. *Analytical Chem.* **33**, 907–910.
4. *ABPI Datasheet Compendium 1991–92.* (1991). Datapharm Publications Ltd, London, pp. 242–244.
5. Trissel, L.A. (1992). *Handbook on injectable drugs*, 7th edn. American Society of Hospital Pharmacists, Bethesda, Maryland, USA.

Prepared by M.C. Allwood

PLICAMYCIN

1 General Details

Approved names: Plicamycin, mithramycin.

Proprietary name: Mithracin.

Manufacturer or supplier: Pfizer Ltd.

Presentation and formulation details: Yellow lyophilized powder in vial, containing 2.5 mg plicamycin. Contains 100 mg mannitol and disodium hydrogen phosphate to adjust pH to 7.0 after reconstitution.

Storage and shelf-life of unopened container: Shelf-life of two years when stored in a refrigerator at 2 to 8°C and protected from light; shelf-life of six months at room temperature.[1]

2 Chemistry

Type: Cytotoxic antibiotic.

Molecular structure:

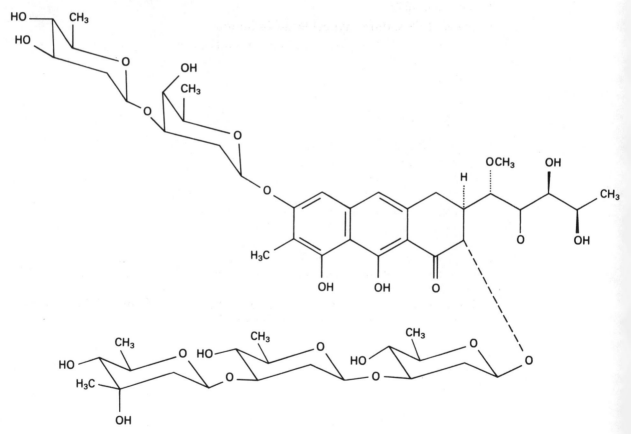

Molecular weight: 1085.2.

Solubility: Soluble in water.

3 Stability Profile

Physical and chemical stability

The dry powder is stable for six months at ambient temperature.[2] The drug in aqueous solution decomposes in acid or alkaline conditions. The pH of an aqueous solution (0.5 mg/ml) is 4.5 to 5.5, although the injection is buffered to pH 7. Losses of about 13% at pH 4 to 5 and ambient temperature after 24 hours have been reported.[3] Solutions at pH 5 to 7.5 are stable for at least two days at 2 to 6°C.[5]

Effect of light: The drug is described as relatively sensitive to light, and direct exposure to strong daylight should be avoided.

Degradation pathways: Acid hydrolysis (below pH 5.0) yields a number of degradation products, including chromomycinone D, mycarose, D olivose and D oliose.[3] The relative toxicity of these compounds is unknown.

Compatibility with containers: Compatible with PVC,[3] and with in-line filters (Ivex-2) during infusion.[4]

Compatibility with other drugs: Plicamycin will chelate metals, such as iron. No further information is available.

Stability in clinical practice

The drug is relatively stable after reconstitution with water for injections and may be stored for two days at 2 to 6°C. The drug may be further diluted in 5% glucose (other infusion fluids are not recommended), although some degradation may occur indicating storage is undesirable. Such dilutions are quite stable (less than 10% loss) for 24 hours at room temperature in either glass or PVC containers, or 48 hours at 2 to 6°C.[3] However, the presence of degradation products is undesirable, so it is recommended the diluted injection be used immediately. It is reported that plicamycin binds to cellulose acetate in-line filters, approximately 14% of the dose being removed during passage of a solution in 5% glucose through an in-line filter.[6]

4 Clinical Use

Type of cytotoxic: Anti-tumour antibiotic.

Main indications: Refractory hypercalcaemia.

Dosage: 25 µg/kg/day for three to four day periods.

5 Preparation of Injection

Dilution: Add 4.9 ml water for injections and shake to dissolve. The solution contains 500 µg/ml plicamycin. It may be stored for short periods at 2 to 6°C, but this is not recommended by the manufacturer.

Bolus administration: Not recommended.

Intravenous infusion: The required volume of the reconstituted injection is added to 1 l of 5% glucose or 0.9% sodium chloride.[7] Inject slowly over four to six hours (200 ml/h). The infusion may be stored at 2 to 6°C for up to 24 hours.

Extravasation: Moderately damaging. There is no known antidote.

Application of moderate heat to the site of extravasation is recommended to disperse the drug and reduce discomfort. (*See* Chapter 9.)

6 Destruction of Drug or Contaminated Articles

Incineration: 1000°C.

Chemical: 10% w/v trisodium phosphate (or 0.1 M sodium hydroxide).

Contact with skin: Wash affected area with copious amounts of water.

References

1. Longland, P.W. and Rowbottom, P.C. (1987). Stability at room temperature of medicines normally recommended for cold storage. *Pharm. J.* **238**, 147–151.
2. Wolfert, R.R. and Cox, R.M. (1975). Room temperature stability of drug products labelled for refrigeration storage. *Am. J. Hosp. Pharm.* **32**, 585–587.
3. Cheng, C.C. and Kwang-Yeun, Z. (1972). Some antineoplastic antibiotics. *J. Pharm. Sci.* **61**, 4.
4. Karke, M. *et al.* (1983). Binding of selected drugs to a 'treated' in-line filter. *Am. J. Hosp. Pharm.* **40**, 1323–1328.
5. Bosanquet, A.G. (1986). Stability of solutions of anti-neoplastic agents during preparation and storage for *in vitro* assays. II. Assay methods, Adriamycin and the other anti-tumour antibiotics. *Cancer Chemother. Pharmacol.* **17**, 1–10.
6. Butler, L.D. *et al.* (1980). Effect of in-line filtration on the potency of low-dose drugs. *Am. J. Hosp. Pharm.* **37**, 935–941.
7. *ABPI Data Sheet Compendium 1991–92.* (1991). Datapharm Publications Ltd, London, pp. 1144–1146.

Prepared by M.C. Allwood

THIOTEPA

1 General Details

Approved names: Thiotepa, thiophosphoramide, TESPA, TSPA.

Proprietary name: Thiotepa.

Manufacturer or supplier: Lederle Laboratories Ltd.

Presentation and formulation details: Lyophilized powder, in vials containing thiotepa 15 mg.

Storage and shelf-life of unopened container: The injection has a shelf-life of 18 months when stored between 2 and 8°C.

2 Chemistry

Molecular structure: 1,1′1″-phosphinothioyldinetris-aziridine.

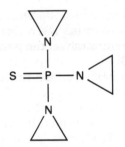

Molecular weight: 189.2.

Solubility: Soluble 1 in 8 in water; 1 in 2 in ethanol; 1 in 2 in chloroform; and 1 in 4 in ether.

3 Stability Profile

Physical and chemical stability

The stability of thiotepa in aqueous solution is pH-dependent; it is least stable in acid solutions. The acid catalysed reaction of thiotepa in the presence of chloride ions yields a series of chloroethyl derivatives (I–III) according to the following scheme:[1]

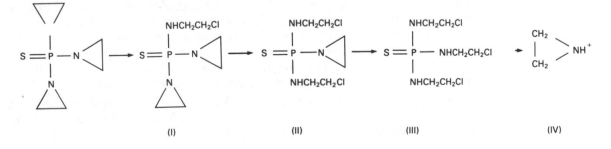

In strong acid solutions and in aqueous solutions at elevated temperatures, thiotepa undergoes P-N cleavage and/or ring-opening to give the azaridinium ion (IV).[2] Thiotepa will also polymerize to form insoluble polymeric derivatives.

At 37°C in pH 4.2 buffer the rate constant for loss of thiotepa is 9.8×10^{-3}/minute giving a $t_{90\%}$ of 10 minutes. At pH 7 degradation was much slower; no breakdown could be detected after two hours at 37°C but longer term data were not available.[3]

Any polymerization reaction is likely to be catalysed by light, reducing the stability of thiotepa.

Compatibility with other drugs: Thiotepa is incompatible in solutions with mitozantrone. When mitozantrone and thiotepa were mixed in 5% glucose in a 10 ml syringe and the solution stored at room temperature protected from light, 10% of the mitozantrone degraded within the first 24 hours and over 50% after seven days.[4]

Stability in clinical practice

The manufacturer indicates that the reconstituted solution has a shelf-life of one day when stored at 2 to 8°C.[6] If a precipitate forms the reconstituted injection must be discarded. The reconstituted solution is in fact reported to be stable for 28 days at 2 to 8°C or seven days at ambient temperature.[6] Solutions of thiotepa, 15 mg in 1.5 ml water for injections, are also reported to be stable when frozen for up to 28 days (temperature not specified).[6] (The previous formulation, containing sodium chloride and sodium bicarbonate, was stable for five days at 2 to 8°C.[5]) Thiotepa solutions reconstituted in water for injections and diluted into 0.9% sodium chloride or 5% glucose infusions to a final concentration of 0.5 mg/ml in PVC bags are stable for 14 days at 2 to 8°C, but losses are more than 10% in seven days at ambient temperature.[6]

When administered as a bladder irrigation it is recommended that up to 60 mg thiotepa in 60 ml sterile water is instilled and the solution retained in the bladder for up to two hours. Thiotepa is, however, unstable in acidic urine at 37°C. At pH 5.5, $t_{90\%}$ is 70 minutes and, at pH 4.0, $t_{90\%}$ is 3.3 minutes with only 2.1% of the initial dose of thiotepa remaining after two hours.[3]

4 Clinical Use

Type of cytotoxic: Thiotepa is a polyfunctional alkylating agent. It releases ethylenimine radicals which disrupt the bonds of DNA.

Main indications: Adenocarcinoma of the breast and of the ovary; for controlling intracavity effusions secondary to diffuse or localized neoplastic disease of various serosal cavities; and for the treatment of superficial papillary carcinoma of the bladder.[5,6] Thiotepa has been effective against lymphosarcoma and Hodgkin's disease but is now largely superseded by other treatments. It has been used also for the post-operative management of pterygium.[8,9]

Dosage: By rapid intravenous infusion, 0.3 to 0.4 mg/kg at one- to four-week intervals. By intracavity instillation, 10 to 65 mg in 20 to 60 ml sterile water. By intravesical administration, up to 60 mg in 30 to 60 ml sterile water.

5 Preparation of Injection

Reconstitution: Reconstitution of the 15 mg vial with 1.5 ml water gives a 10 mg/ml solution. If the thiotepa has polymerized a precipitate will form on reconstitution. Precipitated solutions should be discarded. Large bore needles are recommended to minimize pressure and possible formation of aerosols.

Administration: Thiotepa may be given by intravenous, intramuscular and intrathecal routes. For intracavity instillation first aspirate as much fluid as possible then instil the dose of thiotepa. The same tubing may be used for both aspiration and instillation.

For bladder instillation the patient is dehydrated for eight to 12 hours. The solution is instilled into the bladder and retained there for two hours.

Extravasation: Thiotepa is nonvesicant and non-irritant.

6 Destruction of Drug or Contaminated Articles

Incineration: 800°C.

Chemical: Dilute in large quantities of boiling water.

Contact with skin: Wash off with water.

References

1. Maxwell, J. *et al.* (1974). Behaviour of an aziridine alkylating agent in acid solution. *Biochem. Pharmacol.* **23**, 168–170.
2. Zon, G. *et al.* (1976). Observations of 1,1',1" phosphinothioylidinetris-aziridine (thiotepa) in acidic and saline media. An[1] H-NMR study. *Biochem. Pharmacol.* **25**, 989–992.
3. Cohen, G.E. *et al.* (1984). Effects of pH and temperature on the stability and decomposition of N,N'N" triethylenethio-phosphoramide in urine and buffer. *Cancer Res.* **44**, 4312–4316.
4. Cacek, T. and Weber,R. (1991). Visual and chemical stability of mitoxantrone mixed individually with vincristine, etoposide, thiotepa, metoclopramine and cytarabine in plastic syringes. *ASHP Midyear Clinical Meeting* **25**, 470E.
5. Kirschembaum, B.E. and Latiolais, C.J. (1976). Stability of injectable medications after reconstitution. *Am. J. Hosp. Pharm.* **33**, 767–791.
6. Lederle Laboratories. Personal communication.
7. Uyas, H.M. *et al.* (1987). Drug stability guidelines for a continuous infusion chemotherapy programme. *Hosp. Pharm.* **22**, 685–687.
8. Erlich, D. (1977). The management of pterygium. *Ophth. Surg.* **8**, 23–30.
9. Olander, K. (1978). Management of pterygium: should thiotepa be used? *Ann. Ophthalmol.* **10**, 853–856.

Prepared by M.G. Lee

VINBLASTINE

1 General Details

Approved names: Vinblastine, vincaleukoblastine.

Proprietary name: Velbe (Lilly).

Manufacturers or suppliers: Eli Lilly & Co. Ltd, Lederle Laboratories Ltd, David Bull Laboratories Ltd (DBL).

Presentation and formulation details: Lyophilized powder containing 10 mg vinblastine sulphate. This is supplied with 10 ml aqueous diluent containing 90 mg sodium chloride and 0.2 ml benzyl alcohol (Lilly, Lederle, DBL), or as a solution of 10 mg/ml lyophilized powder (DBL).

Storage and shelf-life of unopened container: The injection has a shelf-life of three years when stored between 0 and 6°C. The solution shelf-life is 18 months.

2 Chemistry

Type: Vinca alkaloid.

Molecular Structure: Vincaleucoblastine.

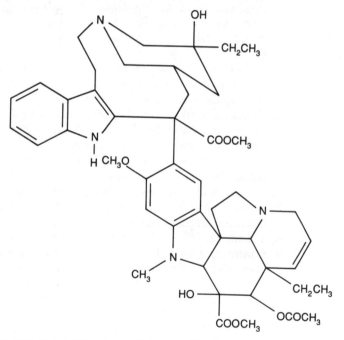

Molecular weight: 811.0 (vinblastine sulphate: 909.0).

Solubility: The base is insoluble in water; soluble in ethanol and chloroform. The sulphate salt is soluble 1 in 10 water; 1 in 1200 ethanol; 1 in 50 chloroform. pKa: 5.4, 7.4.

3 Stability Profile

Physical and chemical stability

Degradation pathways: Aqueous solutions of vinblastine are less stable at lower pH values, 4-desacetylvinblastine is the primary degradation product at pH 2.[1]

More recent studies indicate that the hydrolytic decomposition pathways for vinblastine are more complex. Below pH 1.5 and above pH 10.5, desacetyl-vinblastine has been confirmed as the major degradation product. However, between pH 2.5 and 7.0, the amount of desacetylvinblastine found was neglig-ible and at least three other degradation products were detected.[2] Studies on 1 mg/ml solutions of vinblastine sulphate at pH 4.5 to 5.0 identified up to six breakdown products. The major degradents were tentatively identified as 19'-oxo-vinblastine and an isomer of vinblastine but none of the decomposition products were positively categorized. From the data at 25, 37 and 55°C, $t_{90\%}$ values were estimated to be 16.6 days at 37°C, 150 days at 25°C and 10.7 years at 5°C.[3]

When exposed to direct incandescent light, decomposition is accelerated. At 25°C, the $t_{90\%}$ is approximately seven days and at 30°C, solutions of vinblastine sulphate had lost 10% of their potency after slightly more than one day.[4] The major degradation products were different from those identified in thermal degradation studies but the same pattern of products were identified in both cases.

Vinblastine base is practically insoluble in water and can precipitate from solutions of vinblastine sulphate above pH 6.

Container compatibility: No loss of potency was detected in solutions of vinblastine sulphate (10 mg/ml) stored for 30 days in polypropylene syringes at 4°C or room temperature.[5] There was no significant loss of potency when vinblastine sulphate solution (10 mg in 50 ml) in 5% glucose or 0.9% sodium chloride was filtered through a 0.22 μm cellulose ester membrane filter.[6]

No losses of vinblastine (2.5 mg/10 ml) could be detected to nylon, polysulphone or cellulose ester filters when using a syringe pump driver to deliver the drug. There was, however, significant adsorption to the Pall ELD96 activated nylon filter. A 30–40% loss of potency was detected during the first 30 minutes of infusion with the concentration only returning to its initial value after two to three hours.[7]

Losses of 24% occurred in 24 hours at 37°C from a 1 mg/ml solution of vinblastine sulphate in bacteriostatic 0.9% saline in an Infusaid implantable pump; in 12 days losses totalled 48%. Similar solutions in glass vials exhibited no losses after 24 hours and 20% loss after 12 days at 37°C.[8]

Vinblastine has been shown to be absorbed onto PVC tubing and cellulose proprionate burette chambers. Up to 48% loss was found from a 3 μg/ml solution stored for 48 hours in PVC tubing and up to 20% loss of potency was found in similar solutions stored in cellulose proprionate burette chambers for 48 hours.[9] These results were obtained for a static system and it is difficult to extrapolate them to the dynamic situation of an intravenous administration. Significant losses are likely to occur, however, in PVC administration sets. The absorption losses did not occur in polybutadiene tubing or methacrylate butadeine styrene burettes.[9]

Compatibility with other drugs: Trissel reports studies suggesting that vinblastine may be compatible with a number of drugs.[10]

Stability in clinical practice

The reconstituted injection is chemically stable for at least 28 days at 4°C and at 25°C,[3] provided it is protected from light. When stored at 37°C in the dark, the shelf-life of the reconstituted injection is 14 days. In direct incandescent light, the injection is chemically stable for 7 days at room temperature.[4]

No degradation was detected in vinblastine solution 20 µg/ml in 0.9% sodium chloride, 5% glucose and in Ringer's lactate, stored in polypropylene tubes in the dark, after 21 days at 4°C. At 25°C there was a 2–3% degradation of vinblastine in the three infusion solutions after 21 days.[11]

A 7% degradation has been observed in vinblastine solution ranging from 0.015–0.5 mg/ml 0.9% sodium chloride after storage for 21 days at 4°C + five days at 33°C in a Baxter Infusor. However, the study confirms that degradation is reduced to 5% after 10 days of storage at 4°C followed by five days at 33°C.[12] Vinblastine solution can therefore be stored for ten days at 4°C in a Baxter Infusor prior to being delivered through a one or five day Infusor.

4 Clinical Use

Type of cytotoxic: Vinblastine arrests mitosis at the metaphase and inhibits RNA synthesis.

Main indications: Vinblastine is used in combination with other chemotherapeutic agents for treatment of metastatic testicular carcinoma, Hodgkin's and non-Hodgkin's lymphoma, neuroblastoma, histiocytosis X, mycosis fungoides, Kaposi's sarcoma, advanced breast carcinoma and choriocarcinoma.

Dosage: Usually 4 to 8 mg/m² weekly. Weekly injections starting at 3.7 mg/m² and rising by increments of 1.85 mg/m² up to a maximum of 18.5 mg/m² or until the white cell count has fallen to 3000/mm³ have been used.[13]

5 Preparation of Injection

Reconstitution: Reconstitution of the 10 mg vial with 10 ml of sterile diluent gives a 1 mg/ml solution.

Bolus administration: Intravenously, directly into vein or into the tubing of a running infusion, over a one-minute period.

Intravenous infusion: Vinblastine has also been given as a continuous five-day infusion (1.4 to 2.0 mg/m²/day[14]). Infusions should be administered through a central line.

Since death has resulted from inadvertent intrathecal administration, it is recommended that syringes containing this product, should be labelled 'WARNING – VINBLASTINE FOR INTRAVENOUS USE ONLY'.[15]

Constant ambulatory intravenous infusion has been investigated using a tunnelled subclavian catheter and the Cor-med ML6 infusion pump[16] and the Travenol Infuser system.[17] There are, however, insufficient data to draw reliable conclusions from this work.

Extravasation: Moderate to severe (*see* Chapter 9).

6 Destruction of Drug or Contaminated Articles

Incineration: 1000°C.

Chemical: 10% sodium hypochlorite/24 hours.

Contact with skin: Wash with copious amounts of water.

References

1. Burns, J.H. (1972). *Analytical profiles of drug substance*, Vol. 1, Academic Press, Orlando, Florida, USA, pp. 443.
2. Vendrig, D.E.M.M. *et al.* (1988). Degradation kinetics of vinblastine sulphate in aqueous solutions. *Int. J. Pharm.* **43**, 131–138.
3. Black, J. *et al.* (1988). Studies on the stability of vinblastine sulphate in aqueous solution. *J. Pharm. Sci.* **77**, 630.
4. Black, J. *et al.* (1988). Stability of vinblastine sulphate when exposed to light. *Drug Intell. Clin. Pharm.* **22**, 634.
5. Ireland, D. *et al.* (1990). The chemical stability of cytarabine and vinblastine injections. *Br. J. Pharm. Pract.* **12**, 53–54.
6. Butler, L.D. *et al.* (1980). Effect of in-line filtration on the potency of low-dose drugs. *Am. J. Hosp. Pharm.* **37**, 935.
7. Francombe, M.B. *et al.* (1991). Adsorption of doxorubicin, mitozantrone, vincristine and vinblastine to intravenous filters. *Int. Pharm. J.* **5**, 70.
8. Keller, J.H. and Ensminger, W.D. (1982). Stability of cancer chemotherapeutic agents in totally implanted drug delivery systems. *Am. J. Hosp. Pharm.* **39**, 1321.
9. McElany, J.C. *et al.* (1988). Stability of methotrexate and vinblastine in burette administration sets. *Int. J. Pharm.* **47**, 239–247.
10. Trissel, L.A. (1992). *Handbook on injectable drugs*, 7th edn. American Society of Hospital Pharmacists, Bethesda, Maryland, USA.
11. Beijnen, J.H. *et al.* (1989). Stability of vinca alkaloid anticancer drugs in three commonly used infusion fluids. *J. Parenter. Sci. Technol.* **43**, 84–87.
12. Baxter Healthcare Ltd. Personal communication.
13. Anon. (1986). *Physicians desk reference*, 40th edn. Medical Economics Company, Oradell, New Jersey, USA.
14. Yap, H.Y. *et al.* (1980). Vinblastine given as a continuous five-day infusion in the treatment of refractory advanced breast cancer. *Cancer Treat. Rep.* **64**, 279.
15. *ABPI Data Sheet Compendium 1991–92.* (1991) Datapharm Publications Ltd, London, pp. 829–831.
16. Lokich, J. *et al.* (1982). The delivery of cancer chemotherapy by constant venous infusion. *Cancer* **50**, 2731.
17. Akokoshi, M.P. *et al.* (1987). Safety and reliability of the Travenol Infusor. *J. Pharm. Technol.* (Mar/Apr), 65.

Prepared by M.G. Lee

VINCRISTINE

1 General Details

Approved names: Vincristine, leurocristine.

Proprietary name: Oncovin (Lilly).

Manufacturers or suppliers: David Bull Laboratories Ltd (DBL), Eli Lilly & Co. Ltd, Lederle Laboratories Ltd.

Presentation and formulation details: Lyophilized powder containing lactose in the following proportions of vincristine to lactose: 1 mg–10 mg, 2 mg–20 mg, 5 mg–50 mg*. Supplied with 10 ml of diluent containing 90 mg sodium chloride and 0.2 ml benzyl alcohol (Lilly, Lederle*, DBL).

1 ml, 2 ml and 5 ml (DBL) vials containing vincristine sulphate 1 mg/ml in solution with mannitol 100 mg/ml, methylhydroxybenzoate 1.8 mg/ml and propylhydroxybenzoate 0.2 mg/ml (Lilly), or preservative-free (DBL); also available in prefilled syringes containing 1 mg in 1 ml, 2 mg in 2 ml (DBL).

Storage and shelf-life of unopened containers: When stored at 2 to 8°C, the lyophilized powder has a shelf-life of three years and the solution has a shelf-life of two years in vials or 18 months in syringes.

2 Chemistry

Type: Vinca alkaloid.

Molecular structure: 22-oxo-Vincaleukoblastine (sulphate salt).

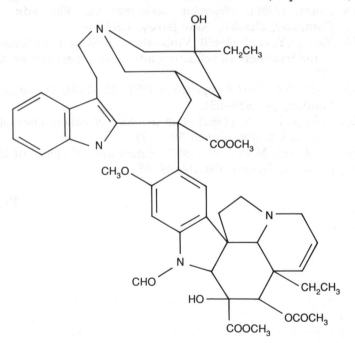

Molecular weight: 825.1 (Vincristine sulphate: 923).

Solubility: Sulphate salt: 1 in 2 of water; 1 in 600 of ethanol; 1 in 30 of chloroform.
pKa: 5.0, 7.4.

3 Stability Profile

Physical and chemical stability

When vincristine sulphate was incubated at 37°C in 0.2 M glycine buffer containing 1% bovine serum albumin, five degradation products could be detected.[1] The major breakdown product was confirmed as 4-deacetyl vincristine. The remaining degradants were postulated to be an isomer of vincristine and of the 4-deacetyl derivative, 4-deacetyl-3-deoxy vincristine and N-formyl-leurosine. The degradation products were formed to the extent of 14%, 44% and 56% of the parent vincristine after incubating at 37°C for 72 hours at pH 4.0, 7.4, and 8.8 respectively.

Studies on the degradation kinetics of vincristine sulphate at 80°C in the pH range 2 to 11 indicate that vincristine is most stable at pH 4.8 and that its stability is comparable to that of vinblastine.[2] A half life of 136 hours is given for vincristine in solutions at pH 4.8 and 80°C with an activation energy of 70–80 kJ/mol, but the data are not easily extrapolated to temperatures of 25°C and below.

The reconstituted injection has a pH of 3.5–5.5. Precipitation can occur at alkaline pHs.

Container compatibility: No losses to plastic containers or syringes have been reported. After filtration through a 0.22 μm cellulose ester filter, 6.5% of a 1 mg/50 ml solution in 5% glucose and 12% of a 1 mg/50 ml solution in 0.9% sodium chloride was bound to the filter.[3] Vincristine sulphate, 1.5 mg in 3 ml, when injected as a bolus through a 0.22 μm nylon filter, and after flushing the filter with 10 ml normal saline, showed losses of 10% of the vincristine to the filter.[4]

No losses of vincristine (0.25 mg/10 ml) could be detected to nylon, polysulphone or cellulose ester filters when using a syringe pump driver to deliver the drug. Significant absorption was found however to the Pall ELD 96 filter. A 30–40% loss of potency could be seen in the first 30 minutes of the infusion, with the concentration only returning to its initial value after two to three hours.[5]

Compatibility with other drugs: Trissel reports studies suggesting that vincristine may be compatible with a number of drugs.[6]

Stability in clinical practice

The manufacturers recommend that the reconstituted injection be discarded after 14 days in the fridge.[7,8] The injection solution has a shelf-life of 18 months at 2–6°C[7,9] and so solutions with a pH of 3.5–5.5 would be expected to be equally stable. The reconstituted injection is chemically stable for 30 days when stored at 2–6°C.[9]

No degradation was detected in vincristine solution 20 μg/ml in 0.9% sodium chloride injection, 5% glucose injection and Ringer's lactate injection when stored at 4°C for 21 days in polypropylene tubes in the dark.[10] At 25°C there was a 5% loss of vincristine in 5% glucose injection after 21 days but losses in the other two infusion solutions were insignificant.

There was no evidence of physical or chemical incompatibility between vincristine and mitozantrone mixed together in 5% dextrose solution contained in 10 ml plastic syringes and stored, protected from light, at room temperature for seven days.[10,11] Admixtures of doxorubicin and vincristine (1.88–2.37 mg/ml and 0.033–0.053 mg/ml respectively) are stable for at least seven days at 37°C in 0.9% sodium chloride injection, or 0.45% sodium chloride and 2.5% glucose injection.[12]

Solutions of vincristine ranging from 0.04 to 0.2 mg/ml, reconstituted with 0.9% sodium chloride, have been shown to be chemically stable for ten days in a Baxter Infusor when stored at room temperature.[13] However, due to the lack of stability data at 33°C, only half-day Infusors should be used.[13]

4 Clinical Use

Type of cytotoxic: Vincristine blocks mitosis with metaphase arrest by binding to tubulin and inhibiting the assembly of microtubules. It is M-phase specific.

Main indications: Vincristine is used, principally in combination chemotherapy regimens, against Hodgkin's and non-Hodgkin's lymphomas, acute lympho-cytic leukaemia, lymphosarcoma, reticulum cell sarcoma, rhabdomyosarcoma, neuroblastoma, Wilms' tumour, advanced breast carcinoma and small-cell lung carcinoma. It has modest to moderate activity in many other malignancies.[14]

Dosage: 1.4 mg/m^2 weekly, up to a maximum of 2 mg. In children weighing less than 10 kg, 0.05 mg/kg weekly is used. Due to the narrow therapeutic range, the dose should be individually adjusted.

5 Preparation of Injection

Reconstitution: Add 1 ml of diluent to a 1 mg vial, 2 ml to a 2 mg vial and 5 ml to a 5 mg vial to give a 1 mg/ml solution.

Bolus administration: By bolus injection or into the tubing of a running intravenous infusion. As it is vesicant, care must be taken to avoid extravasation during administration.

Intravenous infusion: Vincristine has also been administered by continuous infusion[15,16] with reported higher blood concentrations and increased tumour response at a dose of 0.5 mg/m^2 daily for five days in three-week cycles.[15,16]

Since death has resulted from inadvertent intrathecal injection, it is recom-mended that syringes containing this product should be labelled 'WARNING – VINCRISTINE FOR INTRAVENOUS USE ONLY'.[7]

Extravasation: Moderate to severe (*see* Chapter 9).

6 Destruction of Drugs or Contaminated Articles

Incineration: 1000°C.

Chemical: 5% sodium hypochlorite/24 hours.

Contact with skin: Wash with copious amounts of water.

References

1. Sethi, V.S. and Thimmaiah, K.N. (1985). Structural studies on the degra-dation products of vincristine dihydrogen sulphate. *Cancer Res.* **45**, 5386–5389.
2. Vendrig, D.E.M.M. *et al.* (1989). Degradation kinetics of vincristine sulphate and vindesine sulphate in aqueous solutions. *Int. J. Pharm.* **50**, 189–196.
3. Butler, L.D. *et al.* (1980). Effect of in-line filtration on the potency of low-dose drugs. *Am. J. Hosp. Pharm.* **37**, 935–941.

4. Ennis, C.E. *et al.* (1983). *In vitro* study of in-line filtration of medications commonly administered to paediatric cancer patients. *J. Parenter. Enter. Nutr.* **7**, 156–158.

5. Francomb, M.M. *et al.* (1991). Adsorption of doxorubicin, mitoxantrone, vincristine and vinblastine to intravenous filters. *Int. Pharm. J.* **5**, 70.

6. Trissel, L.A. (1992). *Handbook on injectable drugs*, 7th edn. American Society of Hospital Pharmacy, Bethesda, Maryland, USA.

7. *ABPI Data Sheet Compendium 1991–92.* (1991). Datapharm Publications Ltd, London, pp. 785–786, 814–817.

8. David Bull Laboratories. Data Sheet: *Vincristine sulphate.*

9. Vegenbery, F.R. and Souney, P.F. (1983). Stability guidelines for routinely refrigerated drug products. *Am. J. Hosp. Pharm.* **40**, 101–102.

10. Beijnen, J.H. *et al.* (1989). Stability of vinca alkaloid anticancer drugs in three commonly used infusion fluids. *J. Parenter. Sci. Technol.* **43**, 84–87.

11. Cacek, T. and Weber, R. (1990). Visual and chemical stability of mitoxantrone mixed individually with vincristine, etoposide, thiotepa, metoclopramide and cytarabine in plastic syringes. *ASHP Midyear Clinical Meeting* **25**, P-47OE.

12. Beijnen, J.H. *et al.* (1986). Stability of intravenous admixtures of doxorubicin and vincristine. *Am. J. Hosp. Pharm.* **43**, 3022–3027.

13. Baxter Healthcare Ltd. Personal communication.

14. Smith, B.D. Antitumour update: Vinca alkaloids and epipodophyllotoxins. *Hosp. Formul.* **22**, 363–373.

15. Jackson, D.V. *et al.* (1984). Intravenous vincristine infusion. *Cancer* **48**, 2559–2664.

16. Jackson, D.V. *et al.* (1981). Pharmacokinetics of vincristine infusion. *Cancer Treat. Rep.* **65**, 1043–1048.

Prepared by M.G. Lee

VINDESINE

1 General Details

Approved names: Vindesine, desacetyl vinblastine amide.

Proprietary name: Eldisine.

Manufacturer or supplier: Eli Lilly & Co. Ltd.

Presentation and formulation details: Lyophilized powder consisting of 5 mg vindesine sulphate with 25 mg mannitol. Supplied with 5 ml sterile diluent containing sodium chloride 9 mg/ml and 2% benzyl alcohol adjusted to pH 4.2 to 4.5 with hydrochloric acid or sodium hydroxide.[1]

Storage and shelf-life of unopened container: When stored between 2 and 6°C, the injection has a shelf-life of three years.

2 Chemistry

Type: Vinca alkaloid and synthetic derivative of vinblastine.

Molecular structure: 3-(aminocarbonyl)-O-deacetyl-3-de(methoxy-carbonyl)-Vinca-leukoblastine.

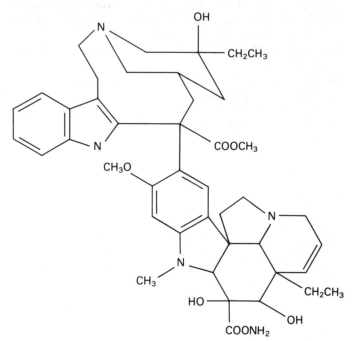

Molecular weight: 753.9 (Vindesine sulphate: 852).

Solubility: The sulphate salt is freely soluble in water. pKa: 5.4, 7.4.

3 Stability Profile

Physical and chemical stability

In studies on the stability of vindesine in buffered serum albumin solution, Thimmaiah *et al.* have found that, when vindesine sulphate (500 mg in 10 ml) is incubated at 37°C in 0.2 M glycine buffer containing 1% bovine serum albumin, two degradation products can be detected.[2] These were tentatively identified as an eneamine/ether derivative of vindesine (I) and 3'4'-epoxyvindesine-N-oxide (II). (*See* Figure 1.)

The degradation products were formed to an extent of about 11, 34 and 39% of the parent vindesine after 72 hours incubation at 37°C at pH 4.0, 7.4 and 8.8 respectively.

Investigations of the degradation kinetics of vindesine sulphate at 80°C in the pH range 2 to 11 indicate that it is most stable at pH 1.9 and that it is more stable than vinblastine and vincristine in aqueous solution.[3] A half life of 690 hours is quoted for vindesine at 80°C and pH 1.9 with an activation energy of 124 kJ/mol, but the data are not easily extrapolated to temperatures of 25°C and below.

Studies of the cell killing efficiency of vindesine solutions used in the human tumour clonogenic assay indicate a deterioration of cytotoxic activity for solutions stored in glass at low concentrations.[4] The lethal efficacy of 60 µg/ml solutions decreased to almost zero when tested after one, two and three weeks storage; a 225 µg/ml solution retained its lethal activity throughout the three-week period. The original reconstituted injection (1 mg/ml), stored in glass under the same conditions, retained its cytotoxic activity when diluted to the test concentrations. This would indicate that the loss of efficacy at low concentrations is not due to chemical inactivation but is more likely a result of sorptive losses to the glass vial.

The reconstituted injection has a pH of 4.2–4.5. Precipitation can occur at alkaline pHs.

Container compatibility: No incompatibilities have been reported with PVC containers and plastic syringes. There is evidence of sorptive losses of 60 µg/ml solutions in borosilicate glass vials.[4]

Compatibility with other drugs: No further information available.

Stability in clinical practice

The reconstituted injection is chemically stable for at least 30 days when stored at 4°C.[1] No degradation was detected in vindesine solution 20 µg/ml in 0.9% sodium chloride injection, 5% glucose injection or Ringer's lactate injection when stored for 21 days at both 4°C and 25°C in polypropylene tubes in the dark.[5]

4 Clinical Use

Type of cytotoxic: Vindesine causes metaphase arrest by binding to tubulin, a substructure of the microtubular spindle apparatus. This leads to inhibition of tubulin polymerization which interrupts mitosis and leads to cell death.[6] For a complete review of the antineoplastic activity of vindesine see Cersosima *et al.*[6]

Main indications: Acute lymphoblastic leukaemia, chronic myelogenous leukaemia in blast crisis, malignant melanoma and advanced breast carcinoma.

Dosage: 3 to 4 mg/m² weekly as a bolus injection, or by four hour[7] or 48 hour infusion.[8] For fuller details of dosage regimens see Cersosima *et al.*[6]

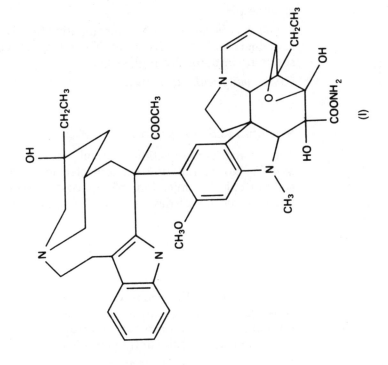

Figure 1: *Two major degradation products of vindesine incubated at 37°C in 0.2 M glycine buffer*

5 Preparation of Injection

Reconstitution: Reconstitute the 5 mg vial with 5 ml of sterile diluent to give a 1 mg/ml solution.

Bolus administration: Inject reconstituted preparation into the tubing of a fast running IV drip.

Intravenous infusion: Prepare in 5% glucose or 0.9% sodium chloride injections. Multielectrolyte infusion solutions, such as lactated Ringer's, are not recommended because of the possibility of precipitation, but this is not a problem for concentrations of less than 20 µg/ml.[5]

Since death has resulted from inadvertent intrathecal administration, it is recommended that syringes containing vindesine should be labelled 'WARNING – VINDESINE SULPHATE FOR INTRAVENOUS USE ONLY'.[4]

Extravasation: Moderate to severe. 1000 units of hyaluronidase in 20 ml saline may aid recovery (*See* Chapter 9).

6 Destruction of Drug or Contaminated Articles

Incineration: 1000°C.

Chemical: 10% sodium hypochlorite/24 hours.

Contact with skin: Wash with copious amounts of water.

References

1. *ABPI Data Sheet Compendium 1991–92.* (1991). Datapharm Publications Ltd, London, pp. 800–801.
2. Thimmaiah, K.N. *et al.* (1990). Chemical characterisation of the *in vitro* degradation products of vindesine sulphate. *Microchem. J.* **42**, 115–120.
3. Vendrig, D.E.M.M. *et al.* (1989). Degradation kinetics of vincristine sulphate and vindesine sulphate in aqueous solution. *Int. J. Pharm.* **50**, 189–196.
4. Yang, L-Y. and Drewinko, B. (1985). Cytotoxic efficacy of reconstituted and stored antitumor agents. *Cancer Res.* **45**, 1511–1515.
5. Beijnen, J.H. *et al.* (1988). Stability of vinca alkaloid anticancer drugs in three commonly used infusion fluids. *J. Parenter. Sci. Technol.* **43**, 84–87.
6. Cersosima, R.J. *et al.* (1983). Pharmacology, clinical efficacy and adverse effects of vindesine sulphate, a new vinca alkaloid. *Pharmacotherapy* **3**, 259–268.
7. Ettinger, L.J. *et al.* (1982). Vindesine – phase II study in childhood malignancies: A report for cancer and leukaemia group. *Med. Pediatr. Oncol.* **10**, 35–44.
8. Mathe, G. *et al.* (1981). Phase II clinical trials with hematogical malignancies. *Anticancer Res.* **1**, 1–10.

Prepared by M.G. Lee

The following monographs on cytokines represent those available on the UK market licensed for use in oncology. The list below contains other cytokines under investigation or awaiting licences in the UK. Many are already available in the United States.

Chemical Group	Approved Name	Company or Producer
Hu-r-GM-CSF	Molgramostim Sargramostim	Schering-Plough, Immunex
Hu-r-M-CSF	–	Eurocetus, Biogen, Immunex, Sandoz, Bristol-Myers Squibb
Interleukin 3	–	Biogen, Eurocetus, Schering-Plough Immunex, Sandoz
Tumour necrosis factor	–	Knoll
Interferon alpha-2c	–	Boehringer Ingelheim
Interferon beta (natural source)	Ferono	Serono, Ferono, Bioferon
Interferon beta (recombinant source)	–	Bristol-Myers Squibb, Boehringer Ingelheim, Eurocetus, Interpharm, Roche, Schering-Plough, Wellcome
Interferon gamma (recombinant source)	–	Biogen

FILGRASTIM

1 General Details

Approved name: Filgrastim.
Proprietary name: Neupogen.
Manufacturer: Amgen Ltd.
Supplier: Roche Products Ltd.
Presentation and formulation details: Filgrastim is a sterile, clear, colourless liquid, formulated in an aqueous sodium acetate buffer, pH 4, containing 4% mannitol and 0.004% polysorbate 80.

It is known chemically as non-glycosylated recombinant methionyl human granulocyte colony-stimulating factor (r-metHuG-CSF), and is produced by recombinant DNA technology using an *Escherichia coli* strain.

Filgrastim contains 30×10^6 IU (300 µg)/ml. Neupogen 30 contains 300 µg of filgrastim in a 1 ml vial. Neupogen 48 contains 480 µg of filgrastim in a 1.6 ml vial.

Storage and shelf-life of unopened container: Filgrastim should be stored at 2–8°C. It should not be frozen. The pack is provided with an indicator to detect possible freezing. Vials that have been frozen (the indicator shows red) should not be used. A single brief period (up to seven days) of exposure to elevated temperatures (up to 37°C) does not affect stability. Unopened vials of filgrastim expire two years from the date of manufacture.[1]

2 Chemistry

Molecular structure: The amino acid composition of the mature r-metHuG-CSF sequence is:

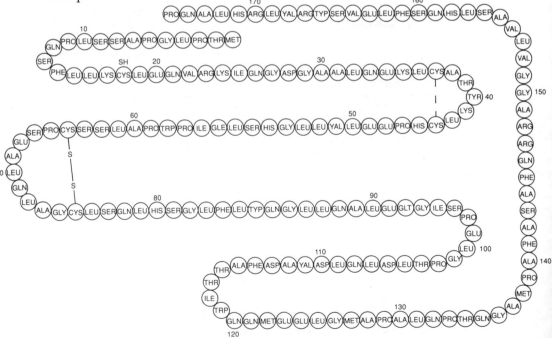

The solution contains filgrastim (r-metHuG-CSF) as a hydrophobic protein comprising 175 amino acids. The recombinant protein differs from natural human G-CSF by virtue of an additional amino terminal methionine residue and the absence of O-glycosylation. There are no potential sites of N-glycosylation on the natural human G-CSF or recombinant G-CSF molecules.

Molecular weight: Approximately 18–22,000 Da.

Solubility: Filgrastim is soluble in aqueous solutions.

3 Stability Profile

pH and physical stability: The pH of filgrastim is 4.0. Low pH and low salt concentration, together with additives, enhance filgrastim stability by preventing protein aggregation. The product should also not be vigorously shaken when diluting in order to avoid the formation of protein aggregates which might induce undesirable effects in the patient (ie formation of antibodies).

Stability on dilution: Diluted filgrastim solutions should not be prepared more than 24 hours before administration and should be stored at between 2 and 8°C. Solutions of filgrastim at concentrations of 15 µg/ml or higher are stable at room temperature for up to one week.[2]

Container compatibility: Filgrastim diluted in 5% glucose or in 5% glucose plus human albumin is compatible with a variety of plastics. These include: PVC, polyolefin (co-polymer of polypropylene and polyethylene) and polypropylene.[2] If filgrastim is to be used as an infusion with the administration set composed of unknown material, human serum albumin (HSA) should always be added as a protective protein to the diluent to a concentration of at least 2 mg/ml. It is not necessary to protect filgrastim from light when the drug is being prepared for administration but it is recommended that filgrastim is stored within the dispensing pack.[2]

Drug compatibility: The compatibility of filgrastim with other products and solutions has not been evaluated, therefore filgrastim should not be given together with any other drugs in the same infusion set and also should not be diluted in any other solution containing sodium chloride.

Stability in clinical practice

Undiluted filgrastim in tuberculin syringes (Becton-Dickinson)[2] is stable for up to 24 hours at controlled room temperature (25°C and not exceeding 37°C) or for up to seven days in the refrigerator 2–8°C. Filgrastim does not contain any preservatives. The manufacturer recommends that, in order to reduce the possibility of bacterial proliferation, filgrastim in syringes should be stored at 2–8°C and used within 24 hours of preparation.[1]

Filgrastim may be diluted in 5% glucose intravenous solution. Very dilute solutions of filgrastim may be adsorbed onto glass and plastic materials. Therefore, dilution to a final concentration of less than 0.2×10^6 IU (2 µg/ml) is not recommended.[2]

For solutions diluted to concentrations below 1.5×10^6 IU (15 µg/ml), HSA should be added to a final concentration of 2 mg/ml, ie in a final injection volume of 20 ml. Total doses of filgrastim less than 30×10^6 IU (300 µg) should be given with 0.2 ml of 20% HSA.[2]

4 Clinical Use

Indications: Filgrastim is indicated for reduction in both the duration of neutropenia and the incidence of febrile neutropenia in patients treated with established cytotoxic chemotherapy for non-myeloid malignancy.[1] This allows the clinician to optimize cytotoxic chemotherapy and reduce the incidence of febrile neutropenia and its clinical sequelae.

Dosage: When filgrastim is administered as an adjunct to standard dose chemotherapy, the recommended dose is 5 µg/kg/day. Individual patients may require dose escalation if the time taken to respond or if the magnitude of the neutrophil response is unacceptable after five to seven days of filgrastim therapy. In such cases, doses may be increased in increments of 5 µg/kg for each chemotherapy cycle.[1] A maximum tolerated dose has not yet been identified. Patients have received doses as high as 115 µg/kg/day with no toxic effects attributable to filgrastim therapy.[1] Filgrastim can be administered either as a bolus subcutaneous injection or as a short (30 minute) or continuous IV or subcutaneous infusion.[1]

Timing of administration: Filgrastim administration should be initiated at least 24 hours after the last dose of chemotherapy and should be discontinued at least 24 hours before the next chemotherapy dose. This is because filgrastim stimulates neutrophil precursor cell proliferation and, since many antineoplastic agents target rapidly proliferating cells, co-administration of filgrastim and antineoplastic therapy may theoretically lead to abolition of neutrophil precursors. Filgrastim administration should be continued throughout the expected chemotherapy-induced nadir until the patient achieves an absolute neutrophil count (ANC) more than or equal to 10,000 cells/ml.[1]

Patients receiving dose-intensified chemotherapy should be continued on filgrastim until two consecutive ANCs register more than 10,000 cells/ml. The time to achieve this ANC level will vary, based on the chemotherapy regimen, the patient's underlying disease, prior treatment history and dose of filgrastim.[1]

5 Preparation of Injection

Reconstitution: Not applicable.

Extravasation: Not irritant; no recommendations available (*see* Chapter 9).

6 Destruction of Drug or Contaminated Articles

Disposal: Excess filgrastim solution may be disposed of into a drain with copious amounts of water. All other waste, including contaminated packaging or cleaning materials and used protective clothing must be placed with clinical waste for incineration. When dealing with broken vials, disposable gloves, eye protection and a face mask should be worn.

Contact with skin: This is thought not to be a serious problem; a general procedure should be adopted of removing contaminated clothing and washing skin thoroughly with soap and water. If the eyes are contaminated, irrigate with water and obtain medical advice.

References

1. *ABPI Data Sheet Compendium 1991–92.* (1991). Datapharm Publications Ltd, London, pp. 1267–1268.
2. Amgen (UK) Ltd. Personal communication.

Prepared by A.P. Stanley

INTERFERON α-2A

1 General Details

Approved name: Interferon α-2a(rbe).

Proprietary name: Roferon-A.

Manufacturer or supplier: Roche Products Ltd.

Presentation and formulation details: Roferon-A vials: Sterile powder for reconstitution in single dose vials, containing 3×10^6, 4.5×10^6, 9×10^6 or 19×10^6 IU of lyophilized interferon α-2a(rbe), 9 mg sodium chloride and 5 mg human serum albumin (European Pharmacopoeia) included as a stabilizer. The solution is reconstituted prior to use by addition of 1 ml of sterile water for injections BP, supplied as solvent. Multiple dosage strengths in solution are 3×10^6 IU in 1 ml, 18×10^6 IU in 3 ml (6×10^6 IU/ml) and 36×10^6 IU in 1 ml.[1]

Storage and shelf-life of unopened container: Unopened vials expire three years from the date of manufacture when stored at or below the recommended maximum storage temperature of 25°C.[2] The interferon α-2a(rbe) solution must be stored between 2 and 8°C.[1] It is likely that storage conditions for all interferons will be standardized in the foreseeable future and that they will recommend refrigeration for all interferons, irrespective of formulation.

2 Chemistry

Interferon α-2a(rbe) is a recombinant interferon. It is a highly purified, sterile non-glycosylated protein containing 165 amino acids with two disulphide bridges between residues 1 and 98 and between 29 and 138.[3] It is produced by recombinant DNA technology using a genetically engineered *Escherichia coli* strain containing DNA that codes for the human protein. It differs from other recombinant interferons by the fact that amino acid 23 is a lysine group and amino acid 34 is a histidine group.

Interferon α-2a(rbe) has been shown to possess many of the activities of 'natural' human α-interferon. It has antiviral, antiproliferative and immuno-modulatory actions.[4]

Molecular weight: Approximately 19,000 Da.

Solubility: Interferon α-2a(rbe) is freely soluble in water.

3 Stability Profile

Physical and chemical stability: Reconstituted vials should not be used after more than 24 hours' storage in a refrigerator (2–8°C) or two hours at room temperature. Reconstituted vials of 3×10^6 IU and 18×10^6 IU interferon α-2a(rbe) in 1 ml of water for injections, frozen immediately after reconstitution to −20°C have shown no physical degradation or loss of chemical activity on thawing at one month.[5] Interferon α-2a(rbe) is sensitive to heat, light and atmospheric oxygen.

Compatibility with other drugs: Data is not available concerning interferon α-2a(rbe) and other compounds, therefore the manufacturer recommends that it is not mixed with other drugs.

Molecular structure:

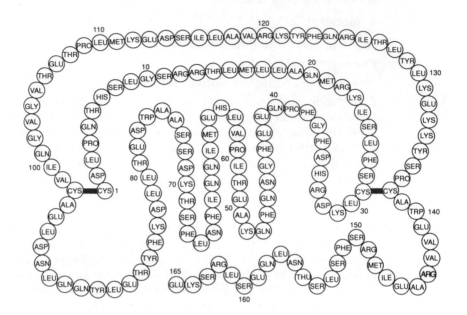

Stability in clinical practice

The recommended maximum storage temperature for interferon α-2a(rbe) vials is 25°C. However, the vials appear stable for up to one month at −20°C when frozen immediately after reconstitution. Reconstituted vials should not be used after more than 24 hours' storage in a refrigerator (2–8°C) or two hours at room temperature.

4 Clinical Use

Type of cytotoxic agent: Activator of natural killer cells.

Main indications: Interferon α-2a is licensed for use as a single agent in the treatment of hairy cell leukaemia, chronic myelogenous leukaemia (specifically in chronic phase Philadelphia chromosome positive disease), recurrent or metastatic renal cell carcinoma and AIDS-related Kaposi's sarcoma in patients without a history of opportunistic infection. It is also indicated for the treatment of adult patients with chronic active hepatitis B who have markers for viral replication.[2]

Interferon α-2a(rbe) has been used in combination regimens with cytotoxics.

Dosage:

▼ AIDS-related Kaposi's sarcoma. Induction dose: 36×10^6 IU intramuscularly daily for four to ten weeks. Maintenance dose: 36×10^6 IU intramuscularly three times per week. Patients should be treated for 30–90 days before the physician determines the possible benefits of continued therapy.

▼ Hairy cell leukaemia. Induction dose: 3×10^6 IU intramuscularly daily for 16–24 weeks.

▼ Recurrent or metastatic renal cell carcinoma. Induction dose: escalation from 3×10^6 IU daily to a maximum of 36×10^6 IU daily by intramuscular injection over ten to 12 weeks.

Schedule:

Days 1–3:	3×10^6 IU daily
Days 4–6:	9×10^6 IU daily
Days 7–9:	18×10^6 IU daily, then continue with 18×10^6 IU daily to maximum 36×10^6 IU daily

Maintenance dose: $18–36 \times 10^6$ IU three times per week. Doses of up to 18×10^6 IU can be given subcutaneously or intramuscularly. Intramuscular injection is recommended for doses of 36×10^6 IU. The maintenance dose should be given until progressive disease is documented unless it is not in the best interest of the patient.

▼ Chronic active hepatitis B. The optimal schedule of treatment has not yet been established. The dose is usually in the range of $2.5–5.0 \times 10^6$ IU/m² body surface area, administered subcutaneously three times per week for four to six months.[2]

5 Preparation of Injection

Reconstitution: The content of Roferon-A vials should be reconstituted with 1 ml of water for injections (supplied as the solvent) and swirled gently. Vigorous shaking should be avoided.

Bolus administration: $2–15 \times 10^6$ IU/m² by subcutaneous injection.

Intravenous infusion: Not recommended due to poor drug stability.

Extravasation: Not irritant; no recommendations available (*see* Chapter 9).

6 Destruction of Drug or Contaminated Articles

Disposal: Excess interferon α-2a(rbe) solution may be disposed of into a drain with copious amounts of water. All other waste, including contaminated packaging or cleaning materials and used protective clothing must be placed with clinical waste for incineration.[6] When dealing with broken vials, disposable gloves, eye protection and a face mask should be worn.[6]

Contact with skin: Remove contaminated clothing and wash skin thoroughly with soap and water. If the eyes are contaminated, irrigate with water and obtain medical advice.[6]

References

1. American Product Information Sheet. (1992). *Am. J. Hosp. Pharm.* **49**, 550–552.
2. *ABPI Data Sheet Compendium 1991–92.* (1991). Datapharm Publications Ltd, London, pp. 1283–1285.
3. Wetzel, R. (1981). Assignment of the disulphide bonds of leukocyte interferon. *Nature* **189**, 606–607.
4. Baron, S. *et al.* (1991). The interferons: Mechanisms of action and clinical applications. *JAMA* **266**, 1375–1383.
5. Roche Products Ltd. Personal communication.
6. Interferon of alfa-2a(rbe). (1992). *COSHH Safety Data Sheet*, prepared by Roche Products Ltd.

Prepared by A.P. Stanley

INTERFERON α-2B

1 General Details

Approved name: Interferon α-2b(rbe).

Proprietary name: Intron-A.

Manufacturer or supplier: Schering–Plough Ltd.

Presentation and formulation details: Vials of lyophilized powder containing 1, 3, 5, 10 and 30 × 10⁶ IU of interferon α-2b(rbe) per vial. The solution is reconstituted just prior to administration by the addition of 1 ml sterile water for injections (supplied as solvent). 10 × 10⁶ IU = 0.05 mg interferon α-2b(rbe) protein.[1]

Interferon α-2b(rbe) 1, 3, 5, 10 and 30 × 10⁶ IU also contains amino-acetic acid, mono and dibasic sodium phosphate, and human albumin.

Storage and shelf-life of unopened container: Store in a refrigerator. The shelf-life is three years from the date of manufacture.

2 Chemistry

Type: Interferon α-2b(rbe) is a recombinant interferon. It is a highly purified, sterile, non-glycosylated single chain protein containing 165 amino acids with two disulphide bridges between residues 1 and 98, and 29 and 138.[2] It is produced by recombinant DNA technology using a genetically engineered *Escherichia coli* strain containing DNA that codes for the human protein. It differs from other recombinant interferons by the fact that amino acid 23 is an arginine group and amino acid 34 is a histidine group.

Molecular structure:

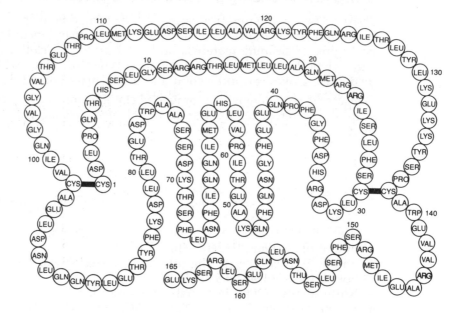

Molecular weight: Approximately 20,000 Da.

Solubility: Interferon α-2b(rbe) is freely soluble, strengths up to 10×10^6 IU/ml are all isotonic when diluted with 1 ml of water for injections; the 30×10^6 IU in 1 ml of water has a tonicity six times normal. Up to 60×10^6 IU will dissolve in 1 ml of water for injections.[2]

3 Stability Profile

Interferon α-2b(rbe) degrades by cleavage of disulphide bridges. The liberated sulphydryl groups form oligomers (dimers and trimers) with other monomers. It is believed that only one disulphide bridge is required for biological activity.

Physical and chemical stability

Interferon α-2b(rbe) is not photosensitive,[2] and is generally chemically unstable after reconstitution.

Effect of pH: Interferon α-2b(rbe) is most stable in the pH range 6.9–7.5.[2]

Container compatibility: No adsorption has been found to occur onto the surface of polypropylene syringes. At low concentrations of less than 0.1×10^6 IU/ml, interferon may bind to PVC, however this is believed to be a non-significant interaction.[2]

Compatibility with other drugs: Interferon α-2b(rbe) should only be reconstituted with water for injections, however, it is known to be compatible with 0.9% sodium chloride, Ringer's solution and lactated Ringer's (Hartmann's) solution; however, it is incompatible with glucose solutions.[2]

Stability in clinical practice

When reconstituted with 1 ml water for injections per vial up to 10×10^6 IU, an isotonic solution is produced which is stable for 24 hours at 2–8°C.[1]

Qualitative gradient-elution HPLC studies[3] on the degradation of aqueous solutions of interferon α-2b(rbe) at a concentration of 430,000 IU/ml have shown significant degradation over five days' storage at 4°C, with measurable degradation products appearing after 48 hours. At 37°C, degradation product peaks were observed after four hours.

However, interferon α-2b(rbe) has been shown to be stable for infusion over a 24-hour period[2] if the following criteria are strictly adhered to:

▼ temperature not greater than 25°C
▼ concentration of interferon α-2b(rbe) greater than 1×10^6 IU/ml
▼ infusion container is glass or PVC (Viaflex).

The stability of interferon α2b(rbe) can be summarized:[2]

Powder in vials	Below 25°C	one month
Powder in vials	45°C	24 hours
Solution in vial or syringe (polypropylene)	2–8°C	one month
Solution in vial	Below 25°C	14 days
Solution frozen in vial or syringe (including four freeze-thaw cycles)	−20°C	two months

4 Clinical Use

Type of cytotoxic agent: Activator of natural killer cells.

Indications: Interferon α-2b(rbe) is licensed for use as a single agent in the treatment of myeloma, chronic myelogenous leukaemia, hairy cell leukaemia, recurrent or metastatic renal cell carcinoma and AIDS-related Kaposi's sarcoma in patients without history of opportunistic infection. It is also indicated for the treatment of adult patients which chronic active hepatitis B who have markers for viral replication and for genital warts.[1] Non-licensed indications for which there are large research programmes include lymphoma,[4] colorectal carcinoma, chronic active hepatitis C and neuroblastoma.[5]

Interferon α-2b(rbe) has been used in combination regimens with cytotoxics.

Dosage:

▼ Hairy cell leukaemia. The recommended dose is 2×10^6 IU/m² Intron A administered subcutaneously three times per week.
▼ Chronic myelogenous leukaemia. The recommended dose is $4–5 \times 10^6$ IU/m² Intron A, administered subcutaneously daily. When the white blood cell count is controlled, the dosage may be administered every other day.
▼ AIDS-related Kaposi's sarcoma. The recommended dose of Intron A is 30×10^6 IU/m² administered subcutaneously three times per week (ie every other day). The regimen should be maintained indefinitely unless the disease progresses rapidly or severe intolerance develops.
▼ Condyloma acuminata. The lesion or lesions to be injected should be cleaned first with a sterile alcohol pad. The intralesional injection should be made at the base of the lesion using a fine needle (30 gauge). Inject 0.1 ml of sterile solution containing 1.0×10^6 IU Intron A into the lesion three times per week on alternate days, for three weeks. As many as five lesions can be treated at one time. The maximum total dose administered weekly should not exceed 15×10^6 IU.[1]

5 Preparation of Injection

Intron A should be reconstituted with 1 ml water for injections (or for condyloma acuminata, with sufficient to produce a concentration of 1×10^6 IU/0.1 ml). The vials should be swirled gently. Vigorous shaking should be avoided.

Bolus administration: $2–15 \times 10^6$ IU/m² injected subcutaneously.

Intravenous infusion: Not recommended due to poor drug stability, unless interferon α-2b(rbe) is being used as part of a high dose protocol, when adherence to the infusion stability criteria and conditions should be observed.

Extravasation: Not irritant; no recommendations available (*see* Chapter 9).

6 Destruction of Drug or Contaminated Articles

Disposal: Excess interferon α-2b(rbe) solution may be disposed of into a drain with copious amounts of water. All other waste, including contaminated packaging or cleaning materials and used protective clothing must be placed with clinical waste for incineration. When dealing with broken vials, disposable gloves, eye protection and a dust mask should be worn.

Contact with skin: Remove contaminated clothing and wash skin thoroughly with soap and water. If the eyes are contaminated, irrigate with water and obtain medical advice.

References

1. *Data Sheet Compendium 1991–92*. (1991). Datapharm Publications Ltd, London, pp. 1390–1391.
2. Schering Corporation, USA. Personal communication.
3. Palmer, A.J. *et al.* (1988). Qualitative studies on interferon alfa-2b in prolonged continuous infusion regimes using gradient elution high performance liquid chromatography. *J. Clin. Pharm. Ther.* **13**, 225–231.
4. Merigan, T.C. *et al.* (1978). Preliminary observations on the effect of human leukocyte interferon in non-Hodgkin's lymphoma. *N. Engl. J. Med.* **199**, 1449–1454.
5. Swada, T. *et al.* (1979). Preliminary report on the clinical use of human leukocyte interferon in neuroblastoma. *Cancer Treat. Rep.* **63**, 2111.

Prepared by A.P. Stanley

INTERFERON α-N1

1 General Details

Approved name: Interferon α-n1(ins).

Proprietary name: Wellferon.

Manufacturer or supplier: Wellcome Medical Division, UK.

Presentation and formulation details: Wellferon is a clear colourless solution in single dose vials, containing 3×10^6 or 10×10^6 IU of purified human lymphoblastoid interferon formulated in 1 ml tris–glycine, buffered saline, with albumin solution (European Pharmacopoeia) at a concentration of 1.5 mg/ml as a stabilizer.

Storage and shelf-life of unopened container: Unopened vials expire three years from the date of manufacture when stored between 2–8°C.

2 Chemistry

Interferon α-n1(ins) is a highly purified blend of natural human α-interferons, which is obtained from human lymphoblastoid cells following induction with Sendai virus. The final product has a purity of at least 95% and contains no detectable DNA (less than 10 pg of Namalwa cell DNA/ml).

Wellferon resembles human leukocyte interferon in that it is a mixture of natural α subtypes; at least 22 have been detected. It also differs from recombinant α-interferon preparations made from bacteria or other genetically engineered cells which contain only a single subtype.[1]

Molecular structure: Not available.

Molecular weight: Approximately 19,000 Da.

Solubility: Interferon α-n1(ins) is supplied as a solution.

3 Stability Profile

Physical and chemical stability

No information is available.

Effect of pH: No information is available.

Effect of light: Interferon α-n1(ins) is sensitive to photodegradation and should therefore be protected from light.[1]

Stability in clinical practice

Due to lack of available information, it is only possible to recommend immediate use of interferon α-n1(ins) after withdrawing the appropriate dose, followed by speedy disposal of any residue.

4 Clinical Use

Main indications: Interferon α-n1(ins) is licensed for use as a single agent in the treatment of hairy cell leukaemia,[1] and for the treatment of adults with chronic active hepatitis B, who have markers for viral replication.

Dosage:

▼ Hairy cell leukaemia. For remission induction, the dose recommended is 3×10^6 IU given daily by intramuscular or subcutaneous injection, the latter being more convenient for patient self-administration. After initial improvement in peripheral haematological indices (commonly 12–16 weeks), the dose may be administered thrice weekly. Prolonged treatment for six months or more may be required to clear hairy cells from the bone marrow.

▼ Chronic active hepatitis B infection. A 12-week course of thrice-weekly intramuscular or subcutaneous injections of $10-15 \times 10^6$ IU (up to 7.5×10^6 IU/m^2 body surface area) is generally recommended. Longer periods of treatment for up to six months at lower doses ($5-10 \times 10^6$ IU thrice wekly or up to 5×10^6 IU/m^2) have been employed and may be preferred for patients who do not tolerate higher doses.[1]

5 Preparation of Injection

Reconstitution: Not applicable.

Bolus administration: $2-7.5 \times 10^6$ IU/m^2 injected subcutaneously or by deep intramuscular injection.

Intravenous infusion: Not recommended.

Extravasation: Not irritant; no recommendations available (*see* Chapter 9).

6 Destruction of Drug or Contaminated Articles

Disposal: Excess interferon solution may be disposed of into a drain with copious amounts of water. All other waste, including contaminated packaging or cleaning materials and used protective clothing must be placed with clinical waste for incineration. When dealing with broken vials, disposable gloves, eye protection and a dust mask should be worn.

Contact with skin: Remove contaminated clothing and wash skin thoroughly with soap and water. If the eyes are contaminated, irrigate with water and obtain medical advice.

References

1. *ABPI Data Sheet Compendium 1991–92.* (1991). Datapharm Publications Ltd, London, pp. 1746–1748.

Prepared by A.P. Stanley

INTERLEUKIN 2

1 General Details

Approved name: Aldesleukin (Proleukin).

Manufacturer or supplier: Eurocetus (UK) Ltd.

Presentation and formulation details: Aldesleukin is a sterile white lyophilized powder for parenteral use containing 1.2 mg (18×10^6 IU/mg) aldesleukin, a recombinant human interleukin-2 (rIL-2), supplied in glass vials (5 ml).

When reconstituted with 1.2 ml water for injections BP each vial delivers 1 ml solution containing 18×10^6 IU (1 mg) aldesleukin, 50 mg mannitol, and 0.2 mg sodium dodecyl sulphate, buffered with sodium phosphates to a pH of 7.5 (range 7.2–7.8).

Storage and shelf-life of unopened container: Unopened vials expire two years from the date of manufacture when stored at 2–8°C.

2 Chemistry

Aldesleukin is produced by recombinant DNA technology using an *Escherichia coli* strain which contains a genetically engineered modification of the human IL-2 gene. This modified recombinant human IL-2 differs from native IL-2 in the following ways:

▼ the molecule is not glycosylated because it is derived from *Escherichia coli*
▼ the molecule has no N-terminal alanine
▼ the molecule has serine substituted for cysteine at amino acid position 125.

The two amino acid changes result in a more homogeneous IL-2 product. The biological activities of aldesleukin and native human IL-2, a naturally occurring lymphokine, are similar; both regulate the immune response. The administration of aldesleukin has been shown to reduce both tumour growth and spread. The exact mechanism by which aldesleukin-mediated immunostimulation leads to antitumour activity is not yet known.

Molecular structure:

Des-alanyl-1, serine-125 human interleukin-2; recombinant interleukin-2

10
Pro-Thr-Ser-Ser-Ser-Thr-Lys-Lys-Thr-Gln-Leu-Gln-Leu-Glu-His-Leu-

20   30
Leu-Leu-Asp-Leu-Gln-Met-Ile-Leu-Asn-Gly-Ile-Asn-Asn-Tyr-Lys-Asn-

40
Pro-Lys-Leu-Thr-Arg-Met-Leu-Thr-Phe-Lys-Phe-Tyr-Met-Pro-Lys-Lys-

50   60
Ala-Thr-Glu-Leu-Lys-His-Leu-Gln-Cys-Leu-Glu-Glu-Glu-Leu-Lys-Pro-

70   80
Leu-Glu-Glu-Val-Leu-Asn-Leu-Ala-Gln-Ser-Lys-Asn-Phe-His-Leu-Arg-

90
Pro-Arg-Asp-Leu-Ile-Ser-Asn-Ile-Asn-Val-Ile-Val-Leu-Glu-Leu-Lys-

100   110
Gly-Ser-Glu-Thr-Thr-Phe-Met-Cys-Glu-Tyr-Ala-Asp-Glu-Thr-Ala-Thr-

120
Ile-Val-Glu-Phe-Leu-Asn-Arg-Trp-Ile-Thr-Phe-Ser-Gln-Ser-Ile-Ile-

Ser-Thr-Leu-Thr

Molecular weight: Approximately 15,600 Da.

Solubility: Aldesleukin is freely soluble in water.

3 Stability Profile

Physical and chemical stability

Store vials of lyophilized aldesleukin (rIL-2) in a refrigerator at 2–8°C. Reconstituted or diluted aldesleukin may be stored at refrigerated and at room temperature (2–30°C).

As rIL-2 is not glycosylated it is less water soluble (more lipophilic) when compared with endogenous IL-2. The more lipophilic properties of rIL-2 make it necessary to use sodium dodecyl sulphate (SDS) during the production and formulation of aldesleukin. SDS is a surface active compound which reversibly binds to rIL-2 and brings the lipophilic molecule into solution. In a solution of reconstituted IL-2 there is an equilibrium between rIL-2 bound SDS and free SDS. The capability for SDS to keep rIL-2 in solution is dependent on the concentrations of SDS and rIL-2. The addition of human serum albumin (HSA) is not needed when the reconstituted IL-2 is further diluted (with 5% glucose) to r-IL2 concentrations of between 100 and 1000 µg/ml, because the SDS concentration is high enough to keep the rIL-2 in solution within this concentration range.

It is also not advisable to use HSA, because its addition to rIL-2 at these high concentrations will result in the binding of HSA to SDS, which disturbs the sensitive equilibrium between the free SDS and the rIL-2 bound SDS. This can result in the precipitation of rIL-2.

However, when the solution is further diluted to concentrations below 100 µg/ml, the addition of HSA (0.1%) is necessary to prevent precipitation of rIL-2.

Human albumin should be added and mixed with 5% glucose injection prior to the additon of IL-2; it is added to protect against loss of bioactivity.

Container compatibility: IL-2 should be administered using infusion bags or syringes composed of one of the following materials: polypropylene syringes (eg Becton-Dickinson Plastipak or Sherwood Monoject), polyvinylchloride bags (eg Viaflex), polyolefine bags (eg PAB-Excel), or glass bottles.

Extension sets composed of polyethylene or standard administration sets can be used.

In-line filters should not be used when administering interleukin.

Effect of light: No information available.

Effect of pH: Stable between pH 7.2–7.8. With time, undergoes hydrolysis outside this range.

Compatibility with other drugs: Reconstitution and dilution procedures other than those recommended may result in incomplete delivery of bioactivity and/or formation of biologically inactive protein.

The use of bacteriostatic water for injections or 0.9% sodium chloride should be avoided because of increased aggregation. Interleukin should not be mixed with other drugs.

Stability in clinical practice

Due to the unstable nature of IL-2, it must be used within 24 hours of preparation and stored refrigerated (2–8°C) until use.

4 Clinical Use

Main indications: Used in the treatment of metastatic renal cell carcinoma, but excluding those patients in whom *all* the following three prognostic factors are present:

▼ a performance status of ECOG 1 or greater
▼ more than one organ with metastatic disease sites
▼ a period of less than 24 months between initial diagnosis of primary tumour and the date the patient is evaluated for IL-2 treatment.

Dosage: Full details of dosage recommendations for each of the licensed indications are provided in the manufacturer's data sheet.[1] Aldesleukin has also been extensively investigated in renal cell carcinoma, melanoma and colorectal tumours using subcutaneous administration schedules to try to minimize the side effects of the rIL-2.[2]

5 Preparation of Injection

Reconstitution: Each vial of IL-2 for injection should be reconstituted with 1.2 ml of water for injections. The diluent should be directed against the side of the vial to avoid excess foaming, and the contents swirled gently until completely dissolved. Do not shake. The resulting solution should be a clear, colourless liquid. When reconstituted as directed, each ml contains 18×10^6 IU (1 mg) aldesleukin.

Extravasation: Not irritant; however may cause local capillary leak syndrome and/or local tissue reaction (*see* Chapter 9).

6 Destruction of Drug or Contaminated Articles

Disposal: Excess IL-2 solution may be disposed of into a drain with copious amounts of water. All other waste, including contaminated packaging or cleaning materials and used protective clothing must be placed with clinical waste for incineration. When dealing with broken vials, disposable gloves, eye protection and a dust mask should be worn.

Contact with skin: Remove contaminated clothing and wash skin thoroughly with soap and water. If the eyes are contaminated, irrigate with water and obtain medical advice.

References

1. *UK Data Sheet January 1992.* Eurocetus (UK) Ltd.
2. Eurocetus (UK) Ltd. Personal communication.

Prepared by A.P. Stanley

This section provides and identifies suitable sources of essential basic information on unlicensed cytotoxic agents known to be of current clinical interest. The interferons, interleukins and related biologically-derived compounds, now all known generically as cytokines, have been intentionally excluded since they do not present to pharmacy staff the same problems of handling as do more conventional cytotoxic agents.

Much of the content draws heavily on information provided by the National Cancer Institute (NCI) of the National Institute of Health of the USA. Copies of two books, *NCI investigational drugs: pharmaceutical data* and *Investigational drugs: chemical data*, which are updated annually, may be obtained by post, free of charge from:

Pharmaceutical Resources Branch
National Cancer Institute
Executive Plaza North
Suite 818
Bethesda, Maryland 20892
USA.

More comprehensive information may also be available from the NCI in clinical brochures for individual drugs, or from investigators currently working with the compounds concerned. For this reason, at the end of each monograph, UK and key overseas centres with a known interest in the compound concerned are identified.

2-CHLORODEOXYADENOSINE

1 General Details

Approved name: 2-chloro-2'-deoxyadenosine (2-CdA).

Proprietary name: None.

Manufacturer or supplier: Initially developed at the Scripps Clinic and Research Foundation. Later the R.W. Johnson Pharmaceutical Institute, Rariton, New Jersey received development rights. Currently the drug is supplied via the National Cancer Institute under protocol number E91-7057.

Presentation and formulation details: 20 ml vials filled with 10 ml of solution. Each ml contains 1.0 mg/ml 2-CdA injectable solution.

Storage and shelf-life of unopened container: The drug should be kept frozen ($-10°C$ to $-20°C$). However, the product may be shipped refrigerated. The drug is stable when subjected to multiple freeze-thaw cycles. It should be protected from light. A product stable at $2-8°C$ may be available shortly.

2 Chemistry

Type: Purine nucleoside analogue (resistant to adenosine deaminase).

Molecular structure: 2-chloro-6-amino-9-(2-deoxy-β-D-erythropento furanosyl) purine.

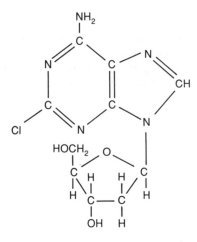

Molecular weight: 287.5.

Characteristics and solubility: A stable white to off-white crystalline powder that is sparingly soluble in water. Dissolves more easily in 0.9% sodium chloride at $60-65°C$.

3 Stability Profile

Physical and chemical stability

Shelf-life surveillance of the intact vials is ongoing. When sterile and non-pyrogenic 2-CdA solution for injection (1.0 mg/ml) is stored at $-20°C$ the product is stable for at least one year. Once the sterile drug solution is thawed, it should be stored at $5°C$ for no more than two weeks. The product should be thawed by storage in a refrigerator or at room temperature. The drug solution has been found to lose less than 5% of activity in seven days at 37°C. The vials contain no preservatives. When diluted to a concentration of 0.15–0.3 mg/ml in 0.9% sodium chloride containing 0.9% benzyl alcohol as the preservative, it is estimated that the solution is chemically stable for at least 14 days at 5°C.

4 Clinical Use

Main indications: Treatment of hairy cell leukaemia. In a multicentre trial a single seven-day infusion gave complete disease remission in 75% of evaluated patients.

Other indications: CLL, non-Hodgkin's lymphoma, cutaneous T-cell lymphoma, ALL, CGL and AML. In addition, patients being prepared for bone marrow transplantation, and those with multiple sclerosis and rheumatoid arthritis have been treated. Overall clinical experience with 2-CdA has demonstrated the drug to be very effective in inducing responses in many patients with lymphoid neoplasms. It has shown greatest promise in CLL, cutaneous T-cell lymphomas and autoimmune haemolytic anaemia.

Dosage regimen: One cycle only–0.1 mg/kg/day for seven days, administered by continuous infusion.

5 Preparation of Injection

The drug is thawed at room temperature or in the refrigerator for up to 24 hours prior to use. Do not thaw by microwave.

Intravenous infusion: 2-CdA is added to 500 ml 0.9% sodium chloride through a supplied Millex filter, and administered intravenously by continuous infusion over 24 hours, daily for seven days. It may also be administered by continuous intravenous infusion, via an ambulatory pump, over seven days.

Extravasation: Non-irritant.

6 Destruction of Drug or Contaminated Articles

Incineration: No specific information.

Chemical: No specific information.

Contact with skin: No specific information.

7 Centres with a Known Interest in this Drug

▼ Scripps Clinic, La Jolla, California, USA.
▼ M.D. Anderson Cancer Hospital, Texas, USA.
▼ Hadassah University Hospital, Jerusalem, Israel.

8 Sources of Information

Beutler, E. Chairman, Dept. of Experimental Medicine, Scripps Clinic, La Jolla, CA, USA. Personal communication.
NCI, Protocol E91-7057-2-CdA.
R.W. Johnson Pharmaceutical Research Institute, Protocol 2-CdA.
Piroet, E. *et al.* (1991). 2 CdA: A potent chemotherapeutic and immunosuppressive nucleoside. *Leuk. Lymph.* **5**, 133–139.
N.I.H. (June 1992). Bulletin on 2–CdA, N.S.C. 105014.

Prepared by Y. Cass

DEOXYCOFORMYCIN

1 General Details

Approved names: Deoxycoformycin, 2-deoxycoformycin, co-vidarabine, pentostatin.

Proprietary names: None.

Manufacturer or supplier: National Cancer Institute.

Presentation and formulation details: Vials of white lyophilized powder containing 10 mg deoxycoformycin. Each vial also contains 50 mg mannitol and sodium hydroxide to adjust pH.

Storage and shelf-life of unopened container: Store at 2 to 8°C. Vials are labelled with an expiry date.

2 Chemistry

Type: Antimetabolite.

Molecular structure: Imidazo (4,5-d d)(1,3)diazepin-8-ol,3-(1-deoxy-β-D-erythro-pentafuranoesyl)-3,4,7,8-tetrahydro-

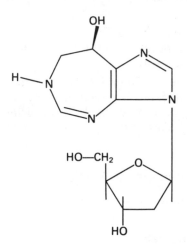

Molecular weight: 268.3.

Solubility: Greater than 30 mg/ml in water.

3 Stability Profile

Physical and chemical stability: Constitution with 0.9% sodium chloride results in a solution which is chemically stable at room temperature (22 to 25°C) for at least 72 hours, exhibiting about 2 to 4% decomposition.

Effect of temperature: When diluted to a concentration of 10 mg in 500 ml 0.9% sodium chloride, or lactated Ringer's Injection, deoxycoformycin is chemically stable for at least 48 hours at room temperature (22 to 25°C), exhibiting less than 5% decomposition.

At a concentration of 10 mg per 500 ml in 5% glucose, approximately 2% decomposition occurs in 24 hours at room temperature. As much as 8 to 10% loss has been reported to occur in 48 hours.

No potency loss was detected in this reconstituted solution or in admixtures in 5% glucose or 0.9% sodium chloride, when refrigerated at 5°C over 96 hours.

4 Clinical Use

Main indications: Treatment of hairy cell leukaemia, chronic lymphocytic leukaemia.

5 Preparation of Injection

Reconstitution: 5 ml of 0.9% sodium chloride is added to provide a solution containing deoxycoformycin 2 mg/ml which has a pH of 6.7 to 8.7.

Bolus administration: IV bolus, slowly over three to five minutes.

Extravasation: Non-irritant.

6 Destruction of Drug or Contaminated Articles

Incineration: No specific information.

Chemical: No specific information.

Contact with skin: No specific information.

7 Centres with a Known Interest in this Drug

▼ The Royal Marsden Hospital, London.
▼ Hammersmith Hospital, London.

8 Source of Information

NCI investigational drug data, 1989.

Prepared by T. Root

FLUDARABINE

1 General Details

Approved names: Fludarabine, fludarabine phosphate, 2-fluoro-adrenine arabinoside-5-phosphate, 2-fluoro-ARA-AMP.

Proprietary names: None.

Manufacturer or supplier: National Cancer Institute. Fludarabine is also manufactured by Triton Biosciences Inc, Alameda, California 94501, USA and by Ben Venue Labs Inc. Bedford, Ohio 44146, USA.

Presentation and formulation details: 5 ml vials of white lyophilized powder containing 50 mg fludarabine. Each vial also contains mannitol 50 mg and sodium hydroxide to adjust pH.

Storage and shelf-life of unopened container: Store at 2 to 8°C (NCI) or at 15 to 30°C (Triton).

2 Chemistry

Type: Antimetabolite.

Molecular structure: 9H-Purine-6-amine, 2-fluoro-9-(5-o-phosphono-β-D-arabino-furanoeyl).

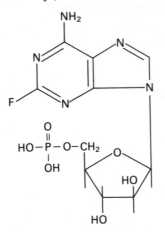

Molecular weight: 401.2.
Solubility: 9 mg/ml in water.

3 Stability Profile

Physical and chemical stability

Shelf-life surveillance of the intact vials is ongoing. One lot has maintained stability after 36 months at room temperature (22 to 25°C) and under refrigeration (2 to 8°C).

Effect of pH: Fludarabine phosphate is relatively stable in aqueous solution. Over a pH range of approximately 4.5 to 8 in aqueous buffer solutions stored at 65°C, less than 4% decomposition occurred in one day and less than 10% occurred in four days. At pH 3 at 65°C, approximately 11% decomposition occurred in one day. From this pH profile, the optimum pH was determined to be approximately 7.6.

Effect of temperature: At a concentration of 25 mg/ml in distilled water stored at room temperature (22 to 25°C) in normal laboratory light, fludarabine phosphate exhibited less than 2% decomposition in 16 days.

Diluted to a concentration of 1 mg/ml in 5% glucose or in 0.9% sodium chloride, less than 3% decomposition occurred in 16 days at room temperature (22 to 25°C) under normal laboratory light.

Diluted to a concentration of 0.04 mg/ml in 5% glucose or in 0.9% sodium chloride in glass bottles and PVC bags, little or no loss occurred in 48 hours at room temperature (22 to 25°C) exposed to normal laboratory light and under refrigeration (about 5°C).

4 Clinical Use

Main indications: Treatment of non-Hodgkin's lymphoma, chronic lymphoblastic leukaemia.

5 Preparation of Injection

Reconstitution: 2 ml of water for injection is added to a 50 mg vial to give a solution of pH 6.5 to 8.5 containing 25 mg fludarabine, 25 mg mannitol and sodium hydroxide.

Bolus administration: Slow bolus in 10 ml 0.9% sodium chloride or infusion in 250 ml 0.9% sodium chloride.

Extravasation: Non-irritant.

6 Destruction of Drug or Contaminated Articles

Incineration: No specific information.

Chemical: No specific information.

Contact with skin: No specific information.

7 Centres with a Known Interest in this Drug

▼ The Royal Marsden Hospital, London.
▼ St Bartholomew's Hospital, London.

8 Source of Information

NCI investigational drug data, 1989.

Trissel, L.A. (1992). *Handbook on injectable drugs,* 7th edn. American Society of Hospital Pharmacists, Bethesda, Maryland, USA.

Prepared by T. Root

LIPOSOMAL DOXORUBICIN

1 General Details

Approved name: Stealth liposomal doxorubicin hydrochloride.

Proprietary name: Doxil.

Manufacturer: Liposome Technology Inc., USA.

Presentation and formulation details: Doxil is supplied in vials containing 20 mg doxorubicin encapsulated in liposomes, as a frozen aqueous suspension. When thawed, the resultant translucent, red suspension has a doxorubicin concentration of 2 mg/ml and should be visually homogeneous.

Storage and shelf-life of unopened container: Store frozen at -10 to $-20°C$ until required for use, protected from light. There is as yet insufficient data on the stability of the product to establish an expiry date. Stability studies are continuing, including the development of a formulation stable at 2–8°C.

2 Chemistry

Type: Cytotoxic anthracycline antibiotic.

Molecular structure: As for doxorubicin, but encapsulated in liposomes coated wth biocompatible polyethylene glycol polymers (Stealth liposomes).

Molecular weight: A particle suspension.

pH: 5.65.

Osmolality: 334 mmol/kg.

Solubility: Soluble in water.

Fluorescence: Orange fluorescence in UV light 284–366 nm.

3 Stability Profile

Doxil is supplied in a frozen state. Vials may be thawed by three methods (in order of increasing rapidity):

▼ place vials in refrigerator (2–8°C)
▼ place vials at room temperature
▼ place vials in 25°C water bath until all frozen material has melted.

The thawed or diluted Doxil may be stored for up to eight hours after dilution at 2–8°C and should then be discarded. Do not re-freeze thawed material. Doxil may be diluted in 0.9% sodium chloride injection or 5% glucose (preferable).

4 Clinical Use

Liposomes are microscopic vesicles made of phospholipids, identical to those found in cell membranes. Liposomes are non-toxic and can safely transport their load through the vascular compartment without dilution or degradation. Thus when the liposomes reach diseased tissues they deliver concentrated doses of medication. Doxorubicin encapsulated in liposomes coated with biocompatible polymers has been shown in animal models to be less toxic and to distribute more selectively to tumours when compared with the same dose of conventional doxorubicin. They are also claimed to evade rapid detection and uptake by cells of the reticuloendothelial system, unlike conventional liposomes that are rapidly cleared from the bloodstream. The treatment rationale for the use of liposome encapsulated doxorubicin is to improve tumour deposition of the drug, thereby improving the disease response rate in solid cancers.

5 Preparation of Injection

The material is thawed as described above. Do not thaw using a microwave, and protect from light. After thawing it should be shaken gently by hand; do not use if it contains a precipitate.

Bolus administration: It may be administered either by bolus injection or infusion over 30 minutes. Dilute with 0.9% sodium chloride or 5% glucose (preferred).

Extravasation: Reported to be less serious than with conventional doxorubicin in animal models (*see* Chapter 9).

6 Destruction of Drug or Contaminated Articles

Disposal: If the raw material is spilled, contain the spill with an absorbant and deactivate with 10% sodium hypochlorite solution until colourless.

Contact with skin: If the material contacts skin or mucous membrane immediately wash thoroughly with soap and water.

7 Centres with a Known Interest in this Drug

▼ University Hospital of South Carolina, USA.
▼ Hadassah University Hospital, Jerusalem, Israel.

8 Sources of Information

Alpar, O. (1989). Liposomes as drug carriers. *Pharm. J.* **243**, 254–355.
Liposome Technology Inc. (1991). Personal communication.
Gabizon, A. Hadassah University Hospital, Sharett Institute of Oncology, Jerusalem. (1991). Personal communication.
Stealth liposomal doxorubicin hydrochloride injection (S-Dox). Liposome Technology Inc. Clinical Study Protocol, April 1991.

Prepared by Y. Cass

ORGANOTELLURIUM

1 General Details

Approved name: Ammonium trichloro(dioxyethylene-O,O')tellurate.

Proprietary names: AS-101, Organotellurium.

Manufacturer or supplier: Wyeth Laboratories Inc. (for Scientific Testing Inc.), Baker Cummins Pharmaceuticals Inc., USA.

Presentation and formulation details: Clear colourless solution of organotellurium in vials containing 100 ml; each ml contains organotellurium (AS-101) 0.05 mg. Each ml also contains sodium chloride 8 mg, dibasic sodium phosphate heptahydrate 2.16 mg, potassium chloride 0.2 mg, monobasic potassium phosphate 0.2 mg, calcium chloride dihydrate 0.13 mg, magnesium chloride hexahydrate 0.1 mg, water for injections (described as 'phosphate-buffered saline', PBS). Hydrochloric acid and/or sodium hydroxide may be added to adjust pH. Organotellurium may also be prepared in citrate buffer.

Storage and shelf-life of unopened container: At 0–5°C, protected from freezing, shelf-life is one year.

2 Chemistry

Type: Synthetic organotellurium compound, a stimulator of lymphokine production.

Molecular structure: Ammonium trichloro(dioxyethylene-O,O')tellurate.

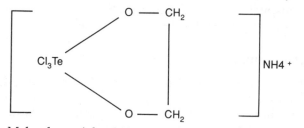

Molecular weight: 311.

Solubility: Soluble in organic solvents. Maximum solubility is 50 mg in 100 ml PBS and 220 mg in 100 ml citrate buffer. It is almost insoluble in water. Organotellurium in aqueous solution is hydrolysed to TeO_2-ethyleneglycol complex which is the active ingredient. This complex is not obtained from TeO_2 and ethyleneglycol separately. In citrate buffer the TeO_2 citrate complex is obtained. This complex is not obtained from TeO_2 in citrate solution.

3 Stability Profile

It is usually administered undiluted or added to 0.9% sodium chloride. Stability studies are continuing but it is recommended that diluted solution should be used within 48 hours. No information on compatibilities with other drugs is available.

4 Clinical Use

Type of drug: It has immunomodulating antiviral and antitumour effects. *In vitro* studies indicate that AS-101 can induce proliferation of human lymphocytes and production of interleukin-2 (IL-2). In mouse spleen cells AS-101 enhances production of IL-2 colony-stimulating factor, gamma interferon and tumour necrosis factor. In cultured mononuclear cells from AIDS patients, AS-101 increases the ratio of OKT4+ to OKT8+ cells. Antitumour activity of AS-101 has been observed in several tumour systems. Phase I and II studies of AS-101 as an antitumour drug are continuing, and also Phase II and III studies of AS-101 alone and in combination with zidovudine in the treatment of HIV infection.

Main indications: Immunomodulator responsive tumours and AIDS.

Dosage: 3–5 mg/m^2, two to three times weekly, every 14 days.

5 Preparation of Injection

Intravenous infusion: The drug is transferred to an infusion solution of 0.9% sodium chloride and given by slow infusion over 15 minutes.

Extravasation: No reported problems.

6 Destruction of Drug or Contaminated Articles

No specific information is available from the manufacturer. Standard procedures should be followed.

7 Centres with a Known Interest in this Drug

▼ Hadassah University Hospital, Jerusalem, Israel.
▼ Bar-Ilan-Tel Hashomer, Tel-Aviv, Israel.

8 Sources of Information

Sredni, B. *et al.* (1987). A new immunomodulating compound (AS-101) with potential therapeutic application. *Nature* **330**, 173.

Sredni, B. *et al.* (1990). Phase I study of AS-101 (an organotellurium compound) in patients with advanced malignancies. In Rubinstein, E., Adam, D., Lewin-Epstein, E., Jerusalem. (eds): *Recent advances in chemotherapy*, pp. 851.1–851.4.

Shani, A. *et al.* (1990). The immunologic effects of the immunomodulator AS-101 in the treatment of cancer patients. *Nat. Immun. Cell Growth Regul.* **9**, 182.

Kalechman Y. *et al.* (1990). The radioprotective effects of the immunomodulator AS-101. *J. Immunol.* **145**, 1512.

Kalechman, Y. *et al.* (1991). Protective and restorative role of AS-101 in combination with chemotherapy. *Cancer Res.* **51**, 1499–1503.

AS-101 Clinical Study Protocol. (1989). Israel.

Prepared by Y. Cass

STREPTOZOCIN

1 General Details

Approved name: Streptozocin.

Proprietary name: Zanosar.

Manufacturer or supplier: In the UK, supplied on a 'named patient' basis through IDIS Ltd.

Presentation and formulation details: Pale-yellow freeze-dried powder containing 1 g streptozocin. Contains sodium hydroxide to adjust pH. Each vial also contains 220 mg citric acid. Contains no preservatives.

Storage and shelf-life of unopened container: Store at 2 to 8°C, protected from light.

2 Chemistry

Type: Nitrosourea.

Molecular structure: 2-deoxy-2-(methyl-nitrosoamino)carbonylamino-(and β)-D-glucopyranose.

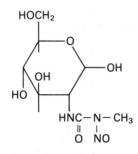

Molecular weight: 265.2.

Solubility: Soluble in water, 0.9% sodium chloride and ethanol.

3 Stability Profile

Physical and chemical stability

Effect of temperature: Streptozocin was reconstituted in 1 l of 20% glucose. The final concentration of the solution was 1 mg/ml. The study indicated less than 10% degradation after 72 hours at both 5°C and 22 to 24°C.

The injection was stable for more than 60 hours at 4 and 25°C when reconstituted with water for injection or 0.9% sodium chloride.

1 g vials were reconstituted with 9.5 ml of 0.9% sodium chloride irrigation, 20% glucose, and deionized water. The vials were stored at 3 and 24°C. pH fell slightly after 48 hours at 24°C, consistent with initial degradation of streptozocin. All solutions were clear, pale-yellow at reconstitution and no colour changes were discernible over 48 hours. No particulates or cloudiness observed in the vials.

Effect of light: A significant loss of potency was observed after 340 days and 740 days of exposure to light.

The freeze-dried product, when stored under conditions of minimal light exposure, did not show significant potency reduction.

Compatibility: Streptozocin may be reconstituted in water for injections, 0.9% sodium chloride or 5% glucose.

Container compatibility: Vials containing 1 g of streptozocin were reconstituted with 9.5 ml of 5% glucose or 0.9% sodium chloride. Aliquots of 10 ml were transferred to 1 l plastic IV bags (Abbott). Samples were assayed for DEHP over a 48-hour period. No leeching of DEHP from the plastic into the streptozocin solution was observed.

4 Clinical use

Main indications: Metastatic islet cell tumours of the pancreas.

5 Preparation of Injection

Reconstitution: Reconstitute each 1 g vial with 9.5 ml of diluent to yield a solution containing 100 mg/ml streptozocin.

Intravenous infusion: In 250 to 500 ml 0.9% sodium chloride or 5% glucose; over 30 to 60 minutes. Bolus not recommended because it is extremely uncomfortable for the patient.

Extravasation: The drug solution is vesicant. No specific recommendations for management (*see* Chapter 9).

6 Destruction of Drug or Contaminated Articles

Incineration: No specific information.

Chemical: No specific information.

Contact with the skin: No specific information.

7 Centres with a Known Interest in this Drug

▼ The Royal Marsden Hospital, London.
▼ Hammersmith Hospital, London.

8 Sources of Information

1. Upjohn (UK) Ltd. (1990). Personal communication.
2. Zanosar Data Sheet.

Prepared by T. Root

TAXOL

1 General Details

Approved name: Taxol, paclitaxel.

Proprietary name: None.

Manufacturer or supplier: Bristol-Myers Squibb, Clinical Cancer Research Department, Bristol-Myers Squibb UK.

Presentation and formulation details: A clear, pale straw-coloured, sterile solution, 6 mg/ml in a 5 ml vial. The vehicle is a 50:50 mixture of polyoxyethylated castor oil (Cremophor EL) and dehydrated alcohol USP and this solution *must* be diluted before administration.

Storage and shelf-life of unopened container: Store at 2–8°C. The vials do not carry an expiry date.

2 Chemistry

Type: A novel drug extracted from the bark of the Pacific yew (*Taxus brevifolia*). It acts at cellular level promoting the assembly of microtubules and stabilizing them against depolymerization.

Molecular structure:

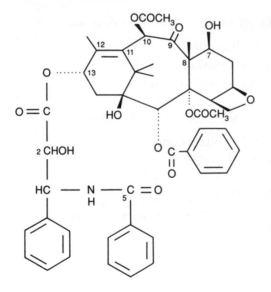

Molecular weight: 853.9.

Solubility: Poorly water soluble.

3 Stability Profile

Physical and chemical stability

Shelf-life studies of the unreconstituted product and of the 'ready-to-use' dilutions for infusion are ongoing. Solutions of taxol diluted to between

0.6 mg/ml and 1.2 mg/ml are both chemically and physically stable for 24 hours and 12 hours respectively (at time of publication).

Taxol, diluted in 0.9% sodium chloride or 5% glucose to concentrations in the range 0.3–1.2 mg/ml are reported to be stable for up to 24 hours in polyolefin or glass. PVC containers are not recommended, as discussed below. Some haziness of solutions has been noted. Care is therefore necessary in applying this data clinically.

4 Clinical Use

Phase I studies began in 1983, and ten have so far been completed. Progress has been slowed by the difficulty of obtaining large quantities of raw material. Phase II studies have been completed or are under way for several tumours including those of the ovary, breast and kidney, and in malignant melanoma.

5 Preparation of Injection

Dilution and administration: Taxol is administered by slow infusion, over one hour or more, in 5% glucose or 0.9% sodium chloride, at a concentration not exceeding 1.2 mg/ml. Several infusion rates are under study. In early studies, a significant incidence of hypersensitivity reactions was seen, but this problem has since been minimized by premedication of the patient with an IV H_2 antagonist, an IV antihistamine and oral dexamethasone.

The infusion containers, administration sets and in-line filters used should not contain PVC, due to the possibility of the leaching out of plasticizers by the Cremophor EL in the vehicle.

One study has shown substantial extraction of DEHP by taxol injection diluted to 0.3–1.2 mg/ml in either 0.9% sodium chloride or 5% glucose from PVC infusion containers and administration sets, and recommends that only glass or polyolefin (eg Polyfusor) containers should be used to administer taxol. Infusion should be through a non-PVC set.

A small number of fibres has been observed in the diluted infusion solution, and the use of a suitable in-line filter (0.22 μm) such as IVEX-2 (cellulose acetate, non-PVC) is strongly recommended. Infusions showing excessive particulate or fibre contamination should not be used.

Extravasation: This has occurred in a few patients being given taxol by peripheral line and, in one case, through a Port-A-Cath. No serious problems resulted.

6 Destruction of Drug or Contaminated Articles

No specific information available.

7 Centre with a Known Interest in this Drug

▼ The Royal Marsden Hospital, London.
▼ MD Anderson Cancer Hospital, Texas, USA.

8 Sources of Information

NCI Investigational Drugs. (1990). Pharmaceutical data.
Bristol-Myers Squibb, Clinical Cancer Research Department.
Waugh, W.N. *et al.* (1991). Stability, compatibility and plasticizer extraction of taxol (NSC-125973) injection diluted in infusion solutions and stored in various containers. *Am. J. Hosp. Pharm.* **48**, 1520–1524.

Prepared by T. Root

TENIPOSIDE

1 General Details

Approved names: Teniposide, VM26, PTG, Thenylidene-Ligan-P.

Proprietary name: Vumon.

Manufacturer or supplier: Bristol-Myers Squibb, Clinical Cancer Research Department, Bristol-Myers Squibb, UK.

Presentation and formulation details: 5 ml ampoules containing a solution of teniposide 10 mg/ml. Each 5 ml also contains benzyl alcohol 150 mg, N,N-dimethylacetamide 300 mg, polyoxyetholated castor oil 2.5 g, absolute alcohol 4.7 g and maleic acid to adjust pH.

Storage and shelf-life of unopened containers: Store at room temperature, protected from light. Ampoules are labelled with an expiry date.

2 Chemistry

Type: Podophyllotoxin derivative.

Molecular structure: Epipodophyllotoxin, 4-demethyl-9-(4,6-*o*-2-thenylidene-β-D-glucopyranoside).

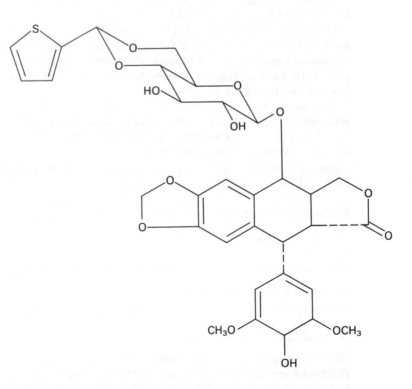

Molecular weight: 656.

3 Stability Profile

Teniposide exhibits physical instability in aqueous solutions in varying periods of time depending on concentration, solution, and container type. The manufacturer recommends the following utility times for dilutions of the drug stored at either 4 or 25°C.

Infusion solution	Container type	Teniposide concentration (μg/ml)	Use within
0.9% sodium chloride	Glass	100	24 hr
	Glass	400	24 hr
	Plastic	100	8 hr
5% glucose	Glass	100	24 hr
	Glass	200	24 hr
Water for injections	Glass	100	24 hr
	Glass	200	24 hr
	Plastic	100	8 hr

More recent work from Amsterdam suggests that, at a concentration of 0.4 mg/ml in 5% glucose or 0.9% sodium chloride, in both glass and PVC infusion containers, teniposide is physically and chemically stable for at least four days at room temperature.

Precipitation may occur frequently in both glass and plastic containers at concentrations greater than those indicated in the table above. Discard solutions that show evidence of a precipitate.

Upon dilution, a slight opalescence may appear due to the surfactant present in the formulation.

Compatibility: 5% glucose and 0.9% sodium chloride.

4 Clinical Use

Main indications: Treatment of acute leukaemia.

5 Preparation of injection

Dilution: Dilute with the appropriate volume of infusion fluid. Refer to protocol.

Administration: Slow IV infusion.

Extravasation: Vesicant. Avoid extravasation. No specific management recommended (*see* Chapter 9).

6 Destruction of Drug or Contaminated Articles

Incineration: No specific information available.

Chemical: No specific information available.

Contact with skin: No specific information available.

7 Centres with a Known Interest in this Drug

None presently known.

8 Sources of Information

NCI investigational drug data, 1989, 1990.

Bristol-Myers Squibb.

Beijnen, J.H. *et al.* (1991). Chemical and physical stability of etoposide and teniposide in commonly used infusion fluids. *J. Parenter. Sci. Technol.* **45**, 108–112.

Trissel, L.A. (1992). *Handbook of injectable drugs*, 7th edn. American Society of Hospital Pharmacists, Bethesda, Maryland, USA.

Prepared by T. Root

Glossary of Drug Names and Synonyms

Aclarubicin	(USAN); Aclarubicin hydrochloride (rINNM); Alacinomycin A hydrochloride. *Aclacin (UK); Aclacinomycine (Fr.); Aclapalstin (Ger.); Jaclacin (Denm.)*
Amsacrine	(BAN, USAN, pINN); AMSA; m-AMSA; Acridinyl; Anisidide. *Amsidine (Fr., UK); Amecrin (Denm., Norw., Swed.) Amsa (Canad.); Amsidyl (Austral., Ger.)*
Asparaginase	(USAN), Colaspase (BAN), Crisantaspase, Erwinia L-aspariginase, L-Asparaginase, L-Asparagine Amidohydrolase. *Erwinase (UK), Crasnitin (Denm., Ger., Ital., Norw., UK); Crasnitine (Belg., Switz.); Elspar (USA); Kidrolase (Canad., Fr.); Laspar (S.Afr.); Leucogen (Spain); Leunase (Austral.)*
Bleomycin	Bleomycin Sulphate (BANM, pINNM) Bleomycin Sulfate (USAN). *Blenoxane (Austral., Canad., S.Afr., USA); Bleo Oil (Jpn); Bleo-S (Jpn); Blocamicina (Arg.); Verbublen (Canad.)*
Carboplatin	(BAN, USAN, rINN); JM8. *Paraplatin (Canad., UK); Paraplatine (Switz.)*
Carmustine	(BAN, USAN, rINN); BCNU. *BiCNU (Canad., Fr., UK, USA); Becenun (Denm., Norw., Swed.,); Carmubris (Ger.); Nitrumon (Ital.)*
Cisplatin	(BAN, USAN, rINN); Cisplatinum, *cis*-DDP; CDDP; Cis-platinum; DDP; Peyrone's Salt. *Cisplatyl (Fr., Swed.); Citoplatino (Ital.); Neoplatin (Spain, UK); Placis (Spain); Platamine (S.Afr.); Platiblastin (Ger.); Platinex (Ger., Ital., UK); Platinol (Austral., Belg., Canad., Denm., Lux., Norw., S.Afr., Swed., Switz., USA); Platistil (Spain); Platistin (Denm., Norw., Swed.) Platosin (UK)*
Cyclophosphamide	(BAN, USAN, rINN); Cyclophospham. *Endoxana (UK); Carloxan (Denm.); Cycloblastin (Austral.); Cyclostin (Ger.); Cyclostine (Switz.); Cytoxan (Canad., USA); Endoxan (Austral., Fr., Ger., Ital., Neth., S.Afr., Switz.); Enduxan (Braz.); Genoxal (Spain); Neosar (USA); Procytox (Canad.); Sendoxan (Denm., Norw., Swed.)*
Cytarabine	(BAN, USAN, rINN); Arabinosylcytosine; Ara-C; Cytosine Arabinoside. *Alexan (Belg., Ger., Ital., Neth., Spain, Switz., UK); Arabitin (Jpn); Aracytin (Arg., Ital.); Cytosar (Austral., Belg., Canad., Denm., Jpn, Neth., Norw., S.Afr., Swed., Switz., UK, USA); Erpalfa (Ital.); Iretin (Jpn); Udicil (Ger.)*
Dacarbazine	(BAN, USAN, rINN); DIC; DTIC; Imidazole Carboxamide. *DTIC-Dome (Austral., Canad., Ital., Neth., NZ, S.Afr., Spain, Swed., Switz., UK, USA); Deticene (Fr., Ger., Ital., Neth., Switz.)*
Dactinomycin	(USAN, rINN); Actinomycin D (BAN); Meractinomycin. *Cosmegen, Lyovac (UK)*
Daunorubicin	Daunomycin Hydrochloride (BANM, USAN, rINNM); Rubidomycin Hydrochloride. *Cerubidin (Austral., Denm., Norw., S.Afr., Swed., UK); Cerubidine (Belg., Canad., Fr., Neth., Switz., USA); Daunoblastina (Ital., Spain)*
Deoxycoformycin	Pentostatin (USAN, rINN); 2'-Deoxycoformycin; Co-vidarabine.

Doxorubicin	Doxorubicin Hydrochloride (BANM, USAN, rINNM); Adriamycin Hydrochloride. *Adriamycin (Austral., Canad., Norw., Swed., UK, USA); Adriblastin (Ger.); Adriblastina (Arg., Belg., Ital., Neth., S.Afr.); Adriblastine (Fr., Switz.); Farmiblastina (Spain)*
Epirubicin	Epirubicin Hydrochloride (BANM, USAN, rINNM); 4'-Epiadriamycin Hydrochloride; 4'-Epidoxorubicin Hydrochloride; Pidorubicin Hydrochloride. *Farmarubicine (Fr.); Farmorubicin (Denm., Ger., S.Afr.); Farmorubicina (Ital., Spain); Farmoribicine (Fr., Switz.); Pharmorubicin (Austral., Canad., UK)*
Etoposide	(BAN, USAN, rINN); EPEG; VP-16; VP-16-213. *Etopol (Jug.); Vepesid (Austral., Canad., Denm., Ger., Ital., Norw., S. Afr., Spain., Swed., Switz., UK, USA)*
Fluorouracil	(BAN, USAN, rINN); 5-Fluorouracil; 5-FU. *Adrucil (Canad., USA); Arumel (Jpn); Carzonal (Jpn); Fluoroplex (Austral., Canad., USA); Fluorouracil (Austral., Belg., Denm., Neth., Norw., S.Afr., Swed., Switz., UK); Fluoro-Uracile (Fr.); Fluroblastin (Ger., S.Afr.); Fluoroblastine (Switz.); Timazin (Jpn); ULUP (Jpn)*
Ifosfamide	(BAN, USAN, rINN); Iphosphamide; Isophosphamide. *Holoxan (Fr., Ger., Ital., Neth., Switz.); Mitoxana (UK); Tronoxal (Spain)*
Interferon alfa	(BAN, rINN); Interferon-; IFN-; Interferon alfa-2a (USAN); *Intron A (UK)*; Interferon alfa-2b (USAN); *Roferon-A (UK)*; Interferon alfa-n1 (USAN); *Wellferon (UK)*
Inteferon gamma	(BAN, rINN); Interferon-; IFN-; Interferon gamma-1b (USAN); Proprietary names of Interferons *Berofor (Ger.); Exovir-HZ (USA); Fiblaferon (Ger.); Frone (Hong Kong, Israel, Ital.); Immuneron; Intron-A (Austral., Canad., Eire, Fr., S.Afr., Switz., UK, USA); Introna (Denm., Swed.); Roferon-A (Fr., Ger., UK, USA); Wellferon (Canad., UK)*
Interleukin-2	Epidermal Thrombocyte Activating Factor; ETAF; IL-2; T-Cell Growth Factor. *Proleukin (Ger., Neth.)*
Melphalan	(BAN, USAN, rINN); PAM; Phenylalanine Nitrogen Mustard. *Alkeran (Austral., Belg., Canad., Denm., Fr., Ger., Ital., Neth., Norw., S.Afr., Swed., Switz., UK, USA); Alkerana (Arg.)*
Mesna	(BAN, rINN); Mesnum. *Ausobronc Mesna (Ital.); Mistabron (Belg., Neth., S.Afr., Switz.); Mistabronco (Ger.); Mucofluid (Belg., Fr., Ger., Ital., Spain); Mucolene (Ital.); Sinomist (S.Afr.); Uromitexan (Fr., Ger., Ital., Spain, Switz., UK)*
Methotrexate	(BAN, USAN, rINN); Amethopterin; Methotrexatum; MTX. *Emtexate (Ger., Switz., UK); Emthexat (Norw., Swed.); Emthexate (Neth.); Farmitrexat (Ger.); Farmotrex (Denm.); Folex (USA); Ledertrexate (Belg., Fr., Neth.); Maxtrex (UK); Methotrexat (Ger.); Metotrexato (Arg.); Metrexan (Denm.); Mexate (USA); Tremetex (Swed.)*
Mithramycin	Plicamycin (BAN, USAN, rINN); Aureolic Acid. *Mithracin (Austral., Norw., UK, USA); Mithracine (Fr., Switz.)*
Mitomycin	(BAN, USAN, rINN); Mitomycin C; Mitomycine C. *Ametycine (Fr.); Mitomycin-C (Austral., S.Afr.); Mitomycin-C Kyowa (UK); Mitomycine (Belg.); Mutamycin (Canad., Norw., Swed., Switz., USA)*
Mitozantrone	Mitozantrone Hydrochloride (BANM); DHAD; Dihydroxyanthracenedione Dihydrochloride; Mitoxantrone Hydrochloride (USAN, rINNM). *Novantron (Ger., Switz.); Novantrone (Austral., Canad., Fr., S.Afr., UK)*
Mustine	Mustine Hydrochloride (BANM); Chlorethazine Hydrochloride; Chlormethine Hydrochloride (rINNM); HN2(mustine); Mechlorethamine Hydrochloride (USAN); Nitrogen Mustard. *Caryolysine (Fr.); Cloramin (Ital.); Erasol (Denm.); Mustargen (Canad., Switz., USA)*

Streptozocin	(USA, rINN); Streptozotocin; *Zanosar (Canad., Fr., USA)*
Taxol	Taxocytol (pINN); Taxol A
Teniposide	(Ban, USAN, rINN); ETP; VM-26; *Vehem (Fr.); Vumon (Austral., Canad., Ital., S.Afr., Spain, Swed., Switz.)*
Thiotepa	(BAN, USAN, rINN); TESPA; Thiophosphamide; Triethylene Thiophosphormide; TSPA. *Ledertepa (Belg., Neth.); Onco tepa (Spain); Tifosyl (Norw., Swed.)*
Vinblastine	Vinblastine Sulphate (BANM, rINNM); Vinblastine Sulfate (USAN); Vincaleucoblastine Sulphate; Vincaleukoblastine Sulphate; VLB (vinblastine). *Velban (USA); Velbe (Arg., Austral., Belg., Canad., Denm., Fr., Ger., Ital., Neth., Norw., S.Afr., Swed., Switz., UK)*
Vincristine	Vincristine Sulphate (BANM, rINNM); 22-Oxovincaleukoblastine Sulphate; Leurocristine Sulphate; Vincristine Sulfate (USAN). *Kyocristine (Jpn); Oncovin (Arg., Austral., Belg., Canad., Denm., Fr., Neth., Norw., Swed., Switz., UK, USA); Pericristine (S.Afr.); Vincasar (USA); Vincrisul (Spain)*
Vindesine	Vindesine Sulphate (BANM, rINNM); Desacetyl Vinblastine Amide Sulfate; Vindesine Sulfate (USAN). *Eldisine (Austral., Canad., Fr., Ger., Ital., S.Afr., Swed., Switz., UK); Enison (Spain)*

ABBREVIATIONS USED IN THIS GLOSSARY

Arg.	Argentina
Aust.	Austria
Austral.	Australia
BAN	British Approved Name
BANM	British Approved Name Modified
Belg.	Belgium
Braz.	Brazil
Canad.	Canada
Denm.	Denmark
Fr.	France
Ger.	Germany
INN	International Nonproprietary Name
Ital.	Italy
Jpn	Japan
Jug.	Yugoslavia
Lux.	Luxembourg
Neth.	The Netherlands
Norw.	Norway
NZ	New Zealand
pINN	Proposed International Nonproprietary Name
pINNM	Proposed International Nonproprietary Name Modified
rINN	Recommended International Nonproprietary Name
rINNM	Recommended International Nonproprietary Name Modified
S.Afr.	South Africa
Swed.	Sweden
Switz.	Switzerland
UK	United Kingdom
USA	United States of America
USAN	United States Adopted Name